Effective Documentation for Occupational Therapy

2nd Edition

Jane D. Acquaviva, OTR/L
Editor

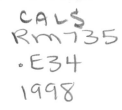
The American Occupational Therapy Association, Inc., Mission Statement

The mission of the American Occupational Therapy Association is to support a professional community for members, and to develop and preserve the viability and relevance of the profession. The organization serves the interests of its members, represents the profession to the public, and promotes access to occupational therapy services.

Disclaimers

"This publication is designed to provide accurate and authoritative information in regard to the subject matter covered. It is sold or distributed with the understanding that the publisher is not engaged in rendering legal, accounting, or other professional service. If legal advice or other expert assistance is required, the services of a competent professional person should be sought."

—From the Declaration of Principles jointly adopted by the American Bar Association and a Committee of Publishers and Associations.

It is the objective of the American Occupational Therapy Association to be a forum for free expression and interchange of ideas. The opinions and positions expressed by the contributors to this work are their own and not necessarily those of either the editors or the American Occupational Therapy Association.

Frances E. McCarrey, AOTA Director of Nonperiodical Publications
Mary C. Fisk, Managing Editor of Nonperiodical Publications
Paul A. Platosh, Production Editor of Nonperiodical Publications
Ethel H. Anagnoson, Copyright Permissions
Designed by RGM Graphics, Inc.

Printed in the United States of America

ISBN 1-56900-091-3

This book is dedicated to all of the therapists who strive daily to communicate the good work of occupational therapy through their documentation, and to those who shared their efforts with me to make this book possible.

J.D.A

Table of Contents

Preface

Since the first edition of *Effective Documentation for Occupational Therapy* was published in 1992, it has assisted thousands of therapists in documenting their services. Over the last 5 years, however, changes in laws and regulations have necessitated the revision of this publication. This second edition is a response to these changes. Many of the original authors have updated their material, and six new authors have been added. Two new chapters address the effects of computerization on documentation and alternatives to documentation. The appendices have been expanded to include essential Medicare forms and AOTA's Uniform Terminology—Third Edition.

J.D.A

Acknowledgments

I would like to thank all the clinicians who responded to my request for forms and sample documentation. Many forms, though extremely valuable, could not be included in this publication.

I would also like to thank Judy Thomas and Denise Mo of the AOTA Government Relations Department for their technical assistance, and Leslie Jackson, Deborah Lieberman, and Marion Scheinholtz of the Practice Department for reviewing chapters. Thanks also goes to Maureen Muncaster, Mary Fisk, and Fran McCarrey of the Nonperiodical Publications department for their assistance.

J.D.A

1. If I Had Known Then What I Know Now...

Dorothy Wilson, OTR, FAOTA

The former director of a large occupational therapy department reflects on the challenges of documentation. Her frustrations are not unusual, as many managers face similar dilemmas. However, the author now has a new vantage point that makes everything clearer. As a consultant to Blue Cross of California, she reviews medical records. She never sees the patient, the therapist, or perhaps even the facility. Her knowledge of the case is only what she can glean from the medical record. Because of her work in medical review, she now understands how she could have helped her staff write more concise notes.

Dorothy J. Wilson is an occupational therapy consultant, Blue Cross of California, Woodland Hills, California.

Creating an environment that facilitates change and guiding the course of that change can be two of the most difficult management tasks. This fact was really brought home to me when I tried to change the documentation methods of a large occupational therapy department in an acute rehabilitation hospital.

The need for change became apparent during my last 4 years as director of this department. The mountains of paper continued to grow, and the documentation consumed more and more of the time that staff should have spent in direct patient care. Although hospital administration approved requests for additional staff to handle both the patient treatment and the documentation, my frustration increased. In spite of the enormous amount of time spent in documentation, the product failed to produce a coherent picture of the occupational therapy services rendered or the patient outcome. Therapists seemed compelled to document every detail so minutely that no one would read it. All the knowledge about occupational therapy services that resulted in improvement in patients' function was lost in verbiage. Computers and word processing software programs were initiated to save time with the process, but the extra time was promptly used to write more.

Although time was not saved by any process initiated, the goal that I hoped to achieve with our documentation was the ability to use the information for assistance in treating patients and as data for clinical research. Unfortunately, several peer review and audit procedures revealed that even this limited goal was not achieved.

New Insights

If a second chance to change documentation methods in this situation were to magically appear, there are several things that could be done differently. Of course, these new ideas come from the genius of hindsight.

The first step would be to develop training programs for the staff members to increase their interview skills. The training would focus on how a therapist uses education, explanation, probing, and questioning during an initial interview with the patient/caregivers to identify realistic, practical, and achievable functional goals. This training would continue until the whole staff had adopted an almost religious focus on patient goals.

This is very difficult for therapists in an acute inpatient setting because most patients who are asked what they would like to achieve during their hospital stay respond with statements such as "get well" or "walk out of here." However, if we are to produce documentation that is concise and relevant, this is where the process must start. If therapists can use their professional skills to initially identify and agree on realistic outcomes that can be achieved through occupational therapy intervention, those goals would shape our documentation.

The next step in the master plan for improved documentation would be to develop and refine therapists' observation skills to their highest possible level. Following the interview, the therapists should identify underlying factors that limit functional performance by observation of the patient's attempt to perform functional tasks.

The third step in this blueprint for change would be easy. It involves expertise already demonstrated by therapists: assessment of the patient's underlying problems that limit performance. Hopefully the amount of testing and other measures used, and the resulting detail, would be cut in half by the focus developed through successful completion of the first two steps. Specific assessment of factors limiting performance should become more efficient if the functional goals and limitations are already clearly defined. The initial assessment gives us the baseline objective measures that will be used to monitor the patient's functional progress.

After selecting the unique occupational therapy media and procedures needed to either alleviate or compensate for the identified deficits, we are finally ready to document. The evaluation or initial assessment report would contain these three major elements:

1. mutually agreed, achievable functional goals
2. problems amenable to occupational therapy intervention
3. the therapy strategy (treatment plan).

These elements could be "garnished" with the length of time predicted to achieve the desired outcome and the frequency of treatment needed to reach the goals by the projected discharge date.

Subsequent progress reports would address how far we have come toward the goals and how far we still have to go. There is no need to repeat the plan of treatment unless goals are changed or new goals are identified.

The rosy glow of hindsight allows one to take advantage of every mistake made or observed during the process of attempting to change a department's documentation methods. However, I am convinced that this blueprint for change would be an effective and less frustrating way to make that change. As therapists add improved interview and observation skills to already excellent assessment and instructional skills, the process of relating functional goals, underlying factors, and the occupational therapy treatment plan in documentation should become the natural course of action. The need to report every detail of our professional process would diminish as we begin to communicate clear, relevant, and meaningful information to physicians, professional colleagues, patients, families, caregivers, third party payers, and each other.

Initial Assessment Report

2. Evolving Health Care Systems: Payment for Occupational Therapy Services

V. Judith Thomas, MGA

An overview of payment sources is provided in this chapter because of the strong link between documentation and payment. Coverage of occupational therapy services by third party payers other than federal programs such as Medicare may vary from state to state and plan to plan. As the author points out, occupational therapists need to investigate local plans, the types of services covered, and any limitations associated with coverage.

V. Judith Thomas is the Director of the Reimbursement Policy Program in the Government Relations Department, American Occupational Therapy Association. In previous positions she managed a health care policy branch in the Health Care Financing Administration's Office of Payment Policy and provided systems analysis support in the development of a managed health care administrative system.

O ccupational therapy practitioners are paid for their services in a variety of ways, often depending on the setting in which they work. They may be employees of, or have contractual arrangements with, a large health care provider, a school system, or another organization. Alternatively they may be in private practice; if so, they receive direct payment for specific services or groups of services either from insurers or from patients who are uninsured or who purchase occupational therapy services not covered under the patients' own insurance contracts. Regardless of payment method, it is important for occupational therapy practitioners to understand the scope of benefits offered by the major public and private health plans in their area. An understanding of payers' rules, coverage limitations, and billing practices allows occupational therapy practitioners to assist their patients and families with care decisions, as well as to develop more effective treatment plans in conjunction with other health care professionals.

Public funds for occupational therapy services are typically available through either insurance or grant programs. Federal and state insurance programs such as Medicare, Medicaid, and workers' compensation generally have structured guidelines specifying which services are covered, in what settings, and by whom. Grant programs such as the Individuals with Disabilities Education Act (1990), the Community Mental Health Centers Act (1963), the Older Americans Act (1965), and Social Security Title XX, the Social Services Block Grant Program (part of the Omnibus Budget Reconciliation Act of 1981), include occupational therapy as part of an overall program for a specific population. Grant programs are more flexible, allowing private, state, or local entities to provide specially designed programs as long as they meet broad national goals.

Under private insurance plans, services are usually provided to groups of individuals through benefit programs offered by employers or other organizations. However, individuals may purchase policies directly from companies, such as Blue Cross/Blue Shield, commercial insurers, and managed care organizations.

This chapter examines the major sources of payment that historically have been available for occupational therapy services. Also, it discusses some of the changes occurring in the United States health care delivery system that may affect future provision and documentation of occupational therapy services.

Federally Administered Systems

MEDICARE – Established by Congress in 1965 as Title XVIII of the Social Security Act, Medicare is by far the largest single payer for occupational therapy services. It provides health insurance coverage for about 14 percent of the total population, including nearly all the nation's elderly (65 years of age and older), over 4 million disabled persons, and over 200,000 persons with end-stage renal disease (Vladeck & King, 1995). With the anticipated increase in the elderly population, it is projected that Medicare will cover nearly 20 percent of the population by 2030 (U.S. Bureau of the Census, 1994). Occupational therapy practitioners provide services to Medicare beneficiaries in a wide range of settings—hospital inpatient and outpatient facilities, physicians' offices, skilled nursing facilities, comprehensive outpatient rehabilitation facilities, hospices, rehabilitation agencies, and clinics—and through home health agencies and private practice. Recent administrative policy and payment changes in the Medicare program are altering both the distribution of occupational therapy practitioners and the decisions that managers and practitioners must make in the provision of care.

The Medicare program, which is administered by the Health Care Financing Administration (HCFA), consists of the Hospital Insurance Program (Part A), which pays for hospital inpatient, skilled nursing facility, home health, and hospice care, and the Supplementary Medical Insurance Program (Part B), which covers hospital outpatient, physician, and other professional services, including occupational therapy services performed by independent practitioners. Table 2.1 explains the basis for Medicare payment to various types of providers.

Generally, occupational therapy is considered a Medicare-covered service under the following circumstances. Services must be

1. prescribed by a physician and furnished according to a written plan of care approved by the physician
2. performed by a qualified occupational therapist, or by an occupational therapy assistant under the general supervision of an occupational therapist
3. reasonable and necessary for the treatment of the person's illness or injury

There are no restrictions on diagnoses (they may be physical or psychiatric or both; no specific diagnosis will automatically prevent payment). There is only the requirement of "an expectation that the therapy will result in a significant practical improvement in the individual's level of functioning within a reasonable period of time" (HCFA, Pub. 13, sec. 3101.9). Medicare manuals containing specific coverage information for each delivery setting are available through the Government Printing Office.

MEDICARE HOSPITAL INSURANCE PROGRAM (PART A) – Occupational therapy services are covered under Part A when they are provided to eligible beneficiaries who are inpatients of hospitals or skilled nursing facilities or patients receiving services under the Medicare home health or hospice benefits. Since October 1993, acute care hospitals have received a *prospective,* or predetermined, rate per inpatient discharge based on established *diagnosis-related groups* (DRGs). This per-case rate covers all inpatient services, including occupational therapy. Individual hospitals determine the mix of services that is appropriate for each patient. Specialty hospitals, such as those offering psychiatric, rehabilitation, pediatric, and long-term care, are at present exempt from the prospective payment system (PPS) applicable to acute care hospitals, as are psychiatric and rehabilitation units of acute care general hospitals. Occupational therapy services are provided to inpatients of psychiatric hospitals or units based on a provision of Part A that requires hospitals to have a sufficient number of "qualified therapists, support personnel, and consultants" to provide comprehensive therapeutic activities for psychiatric inpatients (Public Health, 1986b).

Occupational therapy is also a covered service under Medicare's skilled nursing facility and home health benefits. Patients who receive skilled nursing care must require either skilled nursing or skilled rehabilitation (occupational therapy, physical therapy, or speech-language therapy) on a *daily* basis, defined in Medicare policy as at least 5 days a week. To qualify under the Part A home health benefit, a homebound patient must need intermittent skilled nursing care, physical therapy, or speech-language therapy before receiving occupational therapy. However, Medicare patients may continue to receive occupational therapy under the home health benefit after their need for skilled nursing, physical therapy, or speech-language therapy ends (HCFA, Pub.13, sec. 3132).

Hospice care is a special Part A benefit for eligible Medicare beneficiaries whom a physician has certified as *terminally ill*, defined in the regulations as a medical prognosis of fewer than 6 months to live. A patient who elects to receive hospice benefits must waive inpatient Medicare benefits during the election period. Hospice services may be provided by public agencies or private organizations that are primarily engaged in providing care to terminally ill people.

Medicare regulations for hospices mandate that four core services be available to patients 24 hours a day: counseling, nursing, physicians' services, and social services. The hospice must also provide, as needed, occupational therapy, physical therapy, speech-language therapy, home health aides, homemaker services, and medical supplies, either directly or under a contractual arrangement. Occupational therapy may be provided to control a patient's symptoms or to enable a patient to maintain activities of daily living and basic functional skills. Hospice benefits are paid on a prospective basis. The rates, which are updated annually, are based on four primary levels of care corresponding to the degree of illness and the amount of care required.

MEDICARE SUPPLEMENTARY MEDICAL INSURANCE PROGRAM (PART B) – Occupational therapy services are covered as Part B outpatient services when furnished by or under arrangements with any Medicare-certified provider (i.e., a hospital, a skilled nursing facility, a home health agency, a rehabilitation agency, a clinic, or a public health agency). A provider may furnish outpatient occupational therapy services to a beneficiary in the home or in the provider's outpatient facility, or, under certain circumstances, to a beneficiary who is an inpatient in another institution. Outpatient occupational therapy services are also covered under Part B as comprehensive outpatient rehabilitation facility (CORF) services. A CORF is a public or private institution that is primarily engaged in providing (by or under the supervision of physicians) diagnostic, therapeutic, and restorative services on an outpatient basis for the rehabilitation of injured, sick, or disabled persons. When occupational therapy is provided by or for a certified facility provider, the facility usually bills for the services.

Part B outpatient occupational therapy services also may be furnished to beneficiaries by a Medicare-certified occupational therapist in independent practice (OTIP) when the services are provided by the therapist or under the therapist's direct supervision in his or her office or in the patient's home. OTIPs are paid according to the codes billed (see the later section Billing and Coding for Services). The amount of payment is derived from the Medicare Physicians' Fee Schedule, also known as the Resource Based Relative Value Scale (RBRVS). This fee schedule is used to pay for all physicians' services billed to Medicare. Beginning in 1995, payment for outpatient occupational therapy services furnished by a Medicare-certified OTIP is limited to $900 in incurred expenses annually per beneficiary. (This limit has been increased twice since January 1, 1990, and will increase to $1,500 on January 1, 1999.)

Outpatient occupational therapy services are also covered under Part B of Medicare as incidental to a physician's services when rendered to beneficiaries in a physician's office or a physician-directed clinic. The occupational therapist or therapy assistant providing the services must be employed (either full- or part-time) by the physician or the clinic, and the services must be furnished under the physician's direct supervision (i.e., the physician must be on the premises). The services must be directly related to the condition for which the physician is treating the patient, and they must be included on the physician's bill to Medicare.

Partial-hospitalization services connected with the treatment of a beneficiary with a psychiatric diagnosis (in a hospital-affiliated or community mental health center psychiatric day program) are also covered under Part B of Medicare, but only if the beneficiary would otherwise require inpatient psychiatric care. Under this benefit, Medicare covers occupational therapy services if they are reasonable and necessary for the diagnosis or the active treatment of the beneficiary's condition. They must be reasonably expected to improve or maintain the beneficiary's condition and functional level and to prevent relapse or hospitalization. The course of treatment must be prescribed, supervised, and reviewed by a physician.

THE BALANCED BUDGET ACT (BBA) OF 1997 (P. L. 105-33) – The Balanced Budget Act (BBA) of 1997 (P. L. 105-33) significantly changed the methodologies for payment of Medicare therapy (i.e. occupational and physical therapy and speech-language pathology) services in most settings. Although most provisions will not have been finalized when this chapter is published, Table 2.1 outlines the major legislative revisions affecting occupational therapy. It is incumbent on occupational therapy practitioners to monitor the implementation of these provisions in order to assure compliance with new documentation requirements.

DURABLE MEDICAL EQUIPMENT, PROSTHETICS, AND ORTHOTICS – Expenses incurred by a beneficiary for the rental or the purchase of durable medical equipment (e.g., a wheelchair or a walker) are reimbursable under Part B if the equipment is used in the patient's home and if it is necessary and reasonable to treat an illness or an injury or to improve the functioning of a "malformed body member." Medicare defines *durable medical equipment* as that which can withstand repeated use, is primarily and customarily used to serve a medical purpose, and generally is not useful to a person in the absence of illness of injury. An example is oxygen-assistance breathing equipment. Raised toilet seats, bathtub grab bars, and most types of adaptive equipment are not covered because they are not considered medically necessary.

CERTIFICATION OF PROVIDERS AS MEETING MEDICARE'S CONDITIONS OF PARTICIPATION – All Medicare institutional providers (e.g., hospitals and home health agencies) and individual providers (e.g., OTIPs and physicians) must be certified as meeting Medicare conditions of participation as well as complying

Table 2.1 Selected Medicare Payment Changes Required by the BBA of 1997

Provider Type	BBA Provision	Effective Date
Hospital Outpatient Therapy Services	Payment on a fee schedule basis	Calendar year 1999.
SNF Inpatient Services (Part A — Includes therapy services and applies to free-standing and hospital-based providers)	Payment on a Prospective Payment System basis.	Cost reporting periods beginning on or after July 1, 1998.
SNF Outpatient (Part B) Therapy Services	Fee Schedule*	For services beginning July 1, 1998
Comprehensive Outpatient Rehabilitation Facilities (CORFs) (applies to free-standing and hospital-based providers)	Fee Schedule*	Calendar year 1999.
Outpatient Rehabilitation Providers (rehabilitation agencies, clinics)	Fee schedule*	Calendar year 1999.
Community Mental Health Clinics (CMHCs)	Payment under the outpatient hospital Prospective System Payment basis.	Calendar year 1999.
Outpatient Therapy Services provided by a home health agency (HHA), but not under the HHA benefit	Fee Schedule*	Calendar year 1999.
Occupational therapists in independent practice (OTIPs)	Fee schedule continues, yearly limit raised to $1,500	Calendar year 1999.
HHA Services provided under the home health benefit (includes therapy services and applies to free-standing and hospital-based providers)	Payment on a Prospective System Payment basis.	Cost reporting periods beginning on or after October 1, 1999.

* A $1500 annual limitation on services provided to Medicare beneficiaries will be applied beginning January 1, 1999 where therapy services are provided by providers under the outpatient physical therapy benefit (which includes speech-language pathology services) and occupational therapy benefit.

with all relevant state and local laws and regulations. Before Medicare issues a provider number, providers must either be surveyed by state health agencies and certified using HCFA guidelines, or receive *deemed status* by previously meeting the accreditation standards of a recognized accrediting organization, such as the Joint Commission on Accreditation of Healthcare Organizations or the American Osteopathic Association.

Although in all health care settings, occupational therapy personnel must meet specific state licensure, certification, or other applicable state regulatory requirements, Medicare conditions of participation related to the provision of occupational therapy services differ for various provider settings. For example, in a hospital setting, occupational therapy personnel must meet qualifications "specified by a facility's medical staff that are consistent with state law" (Public Health, 1986a). In home health agencies and comprehensive outpatient rehabilitation facilities, Medicare regulations require that occupational therapy services be provided by occupational therapists or occupational therapy assistants who are eligible for certification by the National Board for Certification in Occupational Therapy (NBCOT), formerly the American Occupational Therapy Certification Board.

MEDICARE MANAGED CARE — The Health Care Financing Administration (HCFA) certifies and awards *cost* or *risk* contracts to health maintenance organizations (HMOs) and other competitive medical plans (CMPs) to provide all Part A and Part B Medicare services (except hospice care) to Medicare enrollees. HCFA pays HMOs and CMPs that participate on a cost basis under a retrospective, reasonable-cost methodology. HCFA pays those that participate under risk contracts a monthly *capitated* amount (an amount per enrolled beneficiary) for each class of Medicare beneficiary. As of February 1996, over 190 plans participated in the Medicare program under risk contracts (HCFA, 1996).

Medicare managed care plans typically cover all preventive, acute, and subacute health services. They must be able to deliver with "reasonable promptness" all medically necessary services that Medicare beneficiaries are entitled to receive and that are available to Medicare beneficiaries who are living in the same geographic area but are not enrolled in a managed care plan (Public Health, 1985). In addition, most plans offer other health care benefits (e.g., coverage of preventive care and prescriptions) that are not included in traditional Medicare coverage. The standard Medicare Part B premium is always required. Although additional cost-sharing levels vary according to policies established by each plan, the beneficiary is often required to pay a supplemental premium for *Medigap* insurance—coverage of Medicare deductibles, Medicare coinsurance, and services not covered by Medicare. Medicare first gave its beneficiaries the option of enrolling in an HMO in 1982. However, fewer than 10 percent had opted for managed care plans by the end of 1995 (Brick, 1996).

HCFA is experimenting with provision of other types of managed care through waivers and demonstration projects, which may be written into future legislation or regulation. For example, in 1995, HCFA announced a new Medicare point-of-service insurance option permitting its HMO enrollees to seek care outside the HMO's provider network, typically at higher cost-sharing levels than those for "in-network" care. HCFA does not mandate that the plan make selected services or providers available outside the network. Instead, each plan specifies the providers and the services that Medicare enrollees may access outside the HMO provider network. The BBA of 1997 also added Medicare managed care options under the new Medicare+ Choice Program effective January 1, 1999.

THE CIVILIAN HEALTH AND MEDICAL PROGRAM OF THE UNIFORMED SERVICES – The Civilian Health and Medical Program of the Uniformed Services (CHAMPUS) is a United States Department of Defense program of health care for the dependents of active-duty members of the armed forces and for retired members. It shares the cost of medical and other health care that eligible beneficiaries receive from civilian sources. For dependents, CHAMPUS is considered secondary to any other health care plan in which a person is enrolled. CHAMPUS, like Medicare, contracts with private health insurers such as Blue Cross/Blue Shield for claim-processing and utilization review services. CHAMPUS regulations provide for a basic health care program and a special program of rehabilitative benefits.

BASIC PROGRAM – Under the basic program, CHAMPUS beneficiaries may obtain both inpatient and outpatient medical and mental health care from civilian sources. To qualify for payment, occupational therapy services must be deemed medically necessary by a supervising physician and must be intended to help the patient overcome or compensate for disability resulting from illness, injury, or the effects of a CHAMPUS-covered condition. The occupational therapist or therapy assistant must be an employee of a CHAMPUS-authorized provider and must render the services in connection with CHAMPUS-authorized care in an organized inpatient or outpatient rehabilitation program. The employing institution must bill for the services. Effective October 28, 1997, occupational therapists in independent practice are recognized as authorized CHAMPUS providers and may receive direct payment under all CHAMPUS programs.

CHAMPUS MANAGED CARE – In November 1995, CHAMPUS implemented a new program for members called TRICARE, which incorporates options and incentives for managed care benefits. Under the TRICARE Prime option, CHAMPUS beneficiaries obtain services through an HMO network. Under TRICARE Standard, a continuation of the old CHAMPUS benefit, enrollees may use either the HMO network providers or choose non-network CHAMPUS providers at a higher out-of-pocket cost. Plans that contract under the TRICARE Prime option may offer benefits beyond the standard CHAMPUS options. Occupational therapists (only therapists will receive direct payment under CHAMPUS) who want to deliver care to CHAMPUS beneficiaries must meet requirements as both CHAMPUS–authorized providers and TRICARE contractors.

SPECIAL PROGRAM OF REHABILITATIVE BENEFITS – The special program of rehabilitative benefits available under CHAMPUS is for seriously physically handicapped and moderately or severely mentally retarded spouses and children of active-duty members. It provides coverage on an inpatient and outpatient basis with a small deductible. However, the qualifying requirements are extremely stringent. CHAMPUS provides a handbook with specific details about this benefit (see "Additional Resources" for the address and the telephone number of CHAMPUS).

FEDERAL EMPLOYEES HEALTH BENEFIT PROGRAM – The Federal Employees Health Benefit Program, which is administered by the Office of Personnel Management, covers federal government employees, retirees, and their dependents. The federal law and regulations governing the scope of benefits that must be offered specify only broad categories, such as hospital, surgical, and medical services. Therefore, coverage of individual types of service, such as occupational therapy, and the settings in which they may be provided is determined by each of the large number of private plans with which the government contracts to administer health care services.

The Federal Employees Health Benefit Program has historically included such insurers as Blue Cross/Blue Shield, Aetna, the Government Employees Hospital Association, and a number of postal worker plans (for example, the Postmasters Benefit Plan and the Mail Handlers Plan). Over the past few years the Office of Personnel Management has contracted with a greater number of national and local managed care organizations (Kaiser Permanente, Principal Health Care, and Healthplus). Most managed care organizations contend that occupational therapy is covered in some settings; however, the scope of coverage is generally restricted, and outpatient visits are usually limited in number and duration. When the Federal Employees Health Benefit Program-Blue Cross/Blue Shield plan expanded coverage of outpatient occupational therapy in 1993, it concurrently imposed a limit of 50 (high option) or 25 (low option) visits yearly, which applies to all outpatient rehabilitation (including occupational therapy, physical therapy, and speech-language therapy) visits.

With the advent of provider networks, occupational therapists often face impediments to participation, such as arbitrary limits on types of providers included in the network or misconceptions about the scope of occupational therapy or the relationship between occupational therapy and physical therapy. In pure managed care plans (for example, HMOs), use of nonaffiliated providers results in a total denial of payment for services, regardless of medical necessity.

Many traditionally fee-for-service plans have introduced managed care options into their packages. For example, the Federal Employees Health Benefit Program-Blue Cross/Blue Shield plan introduced a nationwide preferred provider network in 1993. It did not include occupational therapists until 1996. Use of this network results in lower out-of-pocket costs for federal subscribers.

MEDICAID – Medicaid, Title XIX of the Social Security Act (originally enacted in the Social Security Amendments of 1965, amended in the Social Security Amendments of 1971), is a federal-state program that provides health care to the poor and the *medically indigent*. States have great flexibility in the definition of medically indigent and in the makeup and the administration of the program, so benefits vary significantly from state to state. States must include all recipients of Aid to Families with Dependent Children and most beneficiaries of Supplemental Security

State-Administered Programs

Income. Not all states provide Medicaid coverage for the medically needy. Some states have a spend-down provision under which families with moderately high incomes may become eligible for Medicaid when their medical expenses reduce their income below the state standard.

Medicaid services fall into two categories: mandatory and optional. Mandatory services are ones that a state must provide to qualify for federal matching funds. They include

- hospital services
- laboratory work and X-rays
- skilled nursing facility services
- physicians' services
- early and periodic screening, diagnosis, and treatment (EPSDT) for persons under 21 years of age
- family planning.

States must provide certain services, (including occupational therapy), that are necessary to treat a condition identified during EPSDT. Coverage of these services is required even if they are not normally covered under the state's Medicaid program. Occupational therapy provided as a freestanding discipline is considered an optional service, along with physical therapy, speech-language therapy, drugs, psychiatric care, and others. Nursing home reforms adopted by Congress in 1987 require Medicaid nursing facilities to provide skilled rehabilitation services, including occupational therapy, to patients who require them.

In 1988, Congress approved legislation to allow school systems to bill Medicaid for certain related services, including occupational therapy, provided to children in schools. Implementation of this rule has resulted in the development of various state methods to determine responsibility and pay for occupational therapy services provided to school-age children. The seemingly overlapping language of education and Medicaid laws governing the provision of care for school-age children has given rise to the question of whether services to individual children should be funded as education or health care.

MEDICAID MANAGED CARE – To administer the Medicaid program more efficiently, state governments may apply to the federal government for *waivers,* which allow states flexibility in the types of services and delivery methods that they provide to some or all Medicaid recipients. Most state waivers require that enrollment in managed care plans or use of provider networks be approved by the state. A Section 1915(b) waiver (of the Social Security Act) allows a state to restrict a beneficiary's choice of provider and is often limited to selected geographic regions within a state. A Section 1115 waiver is a more extensive research-and-demonstration project that is usually granted for 5 years. Under Section 1115, states are allowed to test major changes in how Medicaid services are delivered. Under most Section 1115 waivers, the existing benefit packages, including occupational therapy benefits, that were available before the waiver was approved continue to be available through a managed care plan contractor. However, the risk of having services limited is increased when authority for case management, coverage decisions, and utilization review is transferred from the state government to a managed care plan.

To date, most state waivers have focused enrollment in managed care plans on the Aid to Families with Dependent Children population, which primarily comprises women and children with routine care needs, rather than the Supplemental Security Income population, which is primarily made up of disabled beneficiaries with more-expensive chronic care needs. According to a recent major study, "States have been cautious about extending managed care to [Supplemental Security Income] populations, in part because relatively few managed care organizations have developed expertise in managing special needs of these populations" (Lewin–VHI, 1995, p. ES-2). Information on Medicaid coverage of occupational therapy may be obtained from state offices of medical assistance (Medicaid).

WORKERS' COMPENSATION – Workers' compensation programs, developed to compensate employees who have job-related injuries or illnesses, are financed jointly by individual employers or groups of employers and state governments.[1] Each state has a workers' compensation governing board or commission that develops policies regulating whether an employer is required to participate, what the financial responsibility of the employer is, what benefits are provided, which workers are covered, and how the insurance is administered. Workers' compensation insurance may be administered through private insurance plans under contract with the state or through individual employers or groups of employers that administer their own programs (known as self-insuring).

Workers' compensation programs consist of two components, cash benefits and medical benefits. Although the growth of total workers' compensation costs has slowed since 1990 to less than 3 percent a year, medical benefit costs have grown at a rapid rate, leading to initiation of a variety of cost-containment strategies in states.

LIMITS ON CHOICE OF PROVIDERS – States have adopted a number of restrictions on an employee's ability to select an initial provider of care or to change providers during treatment. According to the Workers' Compensation Research Institute (as cited in Burton, 1996), as of January 1995, 14 states allowed an unrestricted initial choice, four states mandated selection from an employer or insurer network, and 13 required use of a managed care organization.

USE OF MEDICAL FEE SCHEDULES – As of 1995, 40 states had adopted some type of fee schedule that prescribed payment amounts for all services performed by health care practitioners for workers' compensation patients. Fee schedules vary in which services are included, what coding scheme is required (see the later section "Billing and Coding for Services"), what formulas are used to calculate the actual dollar amounts, which state entity develops and controls the use, and how

---

[1] This section is based on Burton, J. (1996). *Workers' Compensation, Twenty-Four-Hour Coverage, and Managed Care. Workers' Compensation Monitor, 9*(1), 11–21.

and how often they are updated. A relative value system is used in most jurisdictions, but wide state-to-state variances exist in the compensation for individual procedures.

REGULATION OF HOSPITAL RATES – States have adopted various methods (e.g., fee schedules and discounted charges) to regulate workers' compensation hospital expenditures, often in conjunction with *all-payer* systems that affect payments to all hospitals. Although some states use the DRG-based Medicare system, many of the DRGs do not apply to the workers' compensation population.

UTILIZATION CONTROLS – Because cost and pricing controls alone do not curtail use of services, some states have incorporated various means to address the provision of "unnecessary or inappropriate care." These include retrospective claim review, precertification of services, and case management programs.

WORKERS' COMPENSATION MANAGED CARE – Another approach to controlling costs by states and employers that self-insure has been to contract with HMOs and preferred provider organizations (PPOs) to provide workers' compensation medical care. In this way, workers' compensation programs can take advantage of existing cost-containment strategies used by HMOs, such as case management, utilization review protocols, and return-to-work programs, without having to make incremental changes in state policy.

To date, the few research projects designed to determine whether these strategies actually reduce the cost of care are inconclusive. A more comprehensive approach to the reform of the workers' compensation system is *24-hour coverage*. According to Burton (1996), this term describes "efforts to reduce or eliminate the distinctions between the medical benefits, income benefits, and disability management services provided to disabled workers for work-related injuries and diseases and...[those] provided to disabled workers for non-work-related injuries and diseases" (p. 17). These attempts to coordinate medical, income, and disability benefits from different payment sources vary greatly in configuration and structure. Additional information may be obtained from individual state workers' compensation boards or commissions or the International Association of Industrial Accident Boards and Commissions (see "Additional Resources" for an address and a telephone number).

EDUCATION PROGRAMS AFFECTING CHILDREN WITH DISABILITIES
INDIVIDUALS WITH DISABILITIES EDUCATION ACT – The Education for All Handicapped Children Act (often called Public Law Number 94-142), reenacted in 1990 as the Individuals with Disabilities Education Act (IDEA), provides federal grants to states to ensure that eligible children with disabilities have access to a "free, appropriate public education." This statute has been amended over the years to include preschool-aged children (Education of the Handicapped Amendments of 1986) and additional services such as assistive technology and transition planning (Education of the Handicapped Amendments of 1990). At present it consists of a number of parts that determine the scope of services that states must provide to infants and children with disabilities. Part B of IDEA requires that public school systems and other state agencies involved in educating children with disabilities (ages 3–21) make available "a free

appropriate public education that includes special education and related services to meet their unique needs" (Education, 1977). Under this program, occupational therapy is considered a *related service,* playing a supportive role in helping children benefit from special education (AOTA, 1997).

Part H of IDEA authorizes grant moneys to states "to develop and implement a statewide, comprehensive, coordinated, multidisciplinary, interagency program of early intervention services for infants and toddlers with disabilities and their families" (Education, 1989). Under this early intervention program, for children newborn through 2 years of age, occupational therapy is considered a *primary service.* Under Part B and Part H of IDEA, occupational therapy services must be provided according to an individualized education program (IEP) and an individualized family service plan (IFSP), respectively, by a qualified therapist (as defined by state law).

THE REHABILITATION ACT OF 1973 (SECTION 504) AND THE AMERICANS WITH DISABILITIES ACT (ADA) OF 1990 — Congress enacted the Rehabilitation Act of 1973 (Section 504) and the Americans with Disabilities Act (ADA) of 1990 to protect the rights of persons with disabilities. These civil rights laws may be used to ensure nondiscrimination against students who do not qualify for services under IDEA but need educational support (Copenhaver, 1995). Section 504 includes all institutions that receive federal funding and, with the passage of the ADA, "private institutions" (that is, private schools) with 15 or more employees. There are no federal funding provisions under these acts. Individual states have designated various agencies to administer them.

In 1995, over one-third of all registered occupational therapists in the United States reported that they worked with children in a variety of settings. School systems were the number one employers (either by salary or by contract) of OTRs, and the number two employers of certified occupational therapy assistants (Phyllis Burchman, director of research, AOTA, personal communication, March 1996). Because administrative responsibility for all the programs developed under the IDEA resides with the state governments, occupational therapy practitioners in school settings must work closely with local and state education officials on issues related to funding, human resources, and regulation of services.

Although it is possible to specify the number of private companies offering some type of health insurance, it is impossible to delineate all the variations of plan options offered in the United States. Insurers, especially large companies such as Blue Cross/Blue Shield plans, Aetna, MetLife, and Prudential, have many product lines of health insurance (PPOs, point-of-service plans, indemnity, etc.), including managed care options and often will negotiate unique benefit and premium configurations for a single employer. Therefore, a practitioner can never make assumptions about a person's coverage by plan name alone.

Private Insurance and Managed Care Plans

Because there are no federally mandated requirements for benefits or payment, each state determines the extent of control that it wants to impose on the insurance companies operating within its borders. Also, because employers that self-insure health care benefits are governed not by state insurance codes but by the Employee Retirement Income Security Act (ERISA), there are widely divergent practices across the country. Consistently, traditional indemnity insurers, in addition to administrators of managed care organizations [e.g., HMOs, PPOs, and physician-hospital organizations (PHOs)], are introducing managed care principles into their plans. The following management techniques are often implemented in conjunction with cost-controlling payment strategies, such as use of discounted or capitated rates and preferred provider networks to manage costs and quality more effectively.

1. *Case management.* Especially for long-term or high-cost cases, insurers use case managers, often employed outside the plan, to oversee and designate which group of services will yield the best outcome. Frequently this decision-making power allows a case manager to approve treatments that a plan might not normally cover. Some insurers use the terms *case management* and *managed care* synonymously.

2. *Precertification* or *preauthorization.* The requirement that specific tests, surgical procedures, or categories of services (e.g., mental health) be authorized before they are allowed gives the insurer the opportunity to deny "unnecessary" treatment or substitute lower-cost services.

3. *Mandatory second opinion.* Insisting on a second opinion before approval of any or specific types of surgical procedures serves as a check on a physician's decision regarding the need for surgery. It presents an opportunity for another physician to suggest an alternative, less costly treatment.

4. *Third party administrator.* To obtain the best economies, insurers contract with a private company that specializes in management of various administrative functions (e.g., claims) and managed care responsibilities (e.g., utilization review) of a plan or an employer, if self-insured.

Because state laws and plan philosophies differ, practitioners must research on a very local level the environment in which private insurers operate. Following are questions that occupational therapy managers and practitioners should ask about their patients' health care coverage before providing service. They should also ask these questions about their own policies.

1. What specific types of inpatient and outpatient health care services does the plan cover?

2. Are there limitations in number of visits, sites at which services may be received, or yearly costs for specific services?

3. Is there a network of providers from whom patients must obtain services? Can a patient "opt out" of the network, and if so, what financial disincentives exist?

4. What copayments, deductibles, or other out-of-pocket expenses exist for using non-network providers? Under what circumstances?

5. Does the plan offer case management services for some conditions?

This type of information is essential for practitioners to provide the optimal covered care and to assist patients in making decisions about continuing care that their insurance may not cover. It also provides a basis for managers and practitioners to evaluate the benefits of joining a health plan provider panel or a preferred provider network.

Table 2.2 Tips for using diagnosis and procedure codes

Using Diagnosis Codes (ICD-9-CM)

- Use the most current version of the ICD-9-CM manual, which is updated in October of each year.

- Remember that the patient's condition is key to a medical necessity determination. Justify the care provided by presenting the essential information to assist the payer in determining the need for care.

- Always code as principal diagnosis (the first diagnosis referenced in item 21 on the HCFA-1500 claim and item 67 of the UB-92) the current condition that prompted the patient's visit. Code other conditions or a chronic condition when applicable to the present treatment.

- Relate each service, procedure, or supply to an ICD-9-CM code. Make sure the ICD-9-CM codes on your bill reflect the reasons for each service provided.

Using Procedure Codes (HCPCS)

- Always review the most recent codes and definitions for new code numbers and modified descriptions of services. Level I (CPT) and II HCPCS codes are updated each January.

- Be specific. Always select the code(s) that most closely describe the service(s) provided. Avoid using "unlisted procedure" codes.

- Most CPT codes in the Physical Medicine and Rehabilitation section are defined in 15-minute segments. When coding more than one [15-minute] unit for a single service, indicate the number of units (item 24 G on the HCFA-1500 form). Do not list the same code multiple times.

- List the CPT code and units, where necessary, for each modality and procedure performed. For example, where a modality is used as a precursor to therapy, both the modality and the treatment code can be billed.

- Use modifiers when appropriate with HCPCS codes to describe when a procedure or service has been altered by some specific circumstance but not changed in its definition or code. The modifier indicates to the insurance carrier that the procedure should be manually priced. A complete list of modifiers is contained in the CPT and Level II HCPCS manuals; however, check with the payer to determine local policy in using modifiers.

- Use CPT special service codes (i.e., 99000 to 99199) when appropriate along with the primary procedure code.

Source: Thomas, V.J. (1996, February 8). *"Code It Right," OT Week.*

Billing and Coding for Services

Payment for services provided by both facility and individual providers is usually predicated on proper coding and completion of claim forms. Two common billing forms are

- the Uniform Bill (UB-92; HCFA-1450), used by institutional providers such as hospitals and home health agencies, for Medicaid, CHAMPUS, and Medicare (for most Part A service billing)
- the HCFA-1500 claim form, primarily used by private practitioners such as physicians and occupational therapists in independent practice,[2] for Medicare, CHAMPUS, Medicaid, and workers' compensation in most states.

Public and private payers usually require health care facilities and practitioners to represent their services in terms of diagnosis and procedure codes. Not all payers cover the same range of services or permit use of the same codes. In addition, state regulations or payer policies may establish limitations on the amount paid for a specific code or combination of codes.

DIAGNOSIS CODES – *Diagnosis codes* describe the patient's condition or the medical reason for the patient's requiring services. They are critical to obtaining a favorable determination of coverage. ICD-9-CM (*International Classification of Diseases, 9th Revision, Clinical Modification, 1993*, updated annually) is the most frequently used diagnosis-coding system in the United States. Under the ICD coding system, diseases are categorized primarily by anatomical systems. Also, ICD contains supplementary classifications covering factors influencing health status and external causes of injury and poisoning. An additional volume provides a listing of ICD surgical and medical procedures, which are mainly used to code inpatient hospital services. Table 2.2 offers tips for using diagnosis codes effectively.

PROCEDURE CODES – *Procedure codes* describe specific services performed by health care professionals. One of the most widely used procedure-coding systems is the HCFA Common Procedure Coding System (HCPCS), which includes the American Medical Association's (updated annually) *Physicians' Current Procedural Terminology* (CPT),[3] referred to as Level I HCPCS; the HCFA–developed alphanumeric codes, referred to as Level II HCPCS; and local codes, referred to as Level III HCPCS, created by Medicare and other carriers as needed, when other HCPCS codes do not suffice. Level II HCPCS also contains codes for durable medical equipment, prosthetics, orthotics, and supplies (DMEPOS) and some procedures not found in the CPT system. Table 2.2 also offers tips for using procedure codes effectively.

CURRENT PROCEDURAL TERMINOLOGY – Since 1990, HCFA has contracted with the American Medical Association to use the CPT coding system as the basis for the Medicare Physicians' Fee Schedule (as noted earlier, also known as the Resource Based Relative Value Scale, RBRVS) and to assist with the development of *relative work values* (RVWs) for each code. In May 1993 the American Medical Association invited nine nonphysician practitioner associations to partici-

---

[2] Insurers generally do not recognize occupational therapy assistants for direct payment because they require supervision and do not perform evaluations.

3. CPT five-digit codes and two-digit modifiers are copyrighted by the American Medical Association.

pate in the CPT Editorial Panel and Relative Value Scale Update Committee processes by forming a Health Care Professionals Advisory Committee. AOTA was included in this initial group, along with the American Academy of Physician Assistants, the American Nurses Association, the American Optometric Association, the American Physical Therapy Association, the American Podiatric Medical Association, the American Psychological Association, the American Speech-Language-Hearing Association, and the National Association of Social Workers. In 1995 the American Chiropractic Association joined the committee. These associations, individually and as a group, make recommendations to the annual update of CPT and the relative work values.

The coding system, which is updated annually by the American Medical Association, provides a uniform terminology for each of thousands of medical procedures. Occupational therapists in independent practice use CPT codes to bill Medicare and most other public and private insurers. Although occupational therapists most often use codes in the Physical Medicine section of CPT, under American Medical Association guidelines, physicians and nonphysician practitioners should select the codes that most accurately identify the services performed. Other than the requirement that the service be within the scope of practice of the practitioner, there are no CPT restrictions for use of codes in any section. Occupational therapists should request information on allowable codes, service definitions, and documentation policies before billing a new insurer.

FEE FOR SERVICE – Traditionally, providers have been paid on the basis of *fee for service*, some type of rate per unit of service (e.g., a procedure code or a per diem). This rate may be based on a fee schedule or may be a negotiated discounted rate for a specific treatment or specific groups of treatments. Generally under fee for service, a practitioner is paid for each code or service billed and has no incentive to limit procedures and tests or to examine lower-cost types of treatment. In a fee-for-service system the insurer assumes the primary risk because under the contractual provisions with the employer or another consumer, the insurer must pay for all covered care. For this reason, payers often use cost-saving techniques such as preset service limitations or post-payment utilization reviews to identify overuse by providers.

PROSPECTIVE RATE – Most *prospective rate* formulas are designed to aggregate payment for groups of services necessary for a patient's care for a specific type of injury or illness or over a specific duration of time (e.g., per case or per episode). The Medicare DRG payment is a prospective rate that includes all surgical and medical services (except physicians') required to treat a patient with a specific diagnosis during a specific hospital inpatient stay. Under a prospective payment system, providers have greater flexibility in determining mix of services. However, because a prospective rate is based on the average expense for a particular condition, the provider is at risk for ensuring that costs in the aggregate do not exceed payments.

CAPITATION – In a *capitation* payment system the provider is paid prospectively (usually on a monthly basis), for each member of a specific population (e.g., members of a health plan or Medicaid beneficiaries), regardless of whether any covered health care service is delivered.

Evolving Payment Methodologies

This prospective rate is termed *per member, per month* and is customarily based on the past claim experience of the specific capitated population. Under capitation the provider has the benefit of a predictable revenue source but is at greater financial risk because more service equals less profit. For a provider the per-member-per-month amount is the most important factor in determining the profitability, or even the feasibility, of a capitated contract.

Capitation provisions are primarily found in HMO contracts because this type of managed care organization is the most homogeneous in terms of administrative and utilization controls. However, legal affiliations and payment relationships among hospitals, clinics, laboratories, and other types of health care providers are continually evolving, and other types of networks are using forms of capitated payment. Capitation rates were initially developed for payment of primary care physicians. This payment method is more easily (and equitably) calculated for primary care physicians, who as gatekeepers have the most patient interaction and the most control of services. Additionally, it is easier to project service cost and therefore to set a valid per-member-per-month rate.

PPOs and many HMOs continue to pay specialists—whether physicians, therapists, or other provider types—on a fee-for-service basis. As provider chains and multispecialty organizations continue to grow, however, it becomes easier to estimate statistically the amount of treatment that a prospectively set per-member-per-month rate should cover without the risk of catastrophic loss to the provider. When physicians, independent practice associations, specialty rehabilitation groups, and hospitals are capitated, therapy services are sometimes subcontracted to another entity that may be paid under a different method.

In addition to the per-member-per-month amount, providers should consider all aspects of a contract in evaluating the viability of a capitation arrangement. Table 2.3 presents some of these factors.

Table 2.3 Factors to consider in evaluating the viability of a capitation arrangement

Factor	Consideration
Number of members in capitated population	The greater the number of members, the higher the overall prospectively paid monthly rate from that plan will be.
Member profile	Risk (i.e., use of services) is statistically determined by age, sex, and health care factors relative to type of service provided.
Specific details of plan that affect members' access to and incentives to use services	Benefit package, member deductibles and copayment amounts, referral requirements (e.g., requirements that care be referred by primary care physician), or high copayment for therapy will reduce demand for services. For example, provider may require higher capitation rate to offset low copayment.
Numbers of other similar providers in network	Generally, if there are few providers offering similar services, per-member-per-month rate must be high enough to cover cost of expected large number of referrals.

RISK SHARING AND RISK POOLS – The concept of *risk sharing* and the construction of *risk pools* are critical issues for providers in deciding whether or not to join a capitated network. Risk adjustments can also exist in noncapitated contractual arrangements. A risk pool of dollars is created from a designated amount of money withheld from payments to providers throughout the year, and it is used to meet specified expenses of the pool. On the basis of a predefined "reward" formula, unused funds in the pool are distributed at the end of the year to providers who meet the targeted utilization and cost goals. The design of the pool (e.g., specialties of providers and number per pool) and the way in which it is used during the year determine the risk (i.e., whether there is any money in the pool by the end of the year). An infinite number of arrangements and formulas can be created under the guise of risk sharing. Providers should understand the details of each contract to which they commit.

Conclusion

Payment resources for all health care services are shrinking. Federal and state policymakers are seeking ways to redefine essential services and to provide them at minimal cost. The administrative control of health benefits is gradually shifting to state and local levels and private health insurers. In most states, public programs and private plans are relying on preferred provider networks and managed care strategies to lower costs. With the growth of managed care, the separation between provider and insurer is narrowing as mergers create new health care entities.

For occupational therapy practitioners, these trends argue for better articulation of the value of occupational therapy and development of practice methods that demonstrate more cost-effective ways to provide quality rehabilitation services. For independent practitioners, changing funding methods may require affiliation with larger provider entities that can better negotiate with the health care payers of the future.

Summary

Public funds for occupational therapy services are typically available through either federal or state insurance programs, which generally have structured guidelines specifying which services are covered, in what settings, and by whom; and grant programs, which include occupational therapy as part of an overall program for a specific population. Under private insurance plans, services are usually provided to groups of individuals through benefit programs offered by employers or other organizations. However, individuals may purchase policies directly from companies.

Medicare is by far the largest single payer for occupational therapy services. The Medicare program consists of the Hospital Insurance Program (Part A), which pays for hospital inpatient, skilled nursing facility, home health, and hospice care; and the Supplementary Medical Insurance Program (Part B), which covers hospital outpatient, physician, and other professional services, including occupational therapy services performed by independent practitioners. Generally, occupational therapy is considered a Medicare-covered service if it is

1. prescribed by a physician and furnished according to a written plan of care approved by the physician

2. performed by a qualified occupational therapist, or by an occupational therapy assistant under the general supervision of an occupational therapist

3. reasonable and necessary for the treatment of the person's illness or injury.

The Civilian Health and Medical Program of the Uniformed Services (CHAMPUS) is a United States Department of Defense program of health care for the dependents of active-duty members of the armed forces and for retired members. It shares the cost of medical and other health care that eligible beneficiaries receive from civilian sources. CHAMPUS regulations provide for a basic health care program and a special program of rehabilitative benefits.

The Federal Employees Health Benefit Program covers federal government employees, retirees, and their dependents. Coverage of individual types of services and the settings in which they may be provided is determined by each of the large number of private plans with which the government contracts to administer health care services.

Medicaid is a federal-state program that provides health care to the poor and the medically indigent. Medicaid services fall into two categories: mandatory services, which a state must provide to qualify for federal matching funds; and optional services. Mandatory services include hospital services; laboratory work and X-rays; skilled nursing facility services; physicians' services; early and periodic screening, diagnosis, and treatment (EPSDT) for persons under 21 years of age; and family planning. Occupational therapy provided as a freestanding discipline is considered an optional service.

Workers' compensation programs, developed to compensate employees who have job-related injuries or illnesses, are financed jointly by individual employers or groups of employers and state governments. Each state has a workers' compensation governing board or commission that develops policies regulating whether an employer is required to participate, what the financial responsibility of the employer is, what benefits are provided, which workers are covered, and how the insurance is administered. Workers' compensation programs consist of two components, cash benefits and medical benefits.

The Education for All Handicapped Children Act, reenacted in 1990 as the Individuals with Disabilities Education Act (IDEA), provides federal grants to states to ensure that eligible children with disabilities have access to a "free, appropriate public education." Part B of IDEA requires that public school systems and other state agencies involved in educating children with disabilities (ages 3–21) make available "a free appropriate public education that includes special education and related services to meet their unique needs" (Education, 1977). Under this program, occupational therapy is considered a *related service*. Part H of IDEA authorizes grant moneys to states "to develop and implement a statewide, comprehensive, coordinated, multidisciplinary, interagency program of early intervention services for infants and toddlers with disabilities and their families" (Education, 1989). Under this program, occupational therapy is considered a *primary service.* Under Part B and Part H of IDEA, occupational therapy services must be provided according to an individualized education program (IEP) and an individualized family service plan (IFSP), respectively.

The Rehabilitation Act of 1973, Section 504, and the Americans with Disabilities Act (ADA) of 1990 may be used to ensure nondiscrimination against students who do not qualify for services under IDEA but need educational support (Copenhaver, 1995).

Private insurers have many product lines and will often negotiate unique benefit and premium configurations for a single employer. Four management techniques are often implemented in conjunction with cost-controlling payment strategies: case management, precertification or preauthorization, mandatory second opinion, and third party administrator.

Payment for services provided by both facility and individual providers is usually predicated on proper coding and completion of claim forms. Two common billing forms are the Uniform Bill (UB-92; HCFA-1450) and the HCFA-1500 claim form.

Public and private payers usually require health care facilities and practitioners to represent their services in terms of diagnosis and procedure codes. *Diagnosis codes* describe the patient's condition or the medical reason for the patient's requiring services. *Procedure codes* describe specific services performed by health care professionals.

The concept of risk sharing and the construction of risk pools are critical issues for providers in deciding whether or not to join a capitated network.

References

American Medical Association. (updated annually). *Physicians' current procedural terminology.* Chicago: Author.

American Occupational Therapy Association. (1997). *Guidelines for occupational therapy practice under the Individuals with Disabilities Education Act.* Bethesda, MD: Author.

Americans with Disabilities Act of 1990, Pub. L. No. 101–336, 104 Stat. 327.

Balanced Budget Act (P.L. 105-133).

Brick, L. L. (1996). Medicare HMOs to expand role of rehab, subacute. *Continuing Care, 15*(2), 18–19.

Burton, J. (1996). Workers' compensation, twenty-four-hour coverage, and managed care. *Workers' Compensation Monitor, 9*(1), 11–21.

Community Mental Health Centers Act of 1963, Pub. L. No. 88–164, Title II, 77 Stat. 290.

Copenhaver, J. (1995). *Section 504: An educator's primer.* Logan, UT: Mountain Plains Regional Resource Center. (Address: 1780 North Research Parkway, Suite 112, Logan, UT 84322-9620.)

Education, 34 C.F.R. § 300.1 (1977), redesignated at 45 *Fed. Reg.* 77368 (1980).

Education, 34 C.F.R. § 303.1 (1989), as amended at 56 *Fed. Reg.* 54688 (1991).

Education for All Handicapped Children Act of 1975, Pub. L. No. 94–142, 89 Stat. 773.

Education of the Handicapped Amendments of 1986, Pub. L. No. 99–457, 100 Stat. 1145.

Education of the Handicapped Amendments of 1990, Pub. L. No. 101–476, 104 Stat. 1103.

Employee Retirement Income Security Act of 1974, Pub. L. No. 93–406, 88 Stat. 829.

Health Care Financing Administration. (1996, February). *Medicare prepaid health plans report.* Baltimore: Author.

Health Care Financing Administration. (updated continually). *Medicare intermediary manual.* Baltimore: Author.

Individuals with Disabilities Education Act Amendments of 1991, Pub. L. No. 102–119, 105 Stat. 587.

Individuals with Disabilities Education Act of 1990, Pub. L. No. 101–476, Section 901, 104 Stat. 1103.

International classification of diseases, 9th revision, clinical modification (ICD-9-CM). (1993; updated annually). Salt Lake City, UT: Med-Index Publications; Bethesda, MD: National Center for Health Statistics (Vols. 1–2); Baltimore: Health Care Financing Administration (Vol. 3).

Lewin–VHI, Inc. (1995). *States as payers: Managed care for Medicaid populations.* Washington, DC: National Institute for Health Care Management.

Older Americans Act of 1965, Pub. L. No. 89–73, 79 Stat. 218, as amended.

Omnibus Budget Reconciliation Act of 1981, Pub. L. No. 97–35, 95 Stat. 357.

Public Health, 42 C.F.R. § 417.414 (1985), amended at 58 *Fed. Reg.* 38062 (1993), 60 *Fed. Reg.* 45673, 45677 (1995).

Public Health, 42 C.F.R. § 482.56 (1986a).

Public Health, 42 C.F.R. § 482.62(g)(2) (1986b).

Rehabilitation Act of 1973, Section 504, Pub. L. No. 93–112, 87 Stat. 355.

Social Security Amendments of 1965, Title XVIII, Medicare, Pub. L. No. 89–97, 79 Stat. 206, as amended.

Social Security Amendments of 1971, Title XIX, Medicaid, Pub. L. No. 92–223, 85 Stat. 802, as amended.

Thomas, V.J. (1996, Feburary 8). Code it right. *OT Week*, p. 14.

United States Bureau of the Census. (1994). *Current population reports, 1994.* Washington, DC: Government Printing Office.

Vladeck, B.C., & King, K. M. (1995). Medicare at 30: Preparing for the future. *Journal of the American Medical Association, 274,* 259–62.

Additional Resources

CHAMPUS Information Office, Aurora, CO 80045-6900, telephone 303/361-1000.

Health Care Financing Administration, 7500 Security Boulevard, Baltimore, MD 21244-1850, telephone 410/786-3000.

International Association of Industrial Accident Boards and Commissions, 1575 Aviation Center Parkway, Suite 512, Daytona Beach, FL 32114, telephone 904/252-2915.

Office of Personnel Management, Theodore Roosevelt Federal Building, 1900 E Street NW, Washington, DC 20415, telephone 202/606-1000.

Workers' Compensation Research Institute, 101 Main Street, Cambridge, MA 02142, telephone 617/494-1240.

3. Why We Document

Susan C. Robertson, MS, OTR/L, FAOTA

This chapter provides an overview of the major reasons why we document. It is important to note that, although we have several target audiences when we document, we can use the same strategies to communicate with all of them.

Susan C. Robertson is a mental health specialist in the Rehabilitation Medicine Department of the National Institutes of Health, Bethesda, Maryland.

Documentation is the general term for the communication of information about a patient or client to others. There are many people who request information about the type of service, length of treatment, modalities used, and progress on functional improvement from the service provider. Different information is needed by different people and at different times in the course of treatment. How this information is communicated is the essence of documentation formatting.

The purpose of this chapter is to explore documentation from two critical perspectives. First, the key elements of documentation are outlined. The content to be included in documentation to make it effective is discussed. Second, various approaches to presenting the key information are described. The purpose of this section of the chapter is to articulate the ways in which information may be communicated and the advantages and disadvantages of each approach.

The challenge before every occupational therapy practitioner is to select the key elements to include in the documentation and then to use an existing format or develop one that organizes those key elements into a clear, concise, and comprehensive communication about the occupational therapy outcomes. A system that works well for all kinds of treatment approaches and is easily adaptable for a given individual is worth the time it takes to develop and test a documentation procedure.

Target Audiences

What is documented is contingent on *who* needs the information. Within the managed care system, there is an increased reliance on documentation to communicate among various services along the continuum of care. Decisions about access to services depend on documentation that characterizes the patient's need for health care and prevention programs. Managed care personnel, case managers, and policy makers require clear definition of functional limitations to be addressed, the projected course of treatment, the progress in functional change, and the key decision points to channel services cost effectively.

Briefly, there are several target audiences for typical occupational therapy documentation. First is the *treatment team*. Sharing evaluation results, plans for intervention, progress toward goals, and outcomes is essential to integrated care for the individual. Each member of the treatment team is interested in a different aspect of the occupational therapy program. The physician, for example, may be most interested in physical capacities being developed. On the other hand, the physical therapist may be most interested in successful approaches to achieving functional outcomes so that the occupational and physical therapy programs are complementary.

Another audience in the setting is the individual(s) responsible for *chart review* or *audit*. Occupational therapy charts are reviewed to ensure completeness, that services are appropriate for the diagnosis, and in some cases whether services follow a predetermined clinical path. Occupational therapy documentation provides information used both for retrospective and concurrent review. The record outlines the type and sequence of intervention, length of treatment, outcome, and personnel implementing the program. This information is gathered to evaluate the occupational therapy program and compare it to predetermined criteria for high quality service delivery.

Yet another audience for occupational therapy documentation is the *third party payer*. Before the onset of diagnosis related groups (DRGs), payment for services in hospitals was determined on the basis of what services were provided to achieve predefined goals. The current system of DRGs is based on what length of stay and intervention are considered normal and customary for a given diagnosis. Although the review of inpatient occupational therapy documentation may not occur at the level of the third party payer, but rather at the level of hospital utilization review, it is still essential to the payment for services. In outpatient settings, documentation may be reviewed directly by the third party payer.

An external body that requires good communication about the type and extent of service delivery is the *accrediting agency*. Accredited facilities must meet minimum standards for documentation in order to maintain their accreditation status. This includes not only the content and presentation of records but also the maintenance of records for a certain length of time.

Another significant audience is the *patient* or *client*. The emphasis on patient rights, patient advocacy, and patient autonomy have brought the medical record into the hands of the patient. Careful communication about intervention goals and progress may be integrated into the treatment process and may affect the therapeutic interaction between therapist and patient.

Increasing malpractice litigation has led to another target audience: the *legal system*. The medical record is a legal document often used in court in accident and work injury cases. In the legal system, what is not written in the medical record did not happen. It is essential to write the evaluation protocol and results, treatment goals, modalities, and functional outcomes of occupational therapy intervention.

Documentation is also used by *researchers* interested in evaluating occupational therapy service delivery. Quantitative data gleaned from the medical record may describe the types of diagnoses treated, the range of services provided, the use of types of service providers, and the relationship of modalities to outcomes. The quality of the documentation has a direct effect on the quality of the research and whether the results can be generalized.

Each of these audiences needs different information about the occupational therapy evaluation, goals, progress, and outcomes. It is important for each practitioner to identify the specific individuals and groups that may be interested in the documentation of occupational therapy services. Only then is it clear what information must be communicated and what are the key elements of the documentation.

It is difficult to determine which of the target audiences has the greatest influence on the design and elements of the medical record. Some would argue that the third party payer has the greatest influence because without payment for services provided there would not be an occupational therapy service at all. Others would contend that the treatment team is the most influential because the quality of care is contingent on close coordination of service delivery among related personnel. Still others would argue that the legal system is the most influential because of the high risk and costs associated with malpractice litigation.

Key Elements   There are numerous books and articles written about the content of the medical record. Huffman (1985) has comprehensively described the basic components and specific adaptations suitable for different treatment environments, such as ambulatory care, home care, hospice programs, and long-term care facilities. In each practice setting, the occupational therapist must contribute information to the medical record of the patient or client treated.

Given these considerations, it is possible to identify the following essential elements of the occupational therapy record:

- patient name and patient information
- diagnosis (primary and treatment diagnoses)
- physician referral
- initial evaluation protocol and results (identify prior functional level, functional limitations, and medical conditions)
- place of service
- treatment goals (short-term and long-term, identification of problems)
- progress notes, patient's response to intervention, length of treatment, duration, levels of assistance needed
- reevaluation and results, including changes in treatment goals
- status at discharge (problem resolution, functional status)
- summary of treatment
- name of caregiver
- provider information.

These are the basic components of a comprehensive documentation of occupational therapy services. It is important for each practitioner to ascertain whether these are the only required elements or whether additional items are necessary. There are a number of areas to check to determine whether the documentation is complete.

Some states have specific requirements; some managed care organizations and payers have specific requirements; sometimes the facility has a particular need to include additional information for quality review. In some cases, the nature of the service dictates the information to be included in the occupational therapy record. For instance, documentation for assistive technology often needs very specific technical information.

The key elements of the occupational therapy documentation must be determined by each occupational therapy department and should be reviewed on a regular basis to ensure that the occupational therapy documentation format is correct.

It is critical that these key components of the medical record be consistent between service providers and among facilities. For this reason, it is important to use standard definitions "to facilitate comparison of different data bases across systems and to achieve as much uniformity as possible at the national level" (Public Health Service, 1987, p. 6). To promote consistency, Medicare has developed uniform reporting forms that other third party payers have adopted.

Once the key elements of documentation have been identified, the next step is to design a format for recording information that conveys the key elements, communicates to the various target audiences identified, and is easily usable by the occupational therapy practitioner. This is one of the most creative aspects of documentation—designing a format that includes the necessary information; requires concise, clear, and comprehensive communication; and enables the practitioner to document efficiently and consistently.

Documentation Approaches

Documentation formats may be categorized in many ways. In this chapter, they will be distinguished by their content, authorship, and presentation style. Selecting a general approach to documentation is an essential step in deciding how to organize the information into a particular format.

SOURCE-ORIENTED MEDICAL RECORD — The source-oriented medical record is organized in sections according to the department providing care. All the occupational therapy evaluation, treatment, and progress information is found together in the medical record, arranged in chronological order. It is easy to locate the documentation of the physician, for example, but it is difficult to determine all the patient's problems with the source-oriented medical record.

PROBLEM-ORIENTED MEDICAL RECORD — The problem-oriented medical record, introduced by Lawrence Weed, MD, is organized to reflect the clinical thinking and services provided for specific patient problems. Clinical problems are followed; the efforts of various rehabilitation practitioners in relation to identified problems are noted; and the progress in remediating or minimizing the problem is documented.

The problem-oriented medical record must contain four basic components: the database, a complete list of problems, plans for each problem, and progress notes (Weed, 1971). The database contains the results of the initial evaluation, including how the information was obtained. The data about medical history, social supports, and present illness or complaints yield a list of problems that require further evaluation or intervention. Additions and changes in the problem list are made during the course of treatment. Plans for the problems indicate strategies for how further evaluation will be conducted, how the problem will be treated, and patient education. Progress notes include subjective, objective, assessment, and plan statements commonly known as the SOAP note. The objective is to describe symptoms, report measurements and observations, interpret the data, and develop approaches to remediating or resolving the problems.

The objective, interpretative, and plan sections of the progress notes provide the physician with the opportunity to describe why a particular course of action was taken and why the usual criteria for management of a patient were not followed (Weed, 1971). All of the patient's problems can be viewed as a whole, and the relationship of allied health personnel to the total treatment plan is clearly delineated. The problem-oriented medical record requires a commitment by facility personnel to learn the technique and faithfully follow its protocol.

INTEGRATED MEDICAL RECORD – The integrated medical record is organized in strict chronological order. The information from various sources is mixed throughout the chart. This format enables the reader to define all interventions that were used with a specific phase of the illness, but it is difficult to locate and compare, for example, only the entries of the occupational therapist. This makes it difficult to compare the patient response to treatment over time. Adaptations of the integrated medical record are more commonly seen. The progress notes may take the integrated form, but reports and laboratory results may be found in source-oriented sections of the chart.

Given these three approaches to documenting patient care, there are many variations in the format for communicating information. For instance, the SOAP note from Dr. Weed's system may be used as a way to organize a progress note in the integrated medical record system. The source-oriented note is commonly presented in the narrative form, but it may also be presented in a table or grid. The next section discusses the advantages and disadvantages of various formats for documentation.

Documentation Formats

To this point, the discussion of documentation has centered on the content of the medical record. How the information is presented is another important feature of documentation. Various approaches to the format for communicating information about the patient, evaluation, treatment, and progress are presented.

Before the advent of computers, documentation was done manually—a cumbersome task at best. The literature shows that there were many approaches to organizing and communicating information for the medical record. The earliest form was the narrative. Lengthy descriptions were given of patient complaints, symptoms, function, and intervention. There were no standard protocols for drafting these narratives, and they took many different shapes. Some clearly addressed patient problems, the course of treatment, and outcome. In others, information was not well-organized or clearly descriptive of the course of treatment.

Environmental pressures such as shrinking health resources, increasing productivity standards, and tighter accreditation criteria have influenced the format for documentation. There are numerous examples of charts, grids, tables, flow sheets, and forms that point to widespread efforts in most health disciplines to streamline documentation while ensuring that the professional and legal requirements are met.

While each of these is intended to decrease documentation time and increase legibility and inclusion of necessary content in the medical record, a careful critique will reveal that some formats do not include the information needed for the various target audiences defined in the earlier part of this chapter. The key information is not included or is not presented in a way useful to managed care organizations, third party payers, accrediting bodies, or review agencies. Critics of these formats argue that insufficient information can be included on forms that limit the ability to describe actual intervention. Proponents advocate the use of predesigned and pretested formats to facilitate a consistent, comprehensive, legible communication of the key elements of documentation.

Computers have caused another look at documentation. There are descriptions of computerized documentation strategies as well as critiques of the advantages and disadvantages of computer documentation in the recent literature (Adineh, 1987; Dawdy, Munter, & Gilmore, 1997; Hathaway, 1988; McDonald & Tierney, 1988; Tello, Tuc, & Cosentino, 1995; Wolf, 1987). As with previous formats, the goal is to design a format that provides sufficient communication for targeted audiences and is clear, concise, and comprehensive. Beyond this, "a good computerized care plan system will generate assignment (flow) sheets that specify, for each caregiver, the tasks he or she is to perform in order to achieve the objectives of the plan" (Wolf, 1987, p. 39). Treatment personnel can readily scan the areas to be addressed in the normal course of intervention for a given diagnosis and design a comprehensive treatment plan. The potential for generating reports about the population served, treatment delivered, optimal staffing patterns, and supply requirements is staggering.

The ability to scan and analyze the course of treatment has emerged as a high priority in the managed care climate, and computerization of medical management has become commonplace. Computerized documentation is an asset to examining adherence to clinical pathways or case management plans, since the flow of intervention is more readily followed when documentation from diverse practitioners is entered chronologically.

Computerized documentation, sometimes in the form of a data management system (Sabbo, 1997), is a contributing factor both to outcomes and process audit. Outcomes audit, designed to evaluate the effect of care on health, is used to judge how well standards of care have been met. Process audit focuses on the specific clinical actions, consistent with treatment protocols or clinical pathways, that are assumed to affect overall outcome of intervention (McIntyre, 1995). Documentation, then, can be used to measure improvement in the process of medical care as well as to measure accountability (Solberg, Mosser, & McDonald, 1997).

While computerization of health practices and the effect on functional performance has permeated medical records systems, there are potential risks associated with computerized approaches to documentation. There may be a reduction of emphasis in the medical record on the human element, the real-life problems experienced by the patient or client. When symptoms, functional levels, degrees of assistance needed for independence, and treatment approaches used are predefined by the computer format, it can be difficult to individualize the documentation to reflect the uniqueness of the person being treated. Treatment personnel may rely too heavily on the predefined usual course of treatment and overlook particular manifestations in the individual case. All the components of the medical record cannot be stored in the computer because of the high costs of designing and searching large files.

Computer documentation may also put a burden on the payers and reviewers of claims since standard documentation formats require that the total documentation form be filled in and printed each time a note is generated, even though only a small portion of the documentation may actually change. This can generate a large amount of paperwork and require additional reviewer time to read through the reams of material. Changes in technology alter the computerized documentation system, resulting in increased costs for staff education to use the system. As the computer is used more frequently, additional risks with computerized documentation will come to light.

Selecting an Approach and Format

Formats for documentation are always evolving. It is important for occupational therapy practitioners to update their repertoire of available approaches and routinely reevaluate the usefulness and accuracy of existing formats.

The most important step in selecting an approach to documentation and a format for use by occupational therapy staff is to determine what requirements, if any, the facility uses. Many external influences, such as the Joint Commission on the Accreditation of Healthcare Organizations (JCAHO) and the Commission on Accreditation of Rehabilitation Facilities (CARF) affect how the administration organizes documentation throughout the facility. In addition, internal influences are important. The systems for quality assurance and program evaluation have a great impact on how occupational therapy documentation should be approached. Chapter 4 details how the quality assurance system can influence documentation.

Given that certain elements of documentation are required and that particular information is needed for the target audiences, the way the information is compiled and presented is the creative part of the documentation approach. Each occupational therapy department may have a different format to meet the needs of the various groups with which it communicates.

Selecting the right approach is easy. Following the steps below will ensure success.

- Determine the needs of third party reviewers.
- Determine how the facility is accredited and what information is required by the accrediting agencies.
- Determine what procedures for quality assurance are used in the facility.
- Determine what medical records procedure are used in the facility.
- Meet with occupational therapy staff to decide on the guidelines that should be followed to clearly communicate functional goals.
- Draft a format that incorporates the information that must be communicated.

- Test the instrument and revise as needed.

- Present the instrument in draft form to the groups that would typically use the information: hospital administration, fiscal personnel, physicians, medical records department, quality assurance committee, and other team members.

- Revise the instrument as needed to meet the requirements of these groups.

- Set a time period of 6-8 months to use the instrument. Plan a formal meeting to discuss the instrument, its usefulness, and ability to communicate. Make revisions as needed.

- Keep the instrument fresh by regularly checking to see if the information to communicate is being understood by the target audiences identified.

- Keep current on trends in documentation and payment for health services and adapt the instrument as needed to meet external changes.

Remembering that *form follows function* will help in keeping the paperwork down, designing a useful and usable format, and streamlining the kinds of information that need to be communicated. Monitoring the documentation process may seem to be cumbersome, but doing a thorough job on this aspect of documentation will mean less time overall in documenting practice. The ultimate goal is the provision of high quality care. Documentation is essential to meeting that goal.

References

Dawdy, M. R., Munter, D.W., & Gilmore, R. A. (1997). Correlation of patient entry rates and physician documentation errors in dictated and handwritten emergency treatment records. *American Journal of Emergency Medicine, 15*(2), 115-117.

Huffman, E. K. (1985). *Medical record management.* Berwyn, IL: Physician's Record Company.

McIntyre, N. (1995). Evaluation in clinical practice: Problems, precedents, and principles. *Journal of Evaluation in Clinical Practice, 1*(1), 5-13.

Public Health Service. (1987). *Statistical aspects of physician payment systems.* (DHHS Publication No. PHS 87-1461). Hyattsville, MD: National Center for Health Statistics.

Weed, L. L. (1971). Quality control and the medical record. *Archives of Internal Medicine, 127*, 101-105.

Wolf, S. C. (1987, June). Administration: Computerized care plans a strong management tool. *Provider*, 39-40.

Additional Resources

Acquaviva, J. A., & Steich, T. J. (1988). Occupational therapy documentation in mental health. In S.C. Robertson (Ed.), *Mental health FOCUS: Skills for assessment and treatment* (pp. 1-177). Bethesda, MD: American Occupational Therapy Association.

American Occupational Therapy Association. (1980). *Sample forms for occupational therapy.* Bethesda, MD: Author.

Bair, J., & Gwin, C. (1985). *A productivity systems guide for occupational therapy.* Bethesda, MD: American Occupational Therapy Association.

Butterworth, J. (1997). Clinical pathways for the high-risk patient. *Journal of Cardiothoracic Vascular Anesthesia, 11*(2, supp. 1), 16-18.

Chase, S. K. (1997). Charting critical thinking: Nursing judgments and patient outcomes. *Dimensions of Critical Care Nursing, 16*(2), 102-111.

Corbett, M. W. (1996). Flow chart to benchmark. *Best Practice Benchmarking in Healthcare, 1*(3), 161-166.

Gabriele, E. R. (1973). Medical record system: Acquisition and handling of clinical information. In *Quality assurance of medical care*. Washington, DC: Regional Medical Programs Service, Health Services and Mental Health Administration, U.S. Department of Health, Education, and Welfare.

Gondringer, N. S. (1986). Medical malpractice: The need for documentation/communication. *Journal of the American Association of Nurse Anesthetists, 54*, 490-495.

Gropper, E. I. (1988, March-April). Does your charting reflect your worth? *Geriatric Nursing*. 99-101.

Ibarra, V., Laffoon, T. A., Synder, M., Gambrall, M., & Olson, S. R. (1997). Clinical pathways in the perioperative setting. *Nurse Case Manager, 2*(3), 97-104.

LaRosa-Nash, P., & O'Malley, M. (1997). Streamlining the perioperative process. *Nurse Clinician of North America, 32*(1), 141-151.

Levknecht, L., Schriefer, J., & Maconis, B. (1997). Combining case management, pathways, and report cards for secondary cardiac prevention. *Joint Commission Quality Improvement, 23*(3), 162-174.

Little, A. B., & Whipple, T. W. (1996). Clinical pathway implementation in the acute care hospital setting. *Journal of Nursing Care Quality, 11*(2), 54-61.

Morrissey-Ross, M. (1988). Documentation: If you haven't written it, you haven't done it. *Nursing Clinics of North America, 23*, 363-371.

Murphy, R. N. (1997). Legal and practical impact of clinical practice guidelines on nursing and medical practice. *Nurse Practitioner, 22*(3), 138, 147-148.

Nordstrom, G., & Gardulf, A. (1996). Nursing documentation in patient records. *Scandinavian Journal of Caring Sciences, 10*(1), 27-33.

Rhodes, A. M. (1986). Focus on legal issues: Principles of documentation. *MCN. The American Journal of Maternal Child Nursing, 11*, 381.

Robertson, S. C. (1977). *The development and use of a documentation tool incorporating the occupational therapy outcome criterion in a psychiatric day treatment center*. Unpublished master's thesis, San Jose State University, San Jose, CA.

Tahan, H. A. (1996). A ten-step process to develop case management plans. *Nurse Case Manager, 1*(3), 112-121.

Weed, L. L. (1968). Medical records that guide and teach. *The New England Journal of Medicine, 278*, 593-600.

Weed, L. L. (1968). Medical records that guide and teach (concluded). *The New England Journal of Medicine, 278*, 652-658.

4. Quality Improvement

Deborah L. Wilkerson, MA

This chapter reviews the history of quality improvement systems and the concepts emphasized today. Quality continues to be measured, in part, by reviewing medical documentation. This documentation must report the patient's response to therapy, especially functional gains. Since the focus is also on the consumer, these functional gains must be important to the consumer to maintain consumer satisfaction, another important element of quality improvement.

Deborah L. Wilkerson is the Director, Research and Quality Improvement, for the Rehabilitation Accreditation Commission (CARF), in Tucson, Arizona. She served as Director, Program Evaluation and Outcome Studies, National Rehabilitation Hospital and NRH Research Center, Washington, DC. She earlier served as Administrator, Department of Rehabilitation Medicine, University of Washington in Seattle.

Quality improvement systems, transmutations of quality assurance systems, provide a mechanism for monitoring the quality of care, reviewing the appropriateness and the effectiveness of care, assessing the use of health care resources, and modifying programs and services as a result. It is not sufficient for occupational therapy organizations to assess and monitor outcomes of care. They must apply the knowledge gained to making changes in the system of service delivery. Neither is it sufficient to document that a practitioner has provided quality services to the persons whom he or she serves. As quality improvement systems have evolved, the mandate has become to *improve* the quality of care continually through changes in the processes and the outcomes. What is of importance is the relationship between the processes of care (treatments and interventions, ways of doing things in the organization) and their results (clinical outcomes, consumer satisfaction, and efficiency of operations).

The earlier notion of quality assurance has undergone a transformation during the 1980s and 1990s, based in large part on the spillover of quality improvement concepts from manufacturing industries. The transformation has brought the concept of quality improvement more in line with the long-standing emphasis on program evaluation promoted by CARF for rehabilitation organizations. This chapter discusses quality improvement because of its widespread use in many types of American organizations.[1] Occupational therapists would do well to consider merging the concepts of program evaluation and quality improvement into one effort at providing the highest-quality service possible.

A Definition of Quality Improvement

Quality in occupational therapy and rehabilitation services can and has been described in many ways. At a minimum the highest quality demands that the right things be done, that things be done right, that what is done be done efficiently, that desirable outcomes be achieved, that errors not be made, that decisions be appropriate, and that people be treated well (Crosby, 1979; Deming, 1982). Beyond these basics are many angles on quality specific to occupational therapy and rehabilitation: positive outcomes for recipients of care, individualized care, well-trained staff members, involvement of patients and clients and their families in care decisions, and lack of complications and rehospitalizations (England, Glass, & Patterson, 1989; Johnston & Wilkerson, 1992; National Rehabilitation Hospital, 1992).

Quality improvement (QI) is a system through which better and more efficient processes in an organization continuously raise the levels of performance and the outcomes of all functions, eliminate errors, and reduce cost.[2] All persons in the organization, in all departments, have a responsibility to assess and improve quality. Conceptually very similar to the notion in forma-

[1] The sections of this part titled "Early Lessons in the Importance of Quality Review," "Emergence of Quality Assurance in Health Care," and "Relationship of Quality Improvement to Research and Program Evaluation," are based in part on Joe, B. E. (1992). In Quality Assurance, J. Bair and M. Gray (Eds.), *The Occupational Therapy Manager* (rev. ed., pp. 251-58), Bethesda, MD: American Occupational Therapy Association.

[2] Quality improvement (QI) is sometimes referred to as continuous quality improvement (CQI). The term quality improvement and its abbreviation QI imply continuous improvement of performance, as compared with the notion of improvement of performance to a threshold that need not be altered once it has been reached.

tive program evaluation of using information to improve the program, QI tends to focus more sharply on the processes of care, using outcomes and other information as pointers to areas needing improvement. In addition, as an emerging field, QI has developed well-honed tools for separating processes into their component parts, analyzing where problems exist, and reformatting the processes to improve them. Data on outcomes, cost, and consumers' satisfaction are then used as evidence that the process changes actually created a quality improvement.

EARLY LESSONS IN THE IMPORTANCE OF QUALITY REVIEW – The examination of whether medical treatments really work has evolved through history, but even early observations in quality aimed at reducing error and variation. In the 1860s, nurse Florence Nightingale observed and reported on the deficiencies of health care services provided to those wounded in the war (Huxley, 1975). As the first person to collect and compare mortality statistics from different hospitals, she documented a plunge in the death rate in military hospitals during the Crimean War, from 42 percent to 2.2 percent.

Florence Nightingale's efforts were continued by a physician, Abraham Flexner. His 1910 report on the poor quality of medical education in the United States and Canada was instrumental in closing 60 of 155 United States medical schools then in existence.

In 1912 a revolutionary and prophetic resolution from the Third Clinical Congress of Surgeons of North America began to change health care. The resolution stated:

> Some system of standardization of hospital equipment and hospital work should be developed, to the end that those institutions having the highest ideals may have proper recognition before the profession, and that those of inferior equipment and standards should be stimulated to raise the quality of their work. (Davis, 1960, p. 476)

Five years later the American College of Surgeons initiated the process of hospital accreditation, formulating *Minimum Standards for Hospitals*.

EMERGENCE OF QUALITY ASSURANCE IN HEALTH CARE – In 1951 the American College of Surgeons, in concert with other professional medical groups, established the Joint Commission on Accreditation of Hospitals, now the Joint Commission on Accreditation of Healthcare Organizations (JCAHO). The Joint Commission's quality assurance program evolved over the next several decades. In 1955 the Joint Commission began to stress the importance of medical audits. By 1974 its standards required hospitals to audit medical records and make quarterly reports. In 1981, judging that the audit system was producing good medical records but not necessarily better care, the Joint Commission began urging the introduction of additional *monitors*, or measures of important outcomes of care, and a focus on problem resolution.

As late as 1990, key literature still used the term *quality assurance* (QA), meaning a set of activities designed to monitor the performance of an organization against specified quantitative thresholds of quality. QA had as its hallmark

1. the sampling of case records for review

2. peer study of case records

3. identification of thresholds of performance.

Once performance reached those thresholds, an organization could claim to have met quality screens. Nonetheless, QA was rooted in discovering the relationship between process and outcome.

FROM QUALITY ASSURANCE TO QUALITY IMPROVEMENT – The concepts and the activities surrounding the review and the enhancement of quality health and rehabilitation services have undergone a gradual but major transformation during the 1980s and the 1990s. In the 1980s a quality revolution occurred in American business and manufacturing and began to spread into health care. The concept of *total quality management* (TQM) influenced several key shifts in the paradigm of QA (McLaughlin & Kaluzny, 1990). First, the notion of a quality threshold gave way to the ideas of continuous improvement and zero defects. Second, the notion that quality could be assured gave way to the idea that quality is a matter of perception of the consumer of a service; although quality must be quantified and measured, satisfaction of the consumer is the ultimate demonstration of quality products. Today these ideas are being refined in health care in ways that affect the occupational therapists.

Key Concepts

Several concepts are key to the evolution and the consideration of QI and the design and the implementation of QI systems. Each concept has contributed to modern QI activities.

DONABEDIAN'S FRAMEWORK: STRUCTURE, PROCESS, AND OUTCOME – In 1966, Donabedian proposed a framework for assessing the quality of medical care, and in 1983 and 1988 he elaborated on his now-classic scheme. The framework includes three dimensions: *structure*, or the "attributes of the settings in which care occurs"; *process*, "what is actually done in giving and receiving care"; and *outcome*, "the effects of care on the health status of patients and populations" (1988, p. 1745). These concepts parallel a systems analysis framework (input, process, and output). For a long while, the focus of QA in rehabilitation and occupational therapy was on the structure and the processes of care. The heightened attention to outcomes in health care during the 1980s and the 1990s has brought this third dimension more actively into the QI equation.

The practical implication of the Donabedian framework for QI activities is to focus attention on the relationship between structure, process, and outcome. Causal relationships are difficult to establish, and they must be determined not by QI efforts but by careful prior research (Donabedian, 1988). Yet the assessment of each component of the triad is essential to a thorough review of quality. Organizations are led to include in a quality review all their departments and functions, from clinical program operations (structure and process) and effectiveness (outcome) to support systems (referrals and admissions, finance, housekeeping, food service, and other administrative structures and processes).

TOTAL QUALITY MANAGEMENT – *TQM* is a paradigm for business management that was first developed in the United States by American W. Edwards Deming (1982). Initially ignored in this country, the innovation was adopted by the Japanese manufacturing industry, which subsequently soared to success in the global economy (McLaughlin & Kaluzny, 1990). Central to TQM are 14 points, which emphasize the three TQM themes:

1. Quality, and processes that produce quality products, can always be improved.

2. It is possible for things to be done right the first time, and this should become the standard.

3. Workers at all levels of an organization should be empowered to make improvements and be provided with avenues to take pride in the organization's success.

Health care as an industry has been slower to adopt TQM concepts than business has because of the challenges of translating a paradigm originating in manufacturing into the language of service organizations. However, with JCAHO refocusing its standards on the concepts of TQM (JCAHO, 1995a; McLaughlin & Kaluzny, 1990), health care organizations of all kinds are now implementing TQM strategies and tools to help improve quality.

FOCUS ON THE CONSUMER

CONSUMER SATISFACTION – An important element of TQM is its focus on the consumer's satisfaction with a product. The QI paradigm recognizes that processes of care are successful only to the extent that they result in a high-quality product or service for the consumer and minimize costs to the consumer and the payer. Consequently, consumer satisfaction has become a key new outcomes measure in the tool kit of program evaluation and QI. The implications of this new element for occupational therapist are that they must establish systems for tapping the satisfaction of patients, families, other advocates, and payers, and for incorporating their findings into action plans for quality improvements.

CONSUMER SERVICE – Consistent with the focus on the consumer's satisfaction, QI programs often include specific activities teaching that it is every employee's responsibility to serve the consumer, whether the consumer is internal (other staff members and colleagues) or external (patients, families, referral sources, and payer representatives) to the organization. Occupational therapy managers may find themselves engaged in full-fledged training programs designed to orient staff members to entirely new ways of thinking for a health care organization. Based in the TQM philosophy, a heightened focus on service to consumers is founded on the premise that higher-quality care means meeting the needs of the users of the service. This is in fact a fairly radical shift in medical and health services; traditionally the professional has presumed to know best what is right for the patient, and fee-for-service arrangements have put providers, rather than payers, in charge of what services are rendered. The practice is now changing to place explicit value on including the consumer in decisions about care.

OUTCOMES MANAGEMENT – Paul Ellwood, a leader in outcomes and health policy research, first proposed *outcomes management* in 1988. He defines it as "a technology of patient experience designed to help patients, payers, and providers make rational medical care–related choices based on better insight into the effect of these choices on the patient's life" (p. 1551). It employs four key techniques:

1. use of standards and guidelines to help physicians choose appropriate treatments

2. routine and systematic measurement of patients' functioning and well-being, and of disease-specific outcomes

3. pooling of outcome data and information on the clinical process to form large databases for study

4. analysis and dissemination of results in appropriate form for the use of various decision makers in health care.

Outcomes management forms a link between the traditional arena of program evaluation and the newer notion of QI. At the core is the notion of studying and identifying the relationship between the outcomes of care and the processes that influence those outcomes. Variation in care not attributable to patients' needs should be minimized, and the cost of care should retreat (Berwick, 1989, 1990). The concepts inherent in outcomes management resonate particularly well in the already outcome-oriented field of rehabilitation, to such a degree that CARF adopted the phrase *outcome measurement and management* beginning with its 1995 standards (see above).

An implication of outcomes management for occupational therapy managers is that quality review mechanisms will increasingly include the building of an ongoing database on patients—perhaps in addition to sample case review methods—from which to examine trends in the outcomes of programs. Ongoing data systems are likely to encompass outcomes measures and to be used as a source of evidence that QI efforts are working. Top management will expect occupational therapy managers both to contribute to, and to be able to understand and use information from, an outcomes management system as part of an overall QI initiative.

EFFECTIVENESS, EFFICIENCY, AND VALUE — Many program evaluation and QI systems refer to the twin concepts of effectiveness and efficiency as key indicators of a quality program. *Effectiveness* refers to the outcome dimension: What results are obtained from care? For example, what gains did patients make in functional status? What proportion of clients were able to return to the living arrangements that they enjoyed before incurring a disability? What proportion of consumers received and were able to make use of recommended assistive devices? *Efficiency* considers the resources employed in achieving a certain outcome: What did it cost to obtain certain results of care? How much gain was achieved for a given expenditure of resources? For example, what measurable change in functional status occurred for every thousand dollars of charges?

Value is the principal concept that brings together effectiveness (outcome), cost and price, and efficiency. *Value* is the ratio of quality to price: Although high-quality programs can certainly be provided at high cost, the highest quality for the lowest price is the highest value. A premise of TQM is that quality can be maximized while cost from doing things wrong (error) and doing the wrong things (misfocus) is reduced. The long-range goals of QI and program evaluation are to encourage and communicate value in an organization.

In addition to serving as an organization's means of reviewing and enhancing the value of its services, QI systems are required by external reviewers of quality. As consumers, payers, and the public call on accrediting bodies and peer review organizations to certify the quality of health care providers, those bodies and organizations in turn want assurance that mechanisms are in place to identify problems, find opportunities, and implement strategies for improvement in processes and outcomes, and continually maximize the quality of care provided.

ACCREDITING BODIES

CARF, THE REHABILITATION ACCREDITATION COMMISSION — For more than 2 decades CARF has required that rehabilitation programs use an ongoing, outcome-based program evaluation system to assess effectiveness and efficiency of services. CARF further requires that organizations apply the resulting knowledge to planning and management of clinical programs. Although the CARF standards use terms different from TQM and QI jargon—for example, *program evaluation* and *outcome management*—they describe QI efforts.

JOINT COMMISION ON ACCREDITATION OF HEALTHCARE ORGANIZATIONS — JCAHO heavily influences the QI activities of many provider organizations, and with its 1995 standards it made a major philosophical shift consistent with TQM concepts. Instead of focusing on identifying errors and measuring whether or not a quantitative threshold for quality has been met (as in traditional QA), the agency is now concentrating on improving processes to eliminate errors, and on *continuously* improving quality (eliminating the threshold) (McLaughlin & Kaluzny, 1990).

PEER REVIEW ORGANIZATIONS — *Peer review*, as the name implies, is a system by which professionals review the quality of work of their peers. Berwick (1990) has defined it as "inspection and evaluation of health care structures, practices, or results, conducted or guided by medical professionals" (p. 247). In a peer review model, individual clinicians (physicians, therapists, nurses) are assigned to review sample records of the patients of other professionals in their organization and typically to report to a committee that oversees the enterprise (for example, during a regular morbidity and mortality review).

The Peer Review Improvement Act of 1982 requires each state to designate a single agency as responsible for monitoring the quality of care for Medicare beneficiaries. As a result, provider organizations must review their own work and respond to the inquiries of peer review organizations about the quality of care.

The underlying philosophy of traditional peer review (inspection and sanction by individuals) is in many ways fundamentally at odds with the QI mentality (statistical examination of outcomes, focus on process, and empowerment of individuals). Berwick (1990) suggests, however, that peer review and QI efforts can coexist and complement each other, with peer review professionals playing a role in measurement and information analysis. It is likely that samples of individual case records for peer review will be augmented—and in some organizations replaced—by ongoing clinical information systems and computer databases in which key elements are routinely recorded for statistical analysis.

Occupational therapists can expect to be involved at some level in a peer review activity. Another use of peer review is the monitoring and the improvement of individual clinicians' skills. *Developing, Maintaining, and Updating Competency in Occupational Therapy: A Guide to Self-Appraisal* (AOTA, Commission on Practice, 1995) identifies peer review as one of the methods by which practitioners can achieve competency. The document is the product of a task force established in 1991 by AOTA's Commission on Practice to examine competency issues at all levels and in all practice settings. Establishing, maintaining, and measuring competency is essential for the survival of the occupational therapy profession in today's health care and education systems.

Elements and Steps in Quality Improvement

A number of tools for information management, outcome measurement and monitoring, process analysis, and applied organizational change are available and frequently used in conducting QI programs. Many are drawn from the TQM movement and applied to a health care environment. Occupational therapy managers may well become involved in or be asked to lead QI activities as part of an organizational effort, and therefore should educate themselves on the use of these tools and surrounding structures.

ORGANIZATIONAL INFRASTRUCTURE: QUALITY COUNCILS – A focal point for the activities associated with QI may be an organization's quality council and supporting subgroups responsible for compiling and reviewing plans and data on outcomes and processes of care. Although the specific organizational layout for such councils, committees, and task forces will vary widely (Berwick, 1990), those that are most effective will be guided from the highest levels of the organization (e.g., executive and medical management) and will commit significant time to analyzing findings from the QI reviews and translating findings into actions for improving processes. Occupational therapy managers may well be called on to participate in or report to such groups and should build these activities into their regular work expectations.

DATA COLLECTION – At the core of modern QI efforts is the need to gather data on outcomes, conformance to prescribed standards, and the proportion of persons meeting quality-indicator conditions (Ellwood, 1988; Johnston & Wilkerson, 1992). Methods of data collection may range from retrospective reviews of randomly sampled patients' records to highly automated computer technologies supporting ongoing clinical information systems. Combinations of these methods are likely, depending on the size and the sophistication of the organization. However, even the smallest organizations may have personal computer–based software designed to record and to help analyze outcome and other quality-indicator data.

With the influence of TQM and outcomes management paradigms, QI efforts are placing increased emphasis on the statistical analysis of aggregate data, requiring large databases on

Figure 4.1 Quality evaluation and improvement cycle

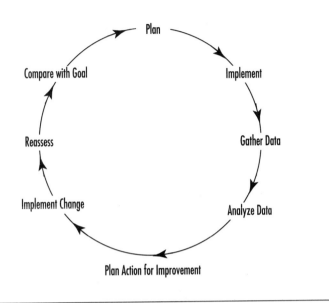

the populations served by the organization. Relying solely on a small peer-reviewed sample of records is inadequate. Thus occupational therapists will benefit from at least a general understanding of what databases and information systems have to offer and the ways in which information must be recorded to accommodate these systems (Lieberman, 1991).

TOOLS AND TECHNIQUES – A variety of tools can be employed to structure an organization's improvement activities, including some described in detail by JCAHO (1992a, 1992b, 1994a, 1994b, 1995b), others stemming from the TQM movement (Plsek, 1993), and program evaluation techniques such as those endorsed by CARF (Commission on Accreditation of Rehabilitation Facilities, 1991a, 1991b, 1991c, 1992. At the core of each is a cycle of planning, implementing, gathering and analyzing data, developing plans for improvement, implementing changes, and reassessing the status of the system in comparison with its status before the change or with the goals for improvement (see figure 4.1).

JCAHO refers to and diagrams this learning-and-change cycle as *plan-do-study-act*, or PDSA. The templates for CARF program evaluation suggest slightly different labels: objective-measurement-performance-action. Occupational therapists should understand that whatever the labels and the organizational placement of QI activity, the goal is a change of processes in order to improve outcomes and consumer satisfaction.

Common tools used in QI efforts include charts and graphs for display of data in formats that facilitate understanding of patterns and trends, and comparisons with external data sources; flow charts that clarify processes and sequences of events; and diagrams that display potential causes of variation and error in processes (Carefoote, 1994; Plsek, 1993). AOTA's

QI Resource Guide (1994) is a valuable publication that will assist occupational therapy managers and practitioners with QI activities. The guide contains an extensive bibliography, a list of resources, and sample forms.

QI teams are also a hallmark of many QI efforts. A task force is convened whose work is temporary but focused on improving a single major process. Based on the premise that persons who do the work know the processes best, QI teams typically involve employees at all levels of the organization and across departments—all those who participate in or use the products of an organization's process. For example, occupational therapy managers or their staff members may be involved with admission personnel, medical records employees, physicians, and administrative representatives on a team to improve the flow of documentation on the care of patients. The potential team member must learn the use of specific tools, as well as understand the overall goals of improving an outcome (in this example, complete and timely documentation of care).

Relationship of Quality Improvement to Research and Program Evaluation

Distinctions have been drawn in the past between quality assurance and research, and skepticism has arisen regarding the validity of decisions based on the relatively unsophisticated early QA activities. The shift from QA to QI and the inherent shift from reviews of small samples of case records to use of population databases move QI toward health services research. Demands on modern systems include valid and reliable outcomes measures, secure and properly used databases, and sound sampling and statistical analysis techniques (Fuhrer, 1987; Johnston, Keith, & Hinderer, 1992). Organization-specific and pooled databases [e.g., the Uniform Data System for Medical Rehabilitation (Hamilton, Granger, Sherwin, Zielzny, & Tashman, 1987)] are the most efficiently designed to meet the needs of QI efforts as well as to provide a foundation for epidemiological and health services research.

Although randomized clinical trials are outside the usual practice of QI projects, *de facto* controls from pre- and post-intervention designs are possible. Analysis of patterns of variation, effectiveness, and efficiency from program evaluation and QI efforts can point to and set the groundwork for more focused and controlled outcomes research. In turn, treatment efficacy suggested by clinical research should be tested in the real-world laboratory of clinical practice. In fact, real-world effectiveness of treatment can often be verified only through outcomes management-type analyses. Research efforts can also lead to changes in practice, clinical guidelines, and evaluation goals. Practice guidelines, which include clinical processes that may be among the targets for improvement, are based in part on efficacy findings from controlled clinical research.

Overcoming of Obstacles to Quality Improvement

Resistance to QI efforts can come from several angles. The culture and the behavior of an organization are being challenged and changed through QI, and people resist change. The flattening of an organizational structure and the empowerment of line staff members that often take place with a TQM philosophy can be very threatening, especially to mid-level managers (Gillem, 1988; McLaughlin & Kaluzny, 1990). Constant change is indeed at the core of continuous improvement. Preparing an organization for change, conveying excitement for better care and service from the top of the organization, and understanding new roles of managers and staff members are critical to a successful QI program (McLaughlin & Kaluzny, 1990).

Managers and staff must also become accustomed to new demands for data collection, which if not implemented carefully can place undue burdens on clinical operations. Involving staff in the design and the use of information systems, as well as on specific teams for quality or process improvement, will help make the information collected and changes recommended meaningful and successful.

Summary

Quality improvement (QI) is a system through which better and more efficient processes in an organization continuously raise the levels of performance and the outcomes of all functions, eliminate errors, and reduce cost. Several concepts are key to QI:

1. Donabedian's (1988) framework for assessing the quality of medical care, which includes three dimensions: *structure*, or the "attributes of the settings in which care occurs"; *process*, "what is actually done in giving and receiving care"; and *outcome*, "the effects of care on the health status of patients and populations" (p. 1745)

2. *Total quality management* (TQM), which emphasizes three themes: continuous quality improvement, doing things right the first time, and empowering workers at all levels to make improvements

3. Focus on the consumer, which includes two elements: consumer satisfaction and consumer service

4. Outcomes management, which employs four key techniques: use of standards and guidelines to help physicians choose appropriate treatments; routine and systematic measurement of functioning, well-being, and disease-specific outcomes; pooling of outcome data and information on the clinical process; and analysis and dissemination of results to decision makers.

Effectiveness refers to the outcome dimension. *Efficiency* considers the resources employed in achieving a certain outcome. Value is the principal concept that brings together effectiveness (outcome), cost and price, and efficiency. *Value* is the ratio of quality to price: The highest quality for the lowest price is the highest value. The long-range goals of QI and program evaluation are to encourage and communicate value in an organization.

QI systems are required by accrediting bodies and peer review organizations. A focal point for QI activities may be an organization's quality council and supporting subgroups. At the core of modern QI efforts is the need to gather data on outcomes, conformance to prescribed standards, and the proportion of persons meeting quality-indicator conditions (Ellwood, 1988; Johnston & Wilkerson, 1992). A variety of tools can be employed to structure an organization's QI activities. At the core of each is a cycle of planning, implementing, gathering and analyzing data, developing plans for improvement, implementing changes, and reassessing the status of the system in comparison with its status before the change or with the goals for improvement. QI teams, also a hallmark of many QI efforts, typically involve employees at all levels of the organization and across departments.

References

American Occupational Therapy Association. (1994). *QI resource guide*. Bethesda, MD: Author.

American Occupational Therapy Association. (1994). Uniform terminology for occupational therapy (3rd ed.). *American Journal of Occupational Therapy*, 48, 1047–54.

American Occupational Therapy Association, Commission on Practice, Competency Task Force. (1995). Developing, maintaining, and updating competency in occupational therapy: A guide to self-appraisal. Bethesda, MD: Author.

Berwick, D. M. (1989). Continuous improvement as an ideal in health care. *New England Journal of Medicine*, 320, 53–56.

Berwick, D. M. (1990). Peer review and quality management: Are they compatible? *Quality Review Bulletin*, 16, 246–51.

Carefoote, R. (1994). Implementing TQM/CQI at rehabilitation hospitals: A survey. *Journal of Healthcare Quality*, 16(3), 34–38.

CARF, The Rehabilitation Accreditation Commission. (1995). 1995 standards manual and interpretive guidelines for medical rehabilitation. Tucson, AZ: Author.

CARF, The Rehabilitation Accreditation Commission. (published annually). Standards manual and interpretive guidelines for behavioral health. Tucson, AZ: Author.

CARF, The Rehabilitation Accreditation Commission. (published annually). Standards manual and interpretive guidelines for employment and community support services. Tucson, AZ: Author.

CARF, The Rehabilitation Accreditation Commission. (published annually). Standards manual and interpretive guidelines for medical rehabilitation. Tucson, AZ: Author.

CARF, The Rehabilitation Accreditation Commission, Board of Trustees. (1995). Quality improvement through measurement and management of rehabilitation outcomes: Tools for application of knowledge of rehabilitation outcomes management [Proposal]. Tucson, AZ: Author.

Commission on Accreditation of Rehabilitation Facilities. (1991a). Program evaluation: A first step. Tucson, AZ: Author.

Commission on Accreditation of Rehabilitation Facilities. (1991b). *Program evaluation: A guide to utilization*. Tucson, AZ: Author.

Commission on Accreditation of Rehabilitation Facilities. (1991c). *Program evaluation: For inpatient medical rehabilitation programs* (1991 ed.). Tucson, AZ: Author.

Commission on Accreditation of Rehabilitation Facilities. (1992). *Program evaluation: Utilization and assessment principles* (1992 ed.). Tucson, AZ: Author.

Crosby, P. B. (1979). *Quality is free*. New York: Mentor/New American Library.

Davis, L. (1960). *Fellowship of surgeons: A history of the American College of Surgeons*. Springfield, IL: Charles C Thomas.

Deming, W. E. (1982). *Out of the crisis*. Cambridge, MA: Massachusetts Institute of Technology, Center for Advanced Engineering Study.

Donabedian, A. (1966). Evaluating the quality of medical care. *Milbank Quarterly, 44*, 166–203.

Donabedian, A. (1983). Quality, cost and clinical decisions. *Annals of the American Academy of Political and Social Science, 468*, 196–204.

Donabedian, A. (1988). The quality of care: How can it be assessed? *Journal of the American Medical Association, 260*, 1743–48.

Ellwood, P. (1988). Outcomes management: A technology of patient experience [Shattuck Lecture]. *New England Journal of Medicine, 318*, 1549–56.

England, B., Glass, R. M., & Patterson, C. H. (Eds.). (1989). *Quality rehabilitation: Results-oriented care*. Chicago: American Hospital.

Flexner, A. (1910). *Medical education in the United States and Canada*. New York: Carnegie Foundation, Merrymount Press.

Fuhrer, M. J. (Ed.). (1987). *Rehabilitation outcomes: Analysis and measurement*. Baltimore, MD: Paul Brookes.

Gillem, T. R. (1988). Deming's 14 points and hospital quality: Responding to the consumer's demand for the best value health care. *Journal of Nursing Quality Assurance*, 2, 70–78.

Hamilton, B. B., Granger, C. V., Sherwin, F. S., Zielzny, M., & Tashman, J. S. (1987). A uniform national data system for medical rehabilitation. In M. J. Fuhrer (Ed.), *Rehabilitation outcomes: Analysis and measurement* (pp. 137–50). Baltimore, MD: Paul Brookes.

Health Care Financing Administration. (1990, September). Medical review (MR) guidelines for OT outpatient services (DHHS Transmittal No. 1489). In *Medicare intermediary manual* (sec. 3906ff, pp. 23–43). Baltimore, MD: Author.

Huxley, E. (1975). *Florence Nightingale*. New York: Putnam.

Joint Commission on Accreditation of Healthcare Organizations. (1992a). *Examples of quality improvement in a hospital setting*. Oakbrook Terrace, IL: Author.

Joint Commission on Accreditation of Healthcare Organizations. (1992b). *Using quality improvement tools in a healthcare setting*. Oakbrook Terrace, IL: Author.

Joint Commission on Accreditation of Healthcare Organizations. (1994a). *Forms, charts, and other tools for performance improvement*. Oakbrook Terrace, IL: Author.

Joint Commission on Accreditation of Healthcare Organizations. (1994b). *Framework for improving performance: From principles to practice*. Oakbrook Terrace, IL: Author.

Joint Commission on Accreditation of Healthcare Organizations. (1995a). *Accreditation manual for hospitals*. Oakbrook Terrace, IL: Author.

Joint Commission on Accreditation of Healthcare Organizations. (1995b). *Leadership skills for performance improvement: Planning for quality*. Oakbrook Terrace, IL: Author.

Johnston, M. V., Keith, R. A., & Hinderer, S. R. (1992). Measurement standards for medical rehabilitation (Work of the American Congress of Rehabilitation Medicine's Task Force on Measurement and Evaluation) [Special supplement]. *Archives of Physical Medicine and Rehabilitation, 73*(supp. no. 12-5).

Johnston, M. V., & Wilkerson, D. L. (1992). Program evaluation and quality improvement systems in brain injury rehabilitation. *Journal of Head Trauma Rehabilitation, 7*, 68–82.

Johnston, M. V., Wilkerson, D. L., & Maney, M. (1993). Evaluation of the quality and outcomes of medical rehabilitation programs. In J. A. DeLisa & B. Gans (Eds.), *Rehabilitation medicine: Principles and practice* (2nd ed., pp. 240–268). Philadelphia: Lippincott.

Lieberman, D. (1991). Foreword. *Occupational Therapy Practice, 2*(2), v–vi.

McLaughlin, C. P., & Kaluzny, A. D. (1990). Total quality management in health: Making it work. *Health Care Management Review, 15*(3), 7–14.

National Rehabilitation Hospital. (1992). Quality in medical rehabilitation: Definitions and dimensions. Washington, DC: Author.

Peer Review Improvement Act of 1982, Pub. L. No. 97–248, 96 stat. 324, § 141.

Plsek, P. E. (1993). Tutorial: Management and planning tools of TQM. *Quality Management in Health Care, 1*(3), 59–72.

Additional Resources

Boon, B. (1995, February 15). Creating an effective results-oriented organization. A Best Practice Presentation at the 1995 CARF Medical Rehabilitation Conference on Standards and Best Practices, Tucson, AZ.

Johnston, M. V., Stineman, M., & Maney, M. (1993, June 17). Improving the reliability and integrity of functional measures in medicine and rehabilitation [Abstract]. West Orange, NJ: Kessler Institute for Rehabilitation.

MacDonell, C. M. (1993, February/March). A tool for the future. *Rehab Management* (Marina del Ray, CA: CurAnt Communications), 6, 112–13.

McNally, D. (1990). *Even eagles need a push*. New York: Delacorte Press.

Wiley, G. (1993, June/July). A scramble for facts. *Rehab Management 6*, 165–67. (Marina del Ray, CA: CurAnt Communications).

Wilkerson, D. L. (1991). Program and outcome evaluation: Opportunity for the 1990s. *Occupational Therapy Practice, 2*(2), 1–15.

Wilkerson, D. L. (1995). Implementing outcomes. *Rehab management 8*, 97–99. Marina del Ray, CA: CurAnt Communications.

Wilkerson, D. L. (1995). Developing outcomes management tools. *Rehab Management 8*, 114–15. Marina del Ray, CA: CurAnt Communications.

Wilkerson, D. L. & Johnston, M. V. (in press). Outcomes research and clinical program monitoring systems: Current capability and future directions. In M. J. Fuhrer (Ed.), *Medical rehabilitation research*. Baltimore, MD: Paul Brookes.

5. Clinical Reasoning for Documentation

Claudia Allen, MA, OTR, FAOTA

This chapter looks at the thinking process behind documentation. Accurate documentation and patient/client intervention are contingent on the selection and synthesis of pertinent information. Information that is useful for keeping the focus on progress toward functional outcomes and safety is identified.

Claudia Allen is Chief of Occupational Therapy, Los Angeles County, Harbor—University of California in Los Angeles Medical Center, Torrance, California.

Documentation is a way of communicating the value of occupational therapy services. The people who read these notes usually refer patients for services or pay for the services provided. To stay in business, therapists must be able to explain the utility, importance, and consequences of the services provided, and that requires a clear understanding of what is expected. The value of occupational therapy services is maximizing a person's remaining ability to function safely. The ability to function is seen while a person is doing an activity. The activity must be meaningful to the individual, given his or her station in life. Occupational therapists are expected to improve the performance of activities that are meaningful to individuals who have experienced a recent loss in their ability to function.

The Clinical Reasoning Process

Keeping track of improvements in activity performance is complicated because the number of underlying factors that can reduce performance is enormous. Sorting through the factors, correcting limitations that can be changed, avoiding limitations that cannot be changed, finding remaining abilities, and negotiating and prioritizing activities with patients and caregivers who may be denying problems is a complex process. This chapter suggests a clinical reasoning process designed to help therapists keep the focus of treatment on the performance of activities that are important to individuals. That clinical reasoning process is outlined in Appendix 1.

Holding therapists accountable for producing an improvement in the quality of activity performance is a relatively recent expectation. While it is true that therapists have always claimed that the value of occupational therapy services was an improved ability to function, the actual outcome of the services provided has been ambiguous. Holding ourselves accountable for specific treatment outcomes is an emerging process with signs of improvement over the years.

This chapter is designed to help therapists orient the way they think about treatment goals. Most of the steps are familiar to experienced therapists. Emphasis is placed on those aspects that are most apt to affect the way therapists think and provide services.

Therapists are expected to help patients improve the performance of activities and prevent potential accidents and injuries. This is aimed at improving the functional outcomes of occupational therapy services. An analysis of the current clinical reasoning process suggests that the improvements can be made by adding two steps to the current process. Current practice has been divided into six steps: steps 1, 4, 5, 6, 7, 8. The additions are described in steps 2 and 3. This clinical reasoning is intended for all specialty areas of practice.

STEP 1: CHART REVIEW – The first step is a prediction of functional outcome based on groups of people with similar problems. The medical diagnosis and the onset set a range for expected change in functional ability. Additional medical diagnoses that could restrict the range or rate of change are noted. The patient's functional history and response to previous occupational therapy treatment can also be used to establish a general prediction of the expected quality of activity performance. From this information an estimate of the discharge placement and the need for assistance can be made. What should be noted here is that predictions of functional outcomes can be made without any consideration of the individual patient, his or her culture, or the social situation. Functional outcomes are largely determined by the pathology and what nature and medicine can do to correct the pathology.

STEP 2: INTERVIEW — The individual patient, his or her culture, and the social situation are factored in step 2. Occupational therapists start with an expected loss in function and begin to explore what that means to the individual. The activities that the person has done in the past, referred to as a *functional history* or *occupational history*, are identified. The therapist is looking for safety hazards that are likely to result from the functional losses that the patient and caregiver may not have considered. Activities that can still be done safely also need to be identified.

The meaning of a loss to individuals, given their stations in life, becomes apparent during the interview. The therapist must begin an educational process about what occupational therapy services can realistically achieve. Many patients and/or caregivers have unrealistic goals in mind. Losses are hard to accept. Step 2 should begin the process of accepting losses that cannot be restored.

Step 2 is a collaborative process. The patient and the caregiver will tell you what the patient used to do before the onset of the diagnosis. The therapist can tell the patient and the caregiver how the loss is apt to affect functional activities (Allen, Earhart, & Blue, 1992). Together you can begin to sketch out activities that are both achievable and meaningful. If the patient is too confused to tell a coherent story and no significant others are available, interview another caregiver.

When an impairment is recent, a denial of the disability is a frequent problem for both the patient and caregiver. A focus on short-term goals is a way of obtaining cooperation during the initial interview, but if this tactic is used, further discussion of long-term goals at a future date is advised. Therapists are often involved in the sad situation of helping people grieve over the loss of former abilities with reduced promises for the future. A neglect of the grief process tends to produce meaningless treatment goals and a sense that occupational therapy services were of no value. Step 2 is painful, but the alternative has been the provision of useless services. Step 2 is completed when the therapist has a list of patient/caregiver goals that are both realistic given the disability and acceptable to the individual.

Long-term goals are set within the context of loss of physical abilities, cognitive abilities, the natural course of the disease, and the available social and physical support systems. The long-term goal is an estimate of the patient's rehabilitation potential to do the activities identified in step 2. The activities selected must be acceptable to the patient and/or the caregiver.

STEP 3: OBSERVE ACTIVITY PERFORMANCE — Step 3 is an observation of the performance of one of the activities requested in step 2. The therapist should observe performance of the requested activity and begin to think about underlying impairments that could explain the patient's difficulties. The purpose of this observation is to select evaluation instruments. Selecting evaluation instruments is a recent change for many therapists who used to go through the same long lists of evaluations for all patients. Lengthy evaluations are expensive and often unnecessary. Therapists should have a rationale for the evaluation administered to each patient. The rationale should explore a hypothesized difficulty that is related to the requested activity. The time saved on unnecessary evaluations makes up for the time spent on steps 2 and 3.

STEP 4: TREATMENT GOALS – Functional treatment goals are aimed at improving the quality of activity performance and protecting the person's safety. The long-term goal is a prediction of the person's rehabilitation potential, stated as the amount of assistance required to do an activity safely. Short-term goals may focus on activities (driving) and underlying impairments (balance). The observations of activity performance in step 3 show the therapist how impairments are related to activities.

Step 4 may be done with acute medical conditions where the final degree of residual loss is ambiguous. The natural course of the disease and the usual response to available medical treatment are predictors of functional outcomes. Recent onset with brain impairments are probably the hardest to predict, and projections of what can be achieved within the next month or two are the most reliable. The fact that most functional change occurs within the first 6 months after brain injury should be explained.

Step 4 establishes the sequence for meeting short-term goals. Changes that involve neuromuscular impairments tend to follow a similar pattern of reducing pain; preventing accidents, injuries, or complications; making neuromuscular changes; and teaching compensations for residual physical disabilities. The sequence of short-term goals for brain impairments probably follows the natural course of recovery from brain injury. Whether short-term goals are following or leading the natural course of recovery is a matter of theoretical debate within occupational therapy that cannot be resolved here (Allen, Earhart, & Blue, 1992).

The issue that does need to be addressed is whether the patient can be expected to improve or not, because that affects payment for occupational therapy services. Payers such as Medicare will pay for two types of treatment goals: improvement and setting up of a maintenance program. The sequence of short-term goals outlined above measures improvement. During the process of developing the Part B guidelines, another form of treatment began to emerge. In Medicare terms, the federal government will pay for setting up a maintenance program but not for carrying out a maintenance program. Setting up a home program is a good example. Treatment goals that ensure safety in a long-term care situation are covered by Medicare. Maintenance programs must be sustainable in the long-term care situation (HCFA, 1989, 390b5a).

Maintenance programs, custodial care, and long-term care are health care needs that are excluded from Medicare coverage and most private insurance policies. The governmental provision of extended care has been the traditional responsibility of the states. The deinstitutionalization of state hospital patients took away the provision of most extended care. Therapists can identify a need for extended care, but very few therapists are employed by institutions that are mandated to provide it.

STEP 5: TREATMENT METHODS – The timing of treatment methods is addressed in step 5. The clinical judgment of the therapist is tested by the need to prioritize, and sequence treatment methods that are logically related to goals make the relationship between goals and methods as explicit as possible in step 3 (McGuire, 1997). A synthesis of the first five steps is required. As treatment progresses, there is a high probability that new information will require a different synthesis with different goals. At this point therapists should note that treatment begins with a mere sketch of a lot of information. Revisions are to be expected. If you seldom revise your treatment goals or observe activity performance, you may be missing the implications of new information you discover during treatment. Changes in the frequency and duration of treatment, as well as in the treatment goals themselves, should be fairly common.

The first five steps of the documentation process may be summarized in the initial note. A tremendous amount of thought, clinical experience, and knowledge is required to set good treatment goals and prioritize methods with the greatest efficiency in reaching goals. The part of practice that needs to be strengthened is negotiating treatment goals with patients and caregivers. The activities are selected by the patients and caregivers. The quality of functional outcome is predicted by the therapist. Treatment effectiveness is based on linking together the patient/caregiver goals, realistic goals predicted by the therapist, and the best methods for achieving goals.

STEP 6: PROGRESS NOTES – Getting into the daily notations and weekly progress notes is a relief after the complex thought required to establish goals and methods. The relief often expresses itself through a natural tendency to avoid changing goals. The easiest goal change occurs when a patient has a period of illness and needs to be placed on hold until he or she is well enough to participate in treatment again. Administrative pressures help us remember to avoid duplicating services and make sure that services are covered. The most difficult error to correct is an inaccurate prediction of what the patient will be able to achieve as a result of our services. An error suggests that the therapist must go back to the treatment planning process and think the whole thing over again. Go back to the initial note and try to find the source of the error. Consult another therapist. When you come up with a new goal to try, be candid in your documentation.

Reassessments and changes in goals are expected. You only look foolish when you adhere rigidly to a goal that is obviously not working, and reimbursement for useless services should be denied. Experience in working with a population is a great help in the early detection of a need to adjust treatment goals.

The design of a maintenance program is also recommended at step 6. Therapists should start setting up a functional maintenance program as soon as improvement begins to slow down. Time is required to instruct the patient and caregiver and to iron out difficulties encountered after a period of use. A home program should be checked for safety and effectiveness, which is a reimbursable part of the stabilization process. An ability to generalize from the treatment setting to the discharge setting should not be assumed with the cognitively disabled (Allen & Earhart, 1992). The most severe and pervasive concerns for safety may be for the cognitively disabled with undiagnosed dementia (Allen, Earhart, & Blue, 1996).

STEP 7: MONTHLY SUMMARY – The monthly summary is a formal reexamination of the treatment goals. The long-term goals may need to be renegotiated with the patient and the caregiver, and a treatment session that is devoted to conducting another interview is a good idea that is seldom seen in current practice. The relationship between long-term goals and short-term goals should also be reexamined at this time. Medical reviewers expect to see necessary adjustments in the monthly summaries. Practicing therapists tend to see monthly summaries as a boring rehash of what they have already done, which is incorrect. Flexibility in adjusting services to the unique needs of the patient and the person's place in life is what is required. By requiring a monthly summary, the insurance industry is recognizing the time that a therapist needs to sit down and think. Use this time to organize your thoughts about this patient and improve your predictions of functional outcomes.

STEP 8: DISCHARGE SUMMARY – The discharge summary helps you to benefit from your experience in working with the patient. The patient's record should identify the factors that contributed to or acted as barriers to treatment effectiveness. Barriers may include medical complications, lack of social or economic support, lack of commitment to stated goals, or an inability to recognize or accept a disability. The reverse may also be true in that the factors contribute to effectiveness. Therapists should make a note of these impacts on treatment for future referral criteria and changes in treatment methods.

Documentation explains the importance of occupational therapy services. Steps 2 and 3 of this clinical reasoning process outline a way to think about meaningful functional outcomes that help people adjust to the realities of living with a disability. Therapists will probably have to repeat these steps several times during the treatment process. The point is that steps 2 and 3 are frequently skipped in current practice and documentation. Therapists often jump in at step 4, with lengthy evaluations of measurable problems. The relationships among these problems, remaining abilities, and activity performance require more thought.

What a problem means to the individual and his or her social support system takes on a sense of significance during activity performance. Occupational therapy documentation should tell individual stories about changes in activity performance. I have yet to see a form or checklist that can capture the essence of what we do. A simple, short narrative note that tells a story about activities can let our readers understand what we do.

Do not be fooled by the words *simple* and *short*. To write simply and concisely is not easy or quick; it is the most difficult form of writing. Try writing a monthly summary that is one paragraph long that any high school graduate could understand. Several drafts will probably be required to eliminate information that may be valuable to you but that your readers do not need or understand. This clinical reasoning process is designed to help you find and keep track of your major points.

The challenge of explaining the value of occupational therapy services is addressed in this chapter. These explanations may be improved by a clinical reasoning process that keeps the therapist's attention focused on making meaningful improvements in activity performance.

References

Allen, C. K., Earhart, C. A., & Blue, T. (1992). *Occupational therapy treatment goals for cognitive and physical disabilities*. Bethesda, MD: American Occupational Therapy Association.

Allen, C. K., Earhart, C. A., & Blue, T. (1996). *Understanding cognitive perfomance modes*. Ormond Beach, FL: Allen Conferences, Inc.

Health Care Financing Administration. (1989). *Medical Review (MR) of Part B intermediary outpatient therapy (OT) bills*. (HHS transmittal no. 1424). Washington, DC: U.S. Government Printing Office.

McGuire, M. J. (1997). Documenting progress in home health. *American Journal of Occupational Therapy*, 51, 436-444.

Appendix 1   Clinical Reasoning Process

Therapist's Long-Term Goals and Changes in Goals

Where OT Documents	What the Therapist Thinks!	What the Therapist Does!	What the OT Documents!
Step 1 Initial note Chart Review Data	**Step 1** Rely on previous knowledge and experience regarding diagnosis and problems Make judgments in response to observations	**Step 1** Literature review as needed Review MD orders and medical record and/or speak with referral source Observes patient <u>Outcome:</u> Predict Natural Course of Disease	**Step 1** Primary diagnosis Treatment diagnosis Date of onset Written physician order Record whether patient has been treated by OT previously
Step 2 Initial note Interview Data	**Step 2** Determine interview/evaluation format Example: use of Canadian Occupational Performance Measure (COPM) **Step 3** Analyze physical and cognitive abilities required to do requested activities	**Step 2** Interview: Patient Patient and Caregiver or Caregiver only Obtain patient/caregiver goals <u>Outcome:</u> Important activities patient wants to perform—along with available social-economic support	**Step 2** Record prior functional level/history Record patient/caregiver goals and available social, economic, and physical supports
Step 3 Initial note Observed Activity Performance	Make initial hypothesis about underlying factors affecting function Begin to formulate problem list Decide whether further evaluation is indicated Yes_____ No_____ If yes, which evaluation tools will be used	**Step 3** Do quick assessment of physical and cognitive activities Screen physical and cognitive Observe performance of activities patient would like to be able to perform Evaluate patient using selected instruments	**Step 3** Record quick assessment Record patient's baseline dysfunctional performance in requested activities Record underlying evaluation results: physical, cognitive, environmental
Step 4 Initial note Treatment Goals	**Step 4** Estimate Long-Term Goals (LTGs) given the following factors • Cognitive Abilities • Physical Abilities • Social & Physical Supports • Natural Course of the Disease Sequence short-term goals (STGs) to: • meet needs and wants of patient • according to the progression of recovery Select treatment plans to: • reduce pain • prevent accidents/injuries • make neuromuscular changes • compensate for physical or cognitive disabilities • teach substitutions • monitor sparing/recovery • etc.	**Step 4** Verify goals with patient/caregiver Establish baseline measure for STGs	**Step 4** Record rehabilitation potential in requested activities, which is the long-term goal Record STGs and expected sequence Record baseline measures

Appendix 1 Clinical Reasoning Process (Continued)

Therapist's Short-Term Goals and Changes in Goals			
Where OT Documents	**What the Therapist Thinks!**	**What the Therapist Does!**	**What the OT Documents!**
Step 5 Initial note Treatment Methods	**Step 5** Estimate frequency and duration of treatment Consider family and other caregivers who provide assistance	**Step 5** Explain the relationship between LTGs and STGs and treatment methods to patient and caregivers Teach assistive techniques to family and caregivers Check estimates of frequency, duration, and degree with other members of the treatment team	**Step 5** Record explicit relationship between short-term and long-term goals and the therapist's treatment methods Record assistive techniques used with family and caregivers Record expected frequency and duration to obtainment of STGs and LTGs

Step 6
Daily notations on chart
Weekly progress note
	Step 6
	Constantly re-assessing goals:
	• Are treatment services covered?
	• Are you duplicating services?
	• Are you providing maintenance care?
	• Are you changing plans as necessary?
	• Also consider:
	  • Should patient be put on hold for a period of time due to illness?
	  • Do you need to design a maintenance program for residual deficits?
		Step 6
		• Chart review
		• Provide treatment
		• Observe performance in requested activities
		• Modify treatment according to patient's response to STG and LTG
		As patient goals change you modify treatment
		• Verify new short-term and long-term goals with patient/caregivers
		• Discontinue patient temporarily if necessary
		• Instruct in-home program
			Step 6
			Record briefly:
			  Date, type, length of treatment
			State change in meeting short-term goals and the effect on long-term goals
			Record changes in goals in weekly or monthly notes
			Every 30 days summarize changes in patient's ability to perform functional activities and changes in underlying factors
			State when patient reaches goals
			• Explanation if patient does not reach goals and how that affects treatment plan
			Record temporary discontinuation of treatment and reason
			Record home program and any follow-up recommendations made

Therapist's Evaluation of Treatment Effectiveness

Where OT Documents	What the Therapist Thinks!	What the Therapist Does!	What the OT Documents!
Step 7 Monthly Summary	**Step 7** Re-examine estimated LTGs for requested activities Re-examine relationship between LTGs, STGs, and treatment methods.	**Step 7** Make note for future LTGs Make note for future LTGs and STGs and treatment methods	**Step 7** Record degree of attainment of LTGs Record explicit relationship between meeting LTGs, STGs, and treatment methods
Step 8 Discharge Summary	**Step 8** Consider other factors that are barriers to treatment: • medical complications • lack of social or economic supports • lack of commitment to change in requested activities • unable to understand or accept disability Consider other factors that contributed to treatment effectiveness: • social and economic support • commitment to change • functional history	**Step 8** Make note for future referral criteria	**Step 8** Record other factors that contributed to or acted as barriers to treatment effectiveness

6. Understanding the Medical Review Process

Claudia Allen, MA, OTR, FAOTA
Mary Foto, OTR, FAOTA
Terry Moon, OTR/L
Dorothy Wilson, OTR, FAOTA
V. Judith Thomas, MGA

This chapter describes the general medical review process used by Medicare fiscal intermediaries and carriers in processing claims. Although other third party payers may not require the technical detail or monthly certification that Medicare requires, many of the concepts of medical review are applicable to all insurers. One of the best methods to improve your own documentation is to review other therapists' documentation and have them review yours. This chapter can be used to develop criteria for just such a review.

Claudia Allen is Chief of Occupational Therapy, Los Angeles, Harbor—University of California in Los Angeles Medical Center, Torrance, California.

Mary Foto is a senior allied health consultant, Blue Cross of California, Woodland Hills, California.

Terry Moon is an occupational therapy consultant, Blue Cross of California, Woodland Hills, California.

Dorothy Wilson is an occupational therapy consultant, Blue Cross of California, Woodland Hills, California.

V. Judith Thomas is Director of the Reimbursement Policy Program in the Government Relations Department of the American Occupational Therapy Association.

This article has been adapted from the December 1989 issue of the *American Journal of Occupational Therapy* and is reprinted here with permission.

Editor's Note: Policies of specifically named insurers are for illustration and may not explicitly apply to all payers.

In a traditional Medicare program, the Health Care Financing Administration (HCFA) contracts with insurance companies to process claims and to ensure that only covered, medically necessary services are paid. Insurance companies that review Medicare Part A and Part B claims submitted by institutional providers (e.g., hospitals, skilled nursing facilities) are referred to as **Fiscal Intermediaries (FIs)**. Carriers are Medicare contractors who process Part B claims submitted by physicians, nonphysician practitioners, including occupational and physical therapists in independent practice (OTIP and PTIP), laboratories, and medical equipment suppliers. HCFA provides guidelines to its contractors to assist in the medical review process. For example, the "Outpatient Occupational Therapy Medicare Part B Guidelines" are included in each Medicare manual to provide instruction for occupational therapy claims review. These and other policy rules are used in the "Focused Medical Review" (FMR) process that targets and directs medical review efforts to claims where there is greatest risk for inappropriate payment for services.

Focused Medical Review

In Focused Medical Review (FMR), fiscal intermediary contractor personnel review aggregate electronic data from similar facilities or practitioners and look for aberrant patterns of service and/or billing. When a facility or practitioner shows an unusual billing pattern, medical review personnel seek additional information to determine if a problem exists or if the variation is appropriate. Occupational therapy notes and other information contained in the medical record may be of critical importance in order to justify treatment protocols, frequency, and duration. Adequate documentation, supported by the Medicare Part B Guidelines, should justify any unusual variations in type or length of treatment. The following overview of Medicare program objectives and requirements will help understand how the FMR process works.

Goals

The overall goal of a Medicare Focused Medical Review is to decrease the receipt of claims for noncovered or unnecessary services. Additionally, the program is expected to protect against inappropriate payment by educating providers, to help improve quality of care, to ensure billing only for covered, necessary services, and to avoid inconvenience to providers who adhere to program requirements.

FMR Process

DATA COLLECTION - Medicare intermediaries and carriers routinely collect Medicare utilization claims data. To identify aberrant procedures, contractors electronically analyze several years of historical data to track patterns and trends in specific areas of practice over a period of time.

DATA ANALYSIS - From the data collected, contractors develop reports that profile providers by comparing national and local utilization by type of service and diagnosis. For instance, a carrier may profile physicians to determine which physicians order significantly greater amounts of therapy services than the norm for specific diagnoses. The FMR program also may perform trend analysis over a period of time for therapy providers to evaluate whether services have increased dramatically, if the number of patients or the number of visits per patient have increased, and if staff has increased commensurate with the increase in visits. With providers such as skilled nursing facilities (SNF), the FMR program might compare the incidence of patients receiving therapy services to the total number of patients among SNFs.

VERIFICATION OF EXISTENCE OF PROBLEMS - The goal of a FMR program is to identify variations in practice patterns and determine the cause. Such variations legitimately may be due to a community's special characteristics such as economic level or a concentration of a specific age group, or they may reflect delivery of inappropriate service or fraudulent practices. *To determine the cause, reviewers will select a sample of cases and review the medical documentation for medical necessity and appropriate utilization.* In the physician example above, the carrier may review a sample of records from those doctors whose numbers of therapy orders are high to determine if the orders meet Medicare's coverage guidelines. If the sample reveals no problem, the review is discontinued.

PROVIDER EDUCATION - Once a problem is identified, the FMR program staff may contact a specific provider to discuss the problem. If there appears to be widespread misunderstanding of a specific coverage policy, the Medicare FI or carrier may issue a provider bulletin or conduct educational seminars for providers.

FISCAL INTERMEDIARY LOCAL MEDICAL REVIEW POLICY (LMRP) DEVELOPMENT - When a problem is identified for which there is no national or local coverage guideline, an FI has the authority to develop local policy as long as it is consistent with national policies and addresses the verified problem. Two intermediaries that have developed LMRPs for occupational therapy are Mutual of Omaha and the Riverbend Government Benefits Administrator (Tennessee). In both cases, the occupational therapy guidelines are more specific than national guidelines and establish "reasonableness" standards based on duration of services. For instance, Mutual of Omaha states, "All transfer training may be covered up to 5 visits. Documentation beyond 5 visits must clearly show why further treatment is medically reasonable or necessary in order for goals to be met."

The Tennessee FI has established guidelines that state that treatment for impairments that are not directly related to the patient's functional limitations are excluded from coverage. Using this rule, a reviewer could deny coverage of occupational therapy for a patient with a Dupuytren's contracture **that does not impede (or is not documented to show that it impedes) hand function**. LMRP guidelines generally establish limitations but should always state that documentation can justify specific patient related needs for therapy beyond these limits. It is the therapist's responsibility to provide the justification.

CARRIER LMRP DEVELOPMENT - Although carriers perform similar FMR analyses of claims to identify aberrant billing behavior, local medical review policy (LMRP) has been developed using a different process than that of FIs.

The Carrier Medical Director (CMD) is responsible for identifying which services require LMRPs. Under Medicare Part B, physicians, OTIPs and PTIPs must submit bills using the HCFA Common Procedural System (HCPCS/CPT) codes. Therefore, data on service frequency by CPT are readily available for analysis from Medicare's national claims history files. In determining targeted services, the CMD also may obtain additional information from state specialty societies, individual practitioners, beneficiary complaint records, model policy developed by national or regional workgroups of CMDs, or other sources. Medicare instructions to carriers regarding LMRP content and format are more explicit than those for FIs, requiring such items as related HCPCS/CPT codes, general indications of when an item or service is covered, coverage limitations, covered ICD-9-CM codes, sources or clinical information used to develop the policy and documentation required to justify coverage.

In 1995, a national Physical Medicine and Rehabilitation (PM&R) workgroup was formed to develop model policy for the PM&R section of CPT codes (i.e., 97000 section). The AOTA presented comments to this group during the development of the model policy that outlines clinical and utilization guidelines for each PM&R CPT codes. The following model policy guideline for CPT code 97770 provides an example of the type of information contained in carrier LMRP.

97770: Development of cognitive skills to improve attention, memory, problem solving, includes compensatory training and/or sensory integrative activities, direct (one-on-one) patient contact by the provider, each 15 minutes.

Clinical Guidelines

1. This procedure may be medically necessary for persons with acquired cognitive defects relating from head trauma, or acute neurologic events including cerebrovascular accidents. It is not appropriate for patients with chronic progressive brain conditions with no potential for restoration. Occupational therapists, speech therapists, or clinical psychologists with specific training in these skills are typically the provider.

2. This procedure may be medically necessary when included in a patient's individual treatment plan aimed at improving or restoring specific functions which were impaired by an identified illness or injury and when expected outcomes that are attainable by the patient are specified in the plan.

Since the PM&R model policy was finalized, a number of Medicare carriers have chosen to incorporate some or all of this model policy into their LMRPs. Carriers must provide a minimum public comment period of 34 days before finalizing a LMRP and the effective date must be at least 30 days after publication of the final policy. Additionally, carriers are instructed not to apply a LMRP retroactively to claims processed prior to the effective date. The Balanced Budget Act of 1997 (P.L. 105-33), contains provisions which require expanded use of CPT codes to bill outpatient Medicare OT services. As these sections of the law are implemented, it is likely that future FI LMRPs for OT will more closely follow the carrier format.

The above information is to help you understand when and why individual medical records may be reviewed. Remember, when a focused medical review is initiated, the review personnel are investigating a variation in practice. This may not mean there is a problem. When your documentation is in line with the Medicare guidelines and demonstrates patient need for occupational therapy, variations can be substantiated. The following information outlines what is required for complete documentation of services.

PATIENT'S MEDICAL HISTORY - These records, which are supplied by the physician or through an interview with the therapist, should provide supportive information to substantiate the need for the stated intervention.

PHYSICIAN'S REFERRAL — A physician's referral should include the following:

- the occupational therapy treatment diagnosis
- the onset date of the treatment diagnosis
- the actual or estimated date of any recent change in level of function
- a request for evaluation or specific orders
- the date and the physician's signature.

If the physician has ordered an evaluation, the therapist should establish a treatment plan (including the type of activity or procedure and the frequency and duration of treatment) at the time of the initial evaluation and sign and date this plan. Any changes or additions to this plan should be in writing and should be signed and dated by the occupational therapist. If the physician has ordered a specific occupational therapy plan, the specific orders must be followed unless the therapist suggests or receives a change in orders from the physician. All telephone orders must be documented and then signed by the physician as required by state law and by facility and occupational therapy department procedures. Common errors in the physician's referral that cause delays or technical denials include incomplete or nonspecific orders (e.g., PRN orders), orders with a span of frequency and duration (e.g., two to three times a week for 4 to 6 weeks), and orders that do not state a specific type of treatment (e.g., activities as needed).

PHYSICIAN CERTIFICATION — Certification for outpatient services is a statement written by the physician at the time treatment is begun indicating that the patient needs occupational therapy services. This certification is good for 30 days from the date of the initial evaluation or the start-of-care date. Blue Cross of California accepts the initial physician's referral as the first certification. On or before the 30th day of treatment and every 30 days thereafter, recertification must be obtained in writing and signed and dated by the physician. The use of a stamp for the physician's signature on orders, certification, or recertification is not valid. The original certification and recertifications with the physician's signature should be kept on file.

Certification or recertification may be in any form but must contain the following key elements:

- a statement that the physician has seen the patient during the 30-day period
- a statement of the need for continuing outpatient occupational therapy
- a statement estimating the length of time services will be needed to achieve the treatment goals
- a statement of the physician's intention to review the case every 30 days.

INITIAL EVALUATION – These records must contain baseline data—both subjective and objective—that measure the relevant recovery factors for that patient's treatment diagnosis. Goals must be clearly stated and must relate directly to the baseline recovery factors.

DAILY DOCUMENTATION FROM THE START-OF-CARE DATE – At a minimum, daily documentation should state the date of treatment, type of treatment, length of the treatment session if the therapist billed by time and procedure, and patient's progress, including documentation of changes whenever they occur. If no changes are occurring, that fact should be documented. To avoid technical denials, we recommend that the occupational therapy department be responsible for reviewing the medical records before they are sent to the intermediary to ensure that they are clear and complete, include all items requested, and reflect the billing period in question. The therapist should include the complete records from the start-of-care date. Determination of the patient's progress for the billing period under review is difficult without the initial evaluation, treatment notes, and summaries from previous billing periods. The intermediary usually does not keep all of the previous medical records on file.

WEEKLY AND MONTHLY PROGRESS NOTES – Brief weekly notes stating changes from the beginning of the treatment week and monthly summaries of changes from the beginning of the treatment month are required. Changes in the patient's ability to perform activities of daily living from one period to the next are summarized.

In daily, weekly, and monthly notes, the therapist should measure and document changes in key factors previously identified as contributing to the patient's decreased function. Relevant factors, such as pain, loss of range of motion, loss of functional ability to follow or retain instruction, and attitude, are frequently related to the patient's performance. The notes should clearly state when the patient reaches a goal. Likewise, if the patient has not reached a goal, an explanation should be provided.

To demonstrate that adequate supervision has been given, the daily notes of all occupational therapy assistants should be cosigned if required by state regulation. Although Medicare's conditions of participation are silent as to cosignature, facility policy may require this practice to demonstrate an adequate level of supervision.

ITEMIZED FINANCIAL LEDGER SHOWING DAILY CHARGES – Itemized services that are billed on the financial ledger must match the daily occupational therapy treatment record. All services billed must be covered by benefits of the Medicare insurance program. Treatments such as biofeedback training for relaxation, driver's education, and case conferences are not covered by the program.

If a claim is questioned because technical requirements are not met, the areas concerning medical necessity are not reviewed. In the medical review process, the quality of a therapist's services may not matter if technical requirements have not been properly addressed. The denial of reimbursement because of technical problems is troubling to a clinician.

Medicare denies coverage for the following basic reasons:

1. *The need for the occupational therapist's unique skills and knowledge is not evident.* Covered treatment must be at a certain level of complexity and sophistication, or the condition of the patient must be such that the treatment can be performed safely and effectively only by a certified occupational therapist or under such a therapist's supervision. If the patient or caregiver could provide the care (e.g., activities of daily living routines, endurance activities, exercises, transfers) or if the treatment consists of instructions that another service could provide, then skilled occupational therapy is considered unnecessary.

2. *The patient would improve naturally without the help of an occupational therapist.* If the general progression of the patient's medical condition would return the patient to a previous level of functioning spontaneously, then skilled occupational therapy intervention is not considered to be medically necessary.

3. *The patient shows no significant improvement within a reasonable and predictable amount of time.* "Reasonable" is considered to mean that there is a greater than 50% probability that the patient will make significant improvement as a consequence of occupational therapy. "Predictable amount of time" is interpreted to mean that the planned frequency and duration of treatments is a knowledgeable estimate of how long it will take the patient to achieve therapy goals in relation to the diagnosis, severity, and prognosis of the condition. If at any point in the course of the treatment it is determined that the expectations will not materialize, occupational therapy services will no longer be considered reasonable. If treatment of underlying factors, such as an increase in endurance, strength, or range of motion, or a decrease in pain, does not improve the performance of functional activities, then improvement is not considered to be significant.

4. *The patient has not demonstrated sustainable gains, is considered to be at a maintenance level and is not expected to show further improvement.* Therapists must document decreased levels of assistance or improved patient responses to assistance provided. Documentation of activity outcomes should be stated in measurable, objective terms.

5. *The occupational therapy services duplicate services provided by other therapists.* If a single discipline, such as physical therapy, occupational therapy, speech therapy, or nursing, could provide the care, only one discipline can bill the charges. For example, if the occupational therapy program provided upper extremity exercises and the physical therapy program provided lower extremity exercises and gait training, then only physical therapy would be covered because physical therapy could also provide upper extremity exercises. If the occupational therapy program included transfers, dressing, and upper extremity exercises and the physical therapy program provided only upper extremity exercises, then only the occupational therapy would be covered. Services are not considered duplicative in cases where both services involved have unique treatment goals that lead to distinct functional outcomes. For example, in *transfer training*, the physical therapy goal is for safe and independent transfers, and the occupational therapy goal is for the appropriate use of transfer techniques in activi-

ties of daily living. In brain injury rehabilitation, the occupational therapy goal is to employ neuromuscular therapies to increase functional use of the upper extremity in dressing or bathing, and the physical therapy goal is to use neuromuscular therapies to assist the patient in the use of the upper extremity during ambulation activities.

Medical Necessity Review

To determine medical necessity, the intermediary reviews the patient's medical records from the start-of-care date. In this review, the intermediary asks: Why does this patient need an occupational therapist now? The therapist's knowledge of disability and activity analysis must be combined with a reasonable expectation for improving functional performance.

The medical reviewer's role is to determine medical necessity on the basis of documentation in the medical records indicating that the patient's condition and level of function required the special knowledge and skill of an occupational therapist. As practicing therapists we focus on the patient's disability, but as medical reviewers we focus on whether the nature of that disability requires a therapist's knowledge to successfully help the patient.

To be covered by the fiscal intermediary, occupational therapy services must be reasonable and necessary. Services are "reasonable" if the patient has a fair or good rehabilitation potential for the established goals. A good rehabilitation potential exists when the patient's function is expected to improve significantly within a limited and predictable amount of time on the basis of the occupational therapist's initial assessment. Services are "necessary" if skilled occupational therapy is required to produce the expected improvement. If the expected improvement is not achieved, the intervening variables that invalidated the therapist's prediction of rehabilitation potential should be identified.

Determining Medical Necessity

Documentation of the presence of a disability alone, however, is not enough. Therapists must identify the specific diagnosis (ICD-9-CM code) that substantiates the need for a skilled occupational therapist's assessment and must prove that the patient could only improve through the application of the therapist's special knowledge of activity analysis and treatment methods.

To document treatment so that the medical reviewer does not need to search for treatment goals and for the patient's progress toward those goals, the therapist can use the following four steps as guidelines:

STEP 1: THE INITIAL EVALUATION — In this step, the therapist asks, "Where are we?" and determines the patient's current levels through an initial evaluation. The initial evaluation begins with an interview of the patient, which is a crucial component of the evaluation and a prerequisite to the establishment of a practical treatment plan. The interview follows a complete review of the medical record and focuses on the perspective of the patient, the caregiver, or both. The interview establishes what activities the patient can perform, how often these activities are performed, and if the patient or caregiver is satisfied or dissatisfied with his or her performance. A successful interview uncovers the patient's perceived problems, physical or cognitive disabilities, relevant medical history, and available family and community support. The interview establishes a request for services by identifying areas in which the patient is doing well or poorly and by screening out activities that are not relevant.

After the initial evaluation, a list of activities requested by the patient or caregiver is developed and improved upon with the special knowledge and skills of an occupational therapist. The therapist should document the patient's current levels for each of the requested activities. This is the starting point for the rest of the documentation.

STEP 2: REHABILITATION POTENTIAL — In this step, the therapist asks, "Where are we going?" and "What are the specific, expected levels of activity for the patient?" The therapist then establishes measurable, realistic goals for the patient. Once the specific activities that can be improved through the intervention of an occupational therapist have been developed and the patient's current activity levels have been documented, the occupational therapist can determine the patient's expected levels. The therapist should write these expected levels as goals for each activity. Such goals must be measurable and must realistically reflect the patient's rehabilitation potential. Each of these goals must be specifically relevant to the performance of functional activities. Ascertaining the patient's potential for improving functional status is a critical assessment decision for the therapist. It not only determines the type of therapy intervention that may be used but also enables the therapist to predict the outcome of the intervention on the patient's task performance.

STEP 3: THE TREATMENT PLAN — In this step, the therapist asks, "How do we get there?" and "What specific treatments will bring the patient to the expected levels?" The therapist determines a specific treatment plan for each expected level identified in Step 2 and states the specific treatment plan and any changes in either the plan or its implementation. Documentation should include a record of treatment activities, modalities, and procedures; the patient's and family's education; the equipment ordered; the need for further evaluation; conferences with others; and discharge plans. The specifics of the discharge plan should be stated—that is, the amount of supervision required, the education of the patient and family that has been accomplished and that is still required, and a tentative discharge date.

STEP 4: ASSESSMENT OF THE PATIENT'S PROGRESS — In this step, the therapist asks, "How are we doing?" The patient's progress is measured. This is the proof that the plan is working, the facts that prove that an occupational therapist is essential to the patient's progress. Each treatment diagnosis has a probable set of outcome alternatives. Once the treatment goal has been established, each progress note must reestablish the appropriateness of these goals and monitor the specific change the patient has made toward the goal.

Progress notes must contain a series of established causes and must measure progress and monitor functional outcome. Each note must reflect progress toward the determined goal. For example, if full range of motion of the shoulder is the underlying component necessary to reach the goal, then the therapist should do the following:

- establish that the causative factor (pain) is being controlled
- measure the shoulder's passive, active, and functional range of motion
- monitor changes in specific tasks, for example, upper extremity dressing.

Alternatively, the therapist could do the following:

- establish that muscle weakness is the underlying cause of shoulder immobility
- measure quantitative changes in strength
- monitor changes in specific tasks (e.g., independence in meal preparation at home).

By establishing causes and measuring progress, the therapist clearly outlines each step toward predetermined goals. This method will help substantiate that the services of an occupational therapist are indeed necessary to secure reimbursement, thus allowing for further treatment for the patient. See Table 6.1 for an example of sufficient and insufficient documentation.

Conclusion

When reimbursement is denied or delayed, it is often due to insufficient documentation—either the documentation lacks technical accuracy or lacks details supporting medical necessity. We recommend that the therapist pay attention to the areas that are screened for accuracy and take the time to review claims before they are sent to a Medicare contractor or private insurance carrier.

Because clerical errors cause the majority of technical errors, we suggest that billing clerks as well as therapists and administrators become familiar with claims coding.

The guidelines presented in this paper to help therapists keep medical records can be used to provide the information necessary for a fair review. By following these guidelines from the beginning of treatment, therapists will have proper documentation when records are requested. Additionally, the four steps of documentation that we provided should help therapists develop a clear image of a patient's progress and should substantiate the need for the specific skills of an occupational therapist, thus helping to establish medical necessity.

References

Blue Cross of California. (1989). PT Medicode+ [Computer program]. Van Nuys, CA: Author.

Mutual of Omaha, Medicare Area. (1997). *Local Medical Review Policy No. 97-1*. Omaha, NE: Author.

Health Care Financing Administration. *Medicare Intermediary Manual* (HCFA Publication No. 13).

Health Care Financing Administration. *Medicare Intermediary Manual* (HCFA Publication No. 14).

Riverbend Government Benefits Administrator. (1997). *Local Medical Review Policy-002-96*. Chattanooga, TN; Author.

Table 6.1. Use of the four documentation steps for a patient with left hemiparesis from a cerebrovascular accident

Documentation Steps	Commonly Used Information (Insufficient)	Specific Information (Sufficient)
Step 1: Initial evaluation	Patient requires assistance with self-care.	The patient requires moderate physical assistance and step-by-step verbal cuing to dress (secondary to left-side neglect, decreased left upper extremity function, and diminished motor planning). The caregiver is not knowledgeable of compensatory dressing techniques and typically performs these tasks for patient.
Step 2: Rehabilitation potential	Instruct the patient in self-care.	The patient will achieve at least a minimum assistance level for dressing with the use of compensatory techniques. The caregiver will learn the proper methods and cues for assisting the patient.
Step 3: Treatment plan	Provide functional activities.	The therapist will provide dressing training and practice with the use of various compensatory techniques to determine the most suitable technique for the patient, combined with instruction of the caregiver to follow through.
Step 4: Assessment of the patient's progress	Patient improved in self-care.	The patient performs dressing with minimum assistance, requiring cuing for left arm placement into sleeve. The caregiver is able to demonstrate appropriate methods of assisting the patient.

7. Writing Functional Goals

Patricia Moorhead, MHCA, OTR/L, and Kathleen Kannenberg, MA, OTR/L

Therapists often say that writing good functional goals is the most difficult part of documentation. Unfortunately, if the goals are not functional and clear, the entire set of notes may not paint a relevent picture of the patient's functional status before, during, and after treatment. This probably explains why the majority of reimbursement problems occur because of inadequate documentation.

Patricia Moorhead is Manager of Rehabilitation Services, Scottsdale Healthcare, Scottsdale, Arizona. She has served as a faculty member for documentation workshops sponsored by the American Occupational Therapy Association.

Kathleen Kannenberg is a private consultant in community mental health, Seattle, Washington. She is the former Mental Health Program Manager for the American Occupational Therapy Association.

Qhanges in health care have had a major impact on documentation requirements over the past 5 years. Occupational therapy practitioners no longer have the luxury of treating patients for an extended period of time or even "as long as progress is being made." Therapists often need to establish goals and begin intervention in the first therapy session and complete the course of therapy quickly. As a result of these changes, documentation has become more streamlined and concise. Further, for occupational therapists and assistants who practice in environments where managed care is predominant, documentation requirements may vary significantly from one payer to another. However, the majority of those who review documentation are still looking for functional goals and outcomes to justify medically necessary therapy services.

The advent of capitation also has changed requirements for documentation. In the past, documentation was essential to justify payment for services. In a capitated environment reimbursement is a set amount. Payment is often per member, per month; accordingly, one may not be looking specifically at documentation to justify payment. However, good documentation continues to be essential in order to clarify the functional outcomes occupational therapy can provide as well as justify the need for continued services.

The cost of health care continues to rise and external mandates for change are driving reform in both reimbursement methods and service delivery options. Third party payers as well as service providers are looking closely at what services they are paying for and the necessity and cost of these services. As hospitals and other providers enter the environment of capitation, both costs of services and client outcomes will be scrutinized closely. Occupational therapy practitioners need to document progress in relationship to functional outcomes in order to demonstrate the need for continued services.

The trend toward cost control within a managed care environment has mandated shifts in documentation requirements. Reviewers are requesting less documentation and are looking more specifically at functional levels, assessments, and goals. Charting forms have been drastically condensed to allow more time for patient treatment and less time for documentation. Streamlined forms and computerized documentation are becoming more common. These efficiency measures will allow for increased time to focus on interventions as well as provide cost effective services and savings in the long run. However, practitioners need to know that reviewers are still looking for individualized documentation; therefore, care needs to be taken when using computerized documentation formats that allow the practitioner to choose information from a menu.

Many reviewers today are using the Medicare Part B Guidelines (see Appendix 1) when looking at documentation for occupational therapy services. The Health Care Financing Administration (HCFA) established the Medicare Part B Guidelines in 1989 in order to clarify what services occupational therapy practitioners can expect to be reimbursed for under Medicare Part B in outpatient settings. Because the Medicare Part B Guidelines are the only comprehensive documentation guidelines in print, they have been used as an accepted standard by payers in a variety of settings to help determine the need for skilled therapy services.

The easiest way to accomplish writing an intervention plan addressing function is to establish functional long-term and short-term goals. The Medicare B Guidelines require that goals be functional, measurable, and objective. In order for a goal to be functional, it must include a functional performance area, e.g., self-care, meal preparation, medication management, or socialization.

One way of documenting measurable and objective goals is to indicate the level of assistance required to accomplish the desired activity. The Medicare B Guidelines include levels of assistance that can be used to measure an individual's progress. The levels of assistance described in the guidelines are also helpful because they include both physical and cognitive levels. Using these levels of assistance can help to justify treating a person who may have not had any physical problems but whose cognitive deficits interfere with functioning and safety in daily life activities. It also can be helpful to use the levels of assistance in conjunction with the patient's identified problem areas in performance on the initial occupational therapy evaluation. Doing this will establish a clear baseline upon which to develop functional goals and measure progress.

When writing functional goals, the therapist should clearly document the functional level the patient is expected to achieve (e.g., "Patient will bathe lower body with minimal assistance," or "Patient will make one purchase from the drug store with moderate assistance"). Depending upon the setting, it may be necessary to document changes in the underlying factors or performance components (e.g., "Patient will attend to cooking task for 20 minutes in order to prepare light meal with standby assistance," or "Patient will demonstrate 90 degrees of shoulder flexion in order to don shirt independently").

Occupational therapists need to document the underlying factors (e.g., range of motion (ROM), sensation, attention span, sequencing, strength, tone, coping skills, or self-control) that are impeding the person's ability to function. Documentation of these factors then must be linked to a functional outcome. For example, documenting limitation in shoulder ROM is not helpful unless it is also clearly documented that the person requires moderate assistance for dressing as a result of the limitation. In the mental health setting, stating that a person is less depressed does not denote a change in function; however, documenting that the person can now dress independently or is now able to follow a daily schedule of daily activities with minimal cueing does demonstrate progress toward a functional outcome.

Occupational therapy practitioners often ask if they can document psychosocial deficits and interventions in the treatment plan for an individual with a nonpsychiatric condition and still be reimbursed. The answer is to clearly identify *any* underlying factors interfering with function in the desired performance area. If psychosocial skills or psychological components, such as self-concept, role performance, social conduct, self-expression, or coping skills, are limiting progress toward performance in daily activities, providing a rationale for inclusion of these factors along with clearly linking them to the functional performance area often will facilitate reimbursement. For example, for a woman whose role as a mother has been disrupted by Guillian-Barre, a functional goal might be to independently prepare an afterschool snack for her son. Underlying factors that might be addressed in this goal would include both physical factors, such as standing endurance and motor control, and psychosocial components such as self-concept, values, self-expression, and role performance. Often, occupational therapy goals have been expressed in terms of changing impairments. However, components themselves do not reflect meaningful changes in a person's life.

Thus, underlying factors that limit performance can include a broad scope, as the components are only a means to the functional outcome and not a goal in and of themselves. Uniform Terminology III defines occupational therapy's domain of concern and can be used as a tool to document outcomes and to help practitioners distinguish between underlying factors or performance components and performance areas when identifying problems and writing goals. By collaborating to develop a mutually desired goal and using activities with relevance and value to the patient, improved progress toward the functional goal may be acomplished.

When occupational therapists begin to evaluate patients, they traditionally look at the underlying factors first: ROM, strength, perception, cognition, and psychosocial skills. However, documenting functional levels in performance areas first and then assessing the limiting factors affecting the person's ability to complete the desired or needed functional activity will serve two purposes. First, there is no need to spend treatment time on particular underlying factors if they have no functional impact. For example, a person may have contractures and limited ROM of the hand but demonstrate independence in all self-care activities. Patients with no functional deficits in performance areas will typically not be approved for occupational therapy services.

Second, by assessing functional activities/abilities first, it is easier to see which underlying factors interfere with performance. For example, by assessing a person during a cooking activity, it is possible to look at several areas of cognition and perception such as sequencing, organization, memory, orientation, depth perception, and apraxia. The next step would be to look more closely at the areas where impairments are evident and conduct an in-depth assessment.

In the same way, after assessing a patient and finding that he or she needs maximum assistance to perform the functional task, it is then necessary to evaluate ROM, strength, cognition, or other factors that limit the person's ability to function. This information assists in writing functional goals that are realistic and measurable (for example "Patient will demonstrate appropriate energy conservation techniques in order to independently prepare a light snack," or "Patient will take a bath 4 times weekly, with prompt of weekly posted schedule").

It may be helpful to structure the occupational therapy initial evaluation summary so that performance areas and functional activities are placed first on the form. This will serve as a reminder to therapists to observe these areas first and then assess the underlying factors. It also provides quickly identified information on functional status for the reviewer. At times, it may seem difficult to relate a goal to a functional outcome. It may be helpful to ask the patient what his or her prior functional level was or what he or she cannot do now that could be accomplished before the illness or injury.

It is also important to ask the patient and caregiver what his or her goals are. If the goals are realistic and appropriate, an intervention plan is established based on goals that are agreed upon between therapist and patient. If the patient's goals seem unrealistic or inappropriate to the setting or diagnosis, it is critical to discuss more fully with the patient and family what that goal means to them, so that the therapist can provide additional education or support to facilitate the establishment of a mutually agreeable intervention plan.

It may seem difficult at times to establish functional goals for patients who function at a higher level (for instance, independent with self-care but unable to live independently in the community). Goals addressing community skills or safety issues are often appropriate in this case. Consider activities where safety is a factor. Patients may also choose to have assistance in personal care areas and concentrate their energies on other performance areas. Referring to a checklist of routine daily activities may be helpful in identifying desired functional goals. The list will vary according to the setting and population and may include such activities as dialing 911 in an emergency, preparing menus, grocery shopping, handling money, balancing a checkbook, writing checks, doing laundry, arranging transportation for appointments, caring for others, managing school assignments, performing job tasks, or participating in valued leisure activities. The generation of such an extensive list of functional activities should assist with establishing goals for clients at all levels.

Goals may also be limited by who the payer is or what the insurance coverage provides (medical insurance such as Medicare does not pay for work or leisure-related goals, and worker's compensation has return to work as its primary focus).

The Treatment Plan

After evaluating the patient and discussing what the patient or family/caregiver needs or wants to be able to do, the next step is to determine the plan of intervention. As we see shorter lengths of stay and fewer therapy services approved with managed care, it is even more essential to involve families, caregivers, and others who may assist in the patient's care, early in the intervention process. Discharge planning should occur at the time of initiation of treatment.

The treatment plan includes both short-term and long-term goals as well as the therapist's plan for specific interventions to accomplish these goals. Long-term goals are written with the intent that they will be achieved at the time of discharge from therapy or discharge to the next appropriate level of care. Short-term goals are intended to be accomplished within the time frame of the long-term goal. Time frames for the short-term goals can range anywhere from 2 days to 1 month or more, depending on the treatment setting. It is best to write short-term goals that include a functional component, keeping in mind that every short-term goal must be associated with a long-term goal.

If the long-term goal states that the patient will be able to shop independently for necessary grocery items, the short-term goal might be that the patient will be able to generate a shopping list with minimal assistance. In this example, it is necessary to achieve the short-term goal prior to achieving the long-term goal of independence with grocery shopping.

Functional goals need to be written to show what the patient will accomplish, not what the therapist will do. Goals such as, "Evaluate for cognitive deficits" or "Teach family car transfers" are part of the therapist's plan, not the patient's goals. If each goal is documented beginning with "Patient will…" or "Patient's family will…", all of the goals will be patient or caregiver goals.

Examples of Functional Goals

Although there is no one perfect format for writing functional goals, the format shown in the following examples may be helpful. Examples are provided from a variety of specialty practice areas.

1. Patient will perform safe transfers on and off the toilet with standby assistance.
2. Patient will create a grocery store list with minimal assistance from pre-planned weekly menus.
3. Patient will demonstrate independence with home exercise program.
4. Patient's daughter will independently transfer patient in and out of the car from the wheelchair.
5. Patient will take a timeout with minimal cueing when angry with peers in order to complete a group school assignment.
6. Child will play with peer without fighting for 10 minutes with minimal prompting.
7. Child will copy a circle with minimal cues.
8. Child will independently play on jungle gym for 5 minutes without falling.
9. Client will independently take bus to weekly support group.

When the focus of intervention is one of the underlying factors, it is important to include these in the functional goals. Examples might include the following

1. Patient will sustain attention to task for 10 minutes to prepare a light snack with standby assistance.
2. Patient will maintain eye contact when greeting visitors at the information desk using cue card with written reminder.
3. Patient will demonstrate 90 degrees shoulder flexion in order to bathe independently using equipment.
4. Patient will demonstrate right wrist extension of 10 degrees in order to operate cash register independently.
5. Patient will use memory log book with minimal assistance in order to follow a daily schedule.
6. Patient's family will demonstrate independence in positioning techniques so the patient can eat with standby assistance.

7. Patient will demonstrate good body mechanics in order to vacuum independently.

8. Using procedure outlined on cue card, client will ask supervisor for help when unable to complete job task in scheduled amount of time.

9. Child will independently use right hand as a functional assist during drawing activities.

10. Client will follow daily schedule and initiate a pre-planned crocheting activity independently.

11. Caregiver will demonstrate independence in laundry set-up so client can complete weekly laundry independently.

12. Patient will demonstrate improved self-concept and beginning acceptance of disability by combing hair and applying makeup independently using tendonesis splint.

Although not every goal needs to include the underlying factors, it is important to identify the underlying factors interfering with the desired performance. Treating the underlying factors may be the major emphasis of the therapist's intervention plan. However, with the changes in managed care, it is critical to know what the reviewers who are looking at the documentation want to see. In some cases the reviewers will want to know specific range of motion measurements or cognitive deficits in order to determine the need for therapy services. Other reviewers will only be concerned with the patient's functional level and will not look for specific information regarding the underlying factors. Often the setting where the therapy services are provided will determine the amount and type of documentation that is required.

Progress notes can be streamlined if documentation focuses on the functional problems and underlying factors. Goal achievement will address the patient's functional improvement in the performance area. Depending upon the documentation requirements, the objective data in the progress notes may identify changes in the underlying factors or address only the functional changes. The assessment section of the progress note should pull it all together by stating how gains in specific areas have increased overall functional performance in the desired area.

Identifying the functional problem and the underlying factors that contribute to the problem assists in the planning of effective goals and interventions. In this way, it becomes clear which areas need to be addressed and how progress will affect function. Patients usually remain in treatment until goals are achieved or no progress is made. It is easier to identify patients who are making progress and those who are not when the goals are measurable, objective, and include functional outcomes. Patients then can be discharged appropriately from occupational therapy services.

Functional goals are appropriate for all settings and individuals requiring occupational therapy services. This includes inpatient acute care and rehabilitation, outpatient facilities, work hardening programs, adult day health programs, skilled nursing facilities, school systems, partial hospital programs, community mental health settings (including, psychosocial rehabilitation programs, clubhouse models, vocational programs), and other community or home health settings. It may be difficult at first to establish functional goals for all patients and to differentiate between underlying factors and performance areas, but this process becomes easier with practice.

Although not all third party payers are requiring that goals be functional, more and more reviewers of documentation are looking for functional progress and outcomes. In order to justify the need for occupational therapy services and ensure payment, all therapists and assistants need to look at their documentation with a critical eye and ask themselves, "Do these services require the skills of an occupational therapy practitioner, and would I pay for these services?"

If therapists write goals that are functional, measurable and achievable, it will help to ensure that the answer to this question is yes.

Resources

American Occupational Therapy Association. (1994). Uniform terminology for occupational therapy (3rd edition). *American Journal of Occupational Therapy, 43,* 793-800.

American Occupational Therapy Association. (1995a). Psychosocial concerns within occupational therapy practice. *American Journal of Occupational Therapy, 49,* 1011-1013.

American Occupational Therapy Association. (1995b). The psychosocial core of occupational therapy. *American Journal of Occupational Therapy, 49,* 1021-1022.

American Occupational Therapy Association. (1995c). Elements of clinical documentation (revised). *American Journal of Occupational Therapy, 49,* 1032-1035.

Hemphill, B., Peterson, C., & Werner, P. (1991). *Rehabilitation in mental health: Goals and objectives for independent living.* Thorofare, NJ: Slack.

8. Special Considerations I: Pediatrics

Barbara E. Chandler, MOT, OTR

In certain areas or settings of practice, special considerations should be highlighted for the purposes of documentation. The areas of pediatrics, home health, and mental health have been selected because they are the most common areas causing difficulties. This chapter focuses on pediatrics, while chapters 9 and 10 address home health and chapter 11 mental health.

Barbara E. Chandler is Assistant Professor, Program in Occupational Therapy, Shenandoah University, Winchester, Virginia. She served as Pediatric Program Manager at the American Occupational Therapy Association

ocumentation for occupational therapy services to pediatric clients shares many similarities with documentation of occupational therapy services for any client. Many of the suggestions for appropriate documentation stated elsewhere in this book are applicable and necessary for documentation for services to pediatric clients. Technical information such as name and insurance number must be correct. The documentation must be organized so that relevant information can be easily located. The services provided must have been skilled services provided by an occupational therapist to increase function. The services must also have been medically necessary. The notes of what occurred during treatment sessions must relate to the goals of the treatment plan. The service should not be a duplication of other services, although clear coordination of efforts with other services is desirable. The documentation must indicate, with some minor exceptions discussed later, steady progression from a dependent to a less dependent or, hopefully, an independent state.

Developmental Considerations

However, there are some important differences to consider when documenting some services for pediatric clients. In general, these differences cluster around two main topics: developmental considerations and educational considerations or relevance.

Many occupational therapists have had experience with submitting claims to third party payers and being informed that the insurance policies did not cover any condition or disability that was developmental in nature. This is a particularly chilling revelation when one considers the vast needs of many children whose functional disabilities are identified early and who could clearly benefit from intervention and require far fewer and less extensive services, if any, later in life.

It may be helpful for occupational therapy practitioners treating children with developmental disabilities to clarify certain points in the documentation process. The difference between the primary medical diagnosis and the secondary treatment diagnosis must be clear. Occupational therapy practitioners do not treat medical diagnoses. They treat the secondary diagnosis or functional disabilities that result from the condition identified in the primary diagnosis.

For example, although occupational therapy practitioners treat many children with cerebral palsy, they do not treat the cerebral palsy. Occupational therapists and COTAs address the functional disabilities that result from the condition, such as inability to feed oneself due to poor manipulation of eating utensils or inability to dress oneself independently. Occupational therapy practitioners may treat the functional disability of poor sequencing skill resulting from seizure activity, but they do not treat the seizures.

Occupational therapy practitioners providing services to children with developmental disabilities must document how the delay in the acquisition of developmental skills leads to functional disability thereby affecting functional abilities.

While age must be considered when setting goals and documenting, it is best not to describe the disability in age terms. One should not say that a child is 2 years behind in dressing skills, or write that the goal is to increase dressing skills to an age-appropriate level. Instead, the goal should be written in functional terms: "By March 1, John will dress himself independently." While this would be an appropriate goal for a 5-year-old, it would not be an appropriate goal for a 2-year-old despite the fact that the developmental delay suggests that this will be a functional disability in the future. A 2-year-old would not be expected to dress independently. A clear indication of progression from a dependent state to a less dependent or independent state should be evident in the documentation. Given the nature of many developmental delays or disabilities, it is advisable to break the goals down into small enough increments so that progress can be clearly indicated within a reasonable time, usually a month.

Sensory integrative dysfunction may be considered a developmental disability by some third party payers or may be considered a condition that is not covered by certain policies or payers. Other payers may say sensory integrative treatment is an educationally related treatment approach. It is important when documenting the treatment provided to children with sensory integrative impairments that the treatment be identified as occupational therapy and that the functional disabilities resulting from the integrative problems be identified and described. Avoiding sensory integrative or developmental terms is advisable. The documentation should describe in functional terms what the individual cannot do as a result of the integrative problems. The purpose of documentation is to communicate, and the majority of individuals reading the documentation, from parents to medical reviewers, is not going to be familiar with the neurological terms so familiar and clear to occupational therapists.

Sensory Integration

The developmental considerations can be summarized in one word: *function*. Occupational therapists treat functional disabilities. The treatment diagnosis, the intervention goals, and the documentation of service delivery must all address functional disabilities and functional goals. If function is the core of the documentation process, it is clearly communicated to anyone who reads the documentation. If function is expressed in terms of moving a child along a continuum from dependence to independence, the question of developmental delay is less likely to arise.

The second major consideration in pediatric documentation and one that is becoming increasingly complex is the issue of educational relevance for occupational therapy services provided in the public schools through an Individualized Education Program (IEP) under Part B of the Individuals with Disabilities Education Act (IDEA). In Part B, IDEA, occupational therapy is defined as a related service to special education. Related services are defined as "...transportation, and such developmental, corrective, and other supportive services as are required to assist a child with a disability to benefit from special education,..." (34 Code of Federal Regulations, §300.16). Since a related service is tied to the need for special education, it is imperative that the occupational therapy intervention be clearly linked to the goals and objectives contained in the current IEP because it is the IEP that delineates what the special education will consist of and what services the child will receive.

Educational Relevance

Many occupational therapists and certified occupational therapy assistants have experienced difficulty in clearly explaining to special educators and other members of an IEP committee how disability and intervention needs identified by the occupational therapist are

Individualized Education Program

related to educational goals and objectives. Often the "OT IEP section" along with the "speech IEP section" and the "adaptive PE IEP section," for example, are all stapled to the back of the educational IEP and presented to the parents as a comprehensive IEP. This is not how an IEP should be developed, and it contributes to the difficulty in explaining how occupational therapy is needed for the child to benefit from special education.

An IEP is developed by an IEP team (whose core members are identified in the Code of Federal Regulations, 34, §300.344). If the occupational therapy evaluation indicates that the child has deficits that interfere with educational functioning, the occupational therapist should attend the IEP meeting and contribute to the development of team consensus goals and objectives. The team consensus goals and objectives may require the services of more than one professional and should reflect the overall needs of the student.

For example, the team consensus goal of increased oral participation in class may require the input of the classroom teacher for management of a language group activity, the input of the speech pathologist to determine the grammatical area that will be focused on, and the input of the occupational therapist to determine an appropriate position to enable the student to do the task. No one professional is going to be able to address this goal and the student's need alone. The occupational therapist may still address areas traditionally thought of as "OT," but should always tie them to the educational (consensus) goal of increased oral participation in class. When an IEP is written and implemented in this way, the link between therapeutic goals and objectives and educational goals and objectives is clear.

Occupational therapy practitioners providing services in the schools should follow the same general guidelines for documentation as those practicing in other settings. A detailed discussion of documenting occupational therapy services in school systems is available in the publication *Occupational Therapy Services for Children and Youth Under the Individuals with Disabilities Education Act* (American Occupational Therapy Association, 1997).

Payment for Services in the Schools

Many school districts are now accessing third party payers for related services that are provided as part of a student's IEP. Since the related service must be educationally necessary and the reimburser covers services that are medically necessary, many questions have arisen about the overlap between these two types of services and the need for documentation that would satisfy the requirements of both the educational and medical systems. School system caseloads, ethics, and common sense dictate that it is impractical to have two sets of documentation for the same service. This apparent dilemma is easily resolved once practitioners providing services in the schools develop their goals and objectives in conjunction with the other members of the IEP committee and focus their goals, objectives, and documentation on functional disabilities and outcomes, as they relate to the educational environment.

It should be noted that there may be services that are educationally necessary but not medically necessary and vice versa. No goals can be said to be clearly educational or clearly medical without considering the context of the child's individual situation. Each decision of medical and/or educational relevance must be based on the child's needs. Occupational therapy services in the schools are based on the individual needs of the child. The decision on whether or how to provide occupational therapy services to a child eligible for special education should never be determined by the availability of a third party to pay for the service. The IDEA clearly states that services are to be provided to students who need the service to benefit from special education. Unlike provisions required by third party payers, there is no requirement that students show progress in order to continue to receive occupational therapy in the school system.

It is important to identify a functional disability and determine a functional goal or objective to address that disability. Documentation should be organized to reflect the relationship between the functional disability and the goal or objective to address that functional disability. The functional disability may be reflected (though not actually described) in the current level of educational functioning, which is a key component of the IEP. The wording of current level of educational functioning should be stated positively, e.g., "Reads four words;" "Identifies six letters of the alphabet;" or "Writes first letter of name." It should not be stated in terms of the functional disability, e.g., "Doesn't read at grade level;" "Doesn't identify 20 letters of the alphabet;" or "Doesn't write first name." **Functional Disability**

A comparison between current level of educational functioning and expected level of educational functioning for age and grade level will indicate educational needs. If the occupational therapist can clearly see a link between the functional disabilities identified through the occupational therapy evaluation and the educational needs, occupational therapy is appropriate as a related service. The occupational therapist would indicate on the IEP how the remediation of the functional disabilities (stated as educationally-related functional goals) would contribute to the educational goal. This is done by including the functional goals as intermediate steps (short-term objectives) toward the annual educational goal. Although the occupational therapist may work on many component parts of the functional goal, the component parts are never identified as the educational goal on the IEP. They are addressed as components and are only included in the therapeutic process because their remediation or improvement contributes to the functional goal (which in turn contributes to the attainment of the educational goal). In some instances, the functional goal and the educational goal may be the same.

The following three examples of parts of this process may help to illustrate these points.

EXAMPLE 1 — Tim is a 6-year-old student enrolled in a regular kindergarten. He is identified as a special needs student who has an orthopedic disability. He is currently dependent in all aspects of self-care and is unable to use any writing instrument. He maneuvers his wheelchair in the school building (level surface) at the rate of 1 foot per minute.

An appropriate educational goal for Tim would be: "Tim will use the toilet independently at school." Short-term objectives for Tim may include the following:

1. Tim will independently alert staff that he needs to go to the toilet.
2. Tim will transfer to the toilet with verbal prompts to sequence the activity.
3. Tim will independently doff and don his pants as needed for toileting.

These goals developed by the IEP team, including the occupational therapist, are educational because they address issues that:

1. allow Tim to function independently in a classroom and during the school day

2. allow Tim to be served in the least restrictive environment, which is a primary goal of special education

3. require less adult supervision or assistance and would promote social interaction with Tim's peers since he would be participating in the same activities in similar, if not the same, ways as his peers

4. indicate progression on the road to independent adult functioning, which is the ultimate goal of public education in general.

All of the above goals are also written in functional terms that would satisfy the requirements of a third party payer.

The actual occupational therapy intervention may consist of activities that address the components or underlying impairments that interfere with the attainment of the functional goal. For example, Tim may need to improve his balance, grip strength, and oral-motor skills before he can feed himself independently. However, documentation of therapy sessions that addressed these component parts would always tie them to the functional goal of self-feeding. Poor mobility and balance, decreased endurance, difficulty sequencing, and inability to manipulate closures may all interfere with the ability to toilet independently. These component parts are appropriate to address in therapeutic intervention, but the intervention notes should always tie the component to the functional goal of more independent toileting.

A common educational goal is to improve handwriting. It may appear on the IEP as a separate annual goal. The therapist may address this by stating it functionally in terms of manipulating objects to perform classroom or learning activities. Zippers, snaps, toys, pencils, utensils, tools, and telephones are all objects that may need to be manipulated in the home, school, or community. The occupational therapy practitioner may need to address underlying muscle tone, grip, tactile perception, and visual-spatial skills to assist Tim in reaching this goal, but the intervention documentation would always link the activities to the functional goal of activity performance such as eating or writing.

Tim needs to be able to move his wheelchair in the school building to get from class to the library, cafeteria, or bus area. The occupational therapy practitioner may need to address poor sustained grip, low endurance, bilateral coordination, and visual-spatial orientation to assist Tim in improving his ability to move around the school in a timely and independent manner. Documentation of the occupational therapy intervention would always tie the treatment interventions and environmental modifications to the functional goal of independent mobility.

EXAMPLE 2 – Sarah, a child with a learning disability, may show tactile defensiveness with high activity level, distractibility, and poor motor planning. The therapeutic functional goal written to demonstrate educational relevance may read as follows:

- Sarah will follow two-step directions in a classroom with six other children present.

That kind of skill is clearly needed in the educational environment and is also a reimbursable functional goal. The skill is needed to learn new tasks, to sequence activities appropriately, to have adequate safety awareness and response, and to participate in social relationships.

The occupational therapist may address the tactile defensiveness as a contributing factor to the poor ability to attend to multiple-step directions, but the intervention documentation should clearly link the intervention focus to the functional, educationally relevant goal.

EXAMPLE 3 – Special education for an older student may need to focus on prevocational or transition activities. Occupational therapy intervention plans that focus on the functional abilities (for example, appropriate work habits or behaviors) that are prevocational in nature and can be generalized to many situations are often covered by third party payers; they are educationally relevant if there is an annual goal in the IEP or ITP (Individualized Transition Plan) that focuses on work habits or behaviors. Supported employment programs, which may be a part of transition programs in the schools, usually focus on vocational skills and are unlikely to be considered medically necessary and, thus, reimbursable.

Linking the occupational therapy intervention to functional goals that contribute to the attainment of educational goals will solve both the problem of articulating how occupational therapy services are related to educational progress and will satisfy the requirements of a third-party payer if one is involved with service delivery in the school system.

Summary

The key to effective documentation in pediatrics is the key to effective documentation in all aspects of occupational therapy. The key is to address occupational functioning.

References

American Occupational Therapy Association. (1979). *Occupational therapy services for children and youth under the Individuals with Disabilities Education Act*. Bethesda, MD: Author.

American Occupational Therapy Association. (1989). *Guidelines for occupational therapy services in school systems* (2nd ed.). Bethesda, MD: Author.

Chandler, B. E. (1989). Fee for service in the public schools. In *Program guide: The AOTA practice symposium* (pp. 34-37). Bethesda, MD: American Occupational Therapy Association.

Code of Federal Regulations, 34, parts 300 to 399. (1990). Washington, DC: U.S. Government Printing Office.

Lewis-Jackson, L. (1994). Third party billing in the public schools. *School Systems SIS Newsletter, 1*(1). Implications for school-based occupational therapy practice.

9. Special Considerations II: Home Health

Velma Reichenbach, MS, OTR/L

This chapter highlights special considerations affecting documentation in home health.

Velma Reichenbach is the former supervisor of acute occupational therapy services, Mercy Hospital, Chicago, Illinois.

The demands on occupational therapists for documentation of service continues to challenge those providing therapy in the home health setting. In order to ensure reimbursement, the documentation must adhere to the rules established by service providers, government agencies, and accreditation organizations while also proving the necessity and uniqueness of occupational therapy as a skilled health care service.

Occupational therapy in home health is an exciting adventure because each patient shows functional performance deficits for a wide variety of reasons. The therapist's role is to search out the sensorimotor, cultural/psychosocial, cognitive, and perceptual dysfunctions that affect the patient's ability to perform. This information is elicited in each treatment session, and the puzzle is gradually documented as hypotheses are made and refined during treatment.

The occupational therapist continues to observe the smallest details and provide the patient with the elements to elicit hope and make progress. Every treatment is an ongoing observation session, and the investigation continually leads to new goals. Hypotheses are switched or elaborated; goals are changed, enhanced, or deleted. In home health this is done superlatively: juggling the patient's sensorimotor, psychosocial/cultural, cognitive, and perceptual deficits with treatment goals, family dynamics, and architectural barriers. Indeed nowhere in occupational therapy practice is there such an opportunity to use a "holistic" approach incorporating a variety of occupational therapy theories.

Even the most experienced and rounded therapist may find documentation a drudgery. However, it is the avenue through which we demonstrate the importance and value of occupational therapy. If documentation is looked upon as the ingredient that allows us to provide needed service and promotion of the profession, it not only becomes tolerable but also challenging and enjoyable. A picture of the patient is painted at the same time that what we do, how we do it, and our anticipated hopes for the patient's future are presented.

Documentation Must Reflect Reimbursement Parameters

One recent article states, "Improper documentation can result in a claim being denied or returned to the provider for additional information thus jeopardizing the patient's access to further treatment" (Allen, Foto, Moon-Sperling, & Wilson, 1989, p. 783). Another source states the following related to the philosophy of documentation, "Every plan of treatment (claim) submitted to an intermediary represents an opportunity to educate a third party payer. Every plan of treatment written and submitted to a third party agency is an act of patient advocacy. The quality of our documentation is a measure of our professional credibility. Clear and accurate documentation reflects sound clinical reasoning" (Gillard & Kern, 1991).

Under Medicare, the patient must be confined to his or her home, under the care of a physician, and in need of skilled nursing services or physical or speech therapy on an intermittent basis.

Coverage under Medicare for home health benefits is reimbursable under both Parts A and B. The need for occupational therapy alone does not qualify a patient for the home health benefit. One of the other services must be required before occupational therapy can be introduced. However, occupational therapy may continue after the other skilled services have discharged the patient. One visit by a nurse to open the case does not constitute "intermittent." However, one visit required of the nurse in a 60-day period would constitute "intermittent."

The patient must be homebound or confined to his or her home. This means that to leave home requires considerable effort or taxing effort and the assistance of another person. Physician appointments are permitted, and an occasional trip to the barber shop might not be questioned. Denials do occur based upon the questioning of homebound status. Care must be taken to provide ongoing documentation indicating the patient is confined to the home.

Other requirements that apply include the following.

- The treatment requires a prescription.

- The treatment must be performed by a qualified occupational therapist or occupational therapy assistant.

- Treatment must be reasonable and necessary.

- Treatment must result in significant practical improvement in functioning in a predictable amount of time based on diagnosis, severity, and prognosis.

- Valid expectation of improvement must exist at the time of assessment although the expectation may not be realized.

- Treatment must not be for maintenance.

- Reevaluation should occur one time per month or as needed to make changes in the program.

- Occupational therapy services can be reimbursed for designing, fabricating, and fitting orthotic and self-help devices.

- A specific "therapy" diagnosis is no longer required for a beneficiary to be eligible for therapy. Only a demonstrated need for therapy is necessary.

- Therapies are not subject to the intermittence rule, and therefore, a one-time-only therapy visit can be made for purposes of safety or instruction.

- Occupational therapy can be provided for patients with psychiatric illness; however, a specific psychiatric diagnosis and the care of a psychiatrist are required. The home care supervisors should be specialized in mental health (Menosky, 1990).

Documentation should always contribute to the overall treatment plan. Keep in mind that under Medicare, therapists are part of a team led by a nurse who may not have much knowledge of occupational therapy practice. Therefore, our documentation statements must provide her or him with the needed words to establish the plan of care.

Insurance and Home Health Organization Parameters

Some insurance companies and health maintenance organizations (HMOs) follow Medicare guidelines, while others have predetermined the number of visits allowed per year or illness.

They may require that documentation notes accompany the billing. In addition, case mangers for the company may also request reports and documentation of the patients. If documentation is not clear, case managers have been known to deny or question an order for activities of daily living training. Items that bring about functional change in performance areas such as dressing, hygiene, or homemaking including muscle reeducation, Cogman exercises, and sensorimotor treatment are reimbursable.

Contents of Documentation Records

As with all documentation, the records must include identification and background information, assessment and reassessment, treatment planning, and implementation and discontinuation of services. Additionally, in the home, the documentation should pay attention to the components needed for restoration of function. It should address safety and the elimination of permanent loss of abilities. This should be done through the *initial evaluation* that includes tests and evaluations administered and results. It should include a summary and analyses of findings as well as reference to pertinent reports and information. It should also include the occupational therapy problem list and recommendations for services. The treatment plan should include measurable goals, activities, and treatment procedures; type, amount, and frequency of treatment; and the anticipated time required to achieve the goals. There should be a statement of the functional outcomes.

Progress notes must be written for each visit. They must reflect activities, procedures, and modalities used; functional goals; and treatment. They must include the functional assessment of progress as well as response to treatment and progress toward goals related in the problem list. Goal modification should be indicated as well as any changes anticipated in the time required to achieve goals. *Discharge notes* should include a summary of the entire occupational therapy intervention process. Goals achieved and functional outcomes should be stated. A comparison should be made of the initial and discharge status. Home program recommendations and follow-up plans should be made.

Assessment/ Evaluation

In the assessment there must be a statement about perceived prognosis; date of onset; prior history and functional status, mental, psychosocial, and emotional condition; as well as environmental, cultural, or architectural barriers. Of course, the assessment of present functional status for activities of daily living, homemaking, or work, including sensorimotor, cognitive, and psychosocial deficits or assets, is routine. Establishing a baseline testing database at the beginning provides the materials necessary for documenting improvement as change occurs during the course of treatment.

Specific Documentation Guidelines

The following short guidelines will be useful in the preparation of documentation.

- Document the need to employ skilled occupational therapy services.
- Indicate the patient is homebound. Each note must stand alone.
- Put the most pertinent diagnosis first; after that, list all the others.
- Reflect specific clinical observations.

- Do indicate frequency and duration plans at the time of assessment.

- Discharge planning is begun at the time of evaluation.

- Do make the problem list compatible with the master list developed by the care team.

- Document the long- and short-term goals and the discussion of treatment procedures with patient, family, or caregivers.

- Do refer to Uniform Terminology for assistance in structuring the framework for documentation of the strengths and deficits identified in assessment and in identifying those for establishing goals.

- Do establish home programs and make copies for patient's chart.

- Do indicate in notes, instruction to patient, family, and/or caregiver.

- Document all health team conferences, whether they occur by telephone or in person.

- Document changes in treatment plans for reaching the stated goals.

- Change goals to match progress or try new approaches to attain progress.

- Indicate the need for aide, family, or caregiver services in your documentation.

- Slow progress must be justified through documentation that the patient will be able to learn and that the results will eventually result in reduced health care costs.

- Do use cost-effective goal statements.

The therapist should be aware that goal statements can often be made into cost-effective goals. For example, a general goal of ability to feed self becomes a cost-effective goal when it is stated: "Patient will become independent in self-feeding so that the home health aide's time may be reduced from 6 hours to 3 hours per day." A goal of training the family in bathing becomes cost-effective when it is stated that the home health aide's time will be reduced by 3 hours. If a patient can become independent in performing toileting, hygiene, and transfers safely; use communication devices; or become capable of using the telephone; a family member may return to work and support the family. This is a cost-effective goal. Goals become cost-effective when the treatment provided is aimed at establishing bed mobility, or ability to reposition self in chair or bed to improve circulation, decrease pain, and prevent decubitus development. Improving patients' functional status and decreasing the amount of work for the spouse may decrease the danger of the caregiver being hospitalized or the potential for both to require nursing home placement. Developing these kinds of goals with the nurse or other members of the team can clearly establish the necessity of services.

The question is often asked: What should be avoided in the documentation? (Or what brings up a "red flag" for a reviewer of Medicare Information Forms?) The following examples are problematic but often would not be if more clearly stated.

One should avoid the word "maintain." It indicates the patient has reached a plateau; Medicare does not pay for maintenance. A statement such as "treatment was provided to maintain

Documentation Tips

function" should be avoided. If there has been a plateau, and new strategies to reverse the plateau have not been successful in short time, then discharge would be advised. However, a therapist may provide treatment for setting up a maintenance program.

The phrase "making slow progress" should be avoided. The words "steady progress" may more accurately describe the client's progress toward functional goals.

One should not say: "Patient is not progressing." It is better to give the reason why progress has been inhibited. The therapist might note that "patient placed on hold" or say that changes in goals and treatment were made as a result of the problem.

The word "prevent" must have a connection with the treatment of the condition. For example, the therapist may realize that unless the patient is taught bed mobility there will be decubitus development, or the caregiver may be so taxed that he or she is in danger of hospitalization because of a back or heart problem. It would be better to describe with words that indicate prevention in the following way: "The patient is responding to sensory stimulation and neurodevelopmental treatment. He or she has ability to perform 1/4 quarter roll to right. Caretaker reports that now there is decreased redness over coccyx area and indications of increased circulation. Caregiver was provided instruction in back or joint protection techniques decreasing pain and the need for increased aide service." In these instances, evidence of the nurse, therapists, and caregiver working as a team toward goals provides further substantiation of the need for services and shows the patient's increased function and the potential for decreasing cost.

Verbs such as "review, reinforce, or reinstruct" should be used carefully because they make it appear that the service is repetitious or that the patient has been noncompliant or was not able to comprehend.

The phrase "unable to learn" should be avoided when there is a learning or cognitive problem. The problem should be addressed indicating goals, treatment techniques, or family or caregiver instructions.

Instead of saying "independent in ambulation using walker" it would be better to say "ambulates with assistance of walker." Care must be taken that documentation statements do not conflict. On occasion a physical therapist will state that the patient is independent with a walker, but the occupational therapist finds that safety is an issue because of loss of balance, perceptual deficit, or impaired safety adherence when attending to other activities such as tasks in the kitchen or bathroom while simultaneously concentrating on ambulation.

Generalized statements such as "generalized weakness" should be replaced by statements of specific functional limitations, such as shortness of breath after climbing a few steps, poor balance, or dizziness or unsteady gait. Generalized weakness is usually thought of in conjunction with an illness where intervention is not required to increase strength or where age is the cause of the weakness.

Other generalized statements that are not objective or measurable include: "healing well," "responding well," and "good endurance." Rather, changes in the patient should be specified.

The therapist should indicate that the patient is in need of skilled services. Case managers or reviewers may look at training in self-dressing or passive range of motion as nonskilled, seeing it as something that could be administered by untrained personnel or a family member, unless there is something in the documentation that shows the uniqueness of your work with the patient. For example, self-ranging may be performed in such a way as to be a part of neurodevelopmental treatment. Dressing may have incorporated proprioceptive neuromuscular facilitation techniques. Backward chaining may be necessary in working with another type of patient, or dressing training may be addressing the perceptual dysfunction.

Duplication of Services

Medicare will not pay for duplication of services. Care must be taken that the documentation proves the disciplines are not duplicating treatments. Transfers training may be done by the physical therapist to determine the level of safety with the technique. The occupational therapist instructs and uses transfer for performance of a daily living skill, such as transfer from wheelchair to bathtub, or wheelchair to toilet with donning and doffing of clothing or toileting hygiene incorporated into this task. The physical therapist may use neurodevelopmental techniques during use of the walker when performing gait training. The occupational therapist may use a similar treatment technique to facilitate increased functional use of the upper extremity in dressing.

In September 1990 the Health Care Financing Administration (HCFA) issued special instructions regarding dysphagia claims. The new guidelines clarify that occupational, physical, or speech-language therapists can evaluate and treat dysphagia patients and be reimbursed if other coverage guidelines specific to their professions are met (Pinson, 1991). Coordination of services with documentation regarding the role of each discipline involved in the case would clarify and prevent problems with reimbursement.

References

Allen, C., Foto, M., Moon-Sperling, T., & Wilson, D. (1989). A medical review approach to Medicare outpatient documentation. *American Journal of Occupational Therapy 43*, 793-800.

Gillard, M., & Kern, S. (1991, June). *Application of AOTA uniform terminology to practice: Guidelines for documentation*. Paper presented at the American Occupational Therapy Association Conference, Cincinnati, OH.

Menosky, J. (1990). Occupational therapy services for the homebound psychiatric patient. *Journal of Home Health Care Practice, 2*(3), 57-67.

Pinson, C. (1991, February 21). Medicare improvements, Medicaid expansions mark progress. *OT Week*, p. 4.

10. Documenting Progress in Health Care

Mary Jo McGuire, MS, OTR/L

The home is an ideal environment for the practice of occupational therapy. However, the tumultuous health care environment of the late 1990s requires practitioners to take special care not only in delivering effective services but also in documenting the delivery of skilled care. Documentation is the bridge between the delivery of occupational therapy services in the home and the approval for reimbursement of services by third party payers. This chapter presents principles for writing reimbursable progress notes for home care that are based on Medicare documents related to occupational therapy. Application of these principles can improve efficiency and excellence in practitioners' documentation skills.

Mary Jo McGuire is Director of Educational Resources for Rehab Educators, Fairlawn, Ohio. This chapter was originally published in the *American Journal of Occupational Therapy, 51,* 436–445, and is reprinted with permission.

The home environment is a virtual paradise for the practice of occupational therapy. Therapeutically selected, adapted, and graded involvement in familiar activities of daily living (ADL) provide a natural form of exercise that can restore health-producing cycles of involvement in self-care, work, play and leisure, and sleep. According to MacRae (1984), "A primary emphasis of home treatment is to assist patients in reconstructing previous activity patterns, which were disrupted by accident or illness, and in developing new patterns, which are compatible with their present condition" (p. 723). The "real" environment of the home provides the ideal context in which to practice habit training, facilitate healthy patterns of temporal adaptation and functional performance, and observe and foster occupational adaptation as described by leaders throughout the history of the occupational therapy profession (Kielhofner, 1985; Meyer, 1922; Reed, 1984; Schkade & Schultz, 1992; Schultz & Schkade, 1992). In contrast to the home atmosphere, which is conducive to the practice of occupational therapy, is the tumult in health care service delivery surrounding the transition from fee-for-service to managed care models. The current atmosphere, which appears threatening, may actually exact from practitioners a purer practice of occupational therapy.

Today, the need for home-based occupational therapy services in the American culture is so real that if the discipline did not currently exist, the pressures of the current health care system would have to create a discipline to provide the services offered by occupational therapy. Since 1983, when the prospective payment system was legislated, increased numbers of persons have been released from hospitals and returned to their homes with needs for professional assistance to enable a return to functional independence. Shorter lengths of stay in the hospital have resulted in greater health care needs in the home. Professional services are needed to adapt the environment or the demands of activities for safety and function; to train caregivers and family members in compensatory methods, the use of adaptive equipment, special handling techniques, and the use and maintenance of personal care devices; to prevent medical complications; to reduce pain; and to maintain function. Occupational therapy practitioners are prepared to provide these skilled services. One of the major challenges facing home care practitioners is the documentation of the delivery of these services so that third party payers recognize them as skilled and medically necessary and agree to pay for them.

Documentation

Many books, articles, and official documents cover the essentials of documentation (Allen, Foto, Moon-Sperling, & Wilson, 1989; American Occupational Therapy Association [AOTA], 1992, 1995; DePaoli & Zenk-Jones, 1984). The purpose of this article is to clarify documentation principles that occupational therapy practitioners can apply to increase efficiency and the potential for reimbursement. It is primarily written to assist practitioners in writing the daily, brief progress notes that must follow each home visit; however, these same principles can be applied in the documentation of occupational therapy services delivered in any setting.

The Target Audience

According to Robertson (1992), the content an occupational therapy practitioner selects for documentation in the medical record depends on the target audience. The target audience may be the treatment team, the client, third party payers, or others. A key to keeping documentation concise and brief is the identification of the target audience. In home health, progress notes are typically written for the practitioner (i.e., to keep track of the intervention plan, to guide plans for the next visit), for the treatment team (i.e., to document communication within and between disciplines, to prevent overlap), for accrediting agencies (i.e., to maintain accreditation status), and for third party payers (i.e., to receive reimbursement).

Kunstaetter (1988) revealed that there was a discrepancy between the treatment provided by home care occupational therapy practitioners and what they documented in the medical record. The surveyed practitioners documented what was reimbursable in areas where they could easily show progress. Kunstaetter warned: "By allowing reimbursement regulations to determine our treatment and documentation needs, we may be gradually diverging from the essence of occupational therapy" (p. 518). As we enter the 21st century, occupational therapy must not permit the changing trends of the health care delivery system to define what the profession has to offer persons with disabilities who are homebound. In understanding current reimbursement guidelines, practitioners must grow in their ability to articulate the importance of occupational therapy services in enabling clients to achieve valued functional outcomes. The application of information related to reimbursement guidelines is intended to assure the delivery of the full scope and potential of occupational therapy services in the home by assisting practitioners in documenting in a manner acceptable to medical reviewers. The concept that documentation of services must be in accordance with reimbursement guidelines should presume only that the content selected for third party payers, as a target audience, is a critical issue.

Third Party Payers

Medicare is the largest third party payer in the United States (Scott & Somers, 1992); private health insurance companies tend to copy the practice of government (Steinhauer, 1984). Because Medicare guidelines continue today to be the dominating standard that private insurance companies use in establishing coverage and medical review criteria, an analysis of the philosophy that underlies the federal documents may help occupational therapy practitioners to document in a manner that meets third party payer standards. To this end, I analyzed the coverage guidelines in the *Medicare Home Health Agency Manual* (Health Care Financing Administration [HCFA], 1996) and *Medical Review of Part B Intermediary Outpatient Occupational Therapy Bills* (HCFA, 1989) guidelines and synthesized basic assumptions that appear to underlie these documents. I also identified principles to assist practitioners in understanding how to write progress notes that comply with these assumptions. Without exception, these principles also reflect excellent standards for occupational therapy documentation in all settings:

- Focus on function
- Focus on underlying causes
- Focus on progress
- Focus on safety
- State expectations for progress

- Explain slow progress or lack of progress
- Summarize skilled services delivered.

Principles for Reimbursement

FOCUS ON FUNCTION

PRIOR LEVEL OF FUNCTION — One of the most critical components of any initial home care occupational therapy evaluation is documentation of the prior level of function. A statement that incorporates environmental clues can connote a level of function beyond simple independence. For example: "Before hospitalization, the client was living independently in a three-story home, was independent in all self-care and homemaking, and used bathroom facilities on the second floor and laundry facilities in the basement."

IDENTIFY AND FOCUS ON MEANINGFUL ACTIVITIES — Probing interview skills are essential for identifying meaningful activities that the client was previously able to perform, that he or she is able or unable to currently perform, and that he or she can be expected to resume. The Uniform Terminology (AOTA, 1994b) provides a careful breakdown of performance areas that can be used to establish long-term or short-term functional goals.

LONG-TERM VERSUS SHORT-TERM GOALS — The classification of goals as long term or short term is determined according to the needs of each client: A long-term goal for one client may be a short-term goal for another. The *Elements of Clinical Documentation* (AOTA, 1995) describes long-term goals as "functional" (p. 1033) and short-term goals as those that "directly relate to long-term functional goals" (p. 1033). There are two major strategies that can be used to

Table 10.1 Example of establishing short-term goals
Long-Term Goal: Independence in Lower-Extremity Dressing

Short-Term Goals Based on Performance Component Deficits Could Be:	Short-Term Goals Based on Task Analysis Could Be:
Trunk flexion and BUE forward reach adequate for LE dressing	Client will be able to properly place trousers over feet for donning.
Cognitive–perceptual skills adequate for positioning clothing for LE dressing	Client will be able to spontaneously dress LLE before RLE.
Endurance adequate for safety and independence in LE dressing	Client will be able to pull up trousers from a supported standing position.
Demonstrate compensatory methods and appropriate use of adaptive equipment for safe, independent LE dressing	Client will be able to demonstrate proper use of sock donner and shoe horn and complete LE dressing in 5 min without becoming SOB.

Note. BUE = both upper extremities; LE = lower extremity; LLE = left lower extremity; RLE = right lower extremity; SOB = shortness of breath.

develop short-term goals: (a) identify performance component deficits that inhibit function or (b) use occupational analysis to identify and sequence segments of the task that must be mastered (see Table 10.1).

ORGANIZE REPORTS BY PERFORMANCE AREAS — The format or organization of the progress note should emphasize the functional goals. Many home care agencies are choosing to develop a checklist format, with functional areas placed in a prominent position. Notes can be organized ADL skill by ADL skill. Occupational therapy practitioners who must use open-narrative-style notes can emphasize function by underlining titles of performance areas and incorporating key information (described in the principles outlined later in this chapter) within each functional category. For example:

> *Bathing:* Client's left hemiparesis, visual skill deficits, and dynamic balance deficits make this task difficult. During an actual performance evaluation, he required moderate assistance of one person to safely enter and exit the tub using a tub-transfer bench. He is expected to progress to needing standby assistance.

RELATE PERFORMANCE COMPONENT DEFICITS TO FUNCTIONAL OUTCOMES — Because performance components can only be addressed (according to reimbursement standards) if improvements are expected to have a major impact on functional outcomes, it may be beneficial to keep the information together in progress notes. For instance, to extend the previous example, the practitioner's next visit could include the following:

> *Bathing:* Client's need for moderate assistance in bathing is associated with an impairment in dynamic balance. He was involved in activities to challenge the development of postural control in dynamic sitting and standing and was instructed in proper biomechanics necessary for safe transfer into the tub.

RELATE PERFORMANCE COMPONENT GOALS TO FUNCTIONAL OUTCOMES — In the not-too-distant past, including a quantifiable component in a goal assured good quality. For instance, "Increase active RUE [right upper extremity] shoulder flexion from 110° to 140°" would have been considered a good measurable goal. However, in the socioeconomic climate of the late 1990s, such a goal is inadequate. The questions that third party payers ask are: For what purpose? Why? or What will the consumer be able to do (functionally) with the increased shoulder flexion? Performance component deficits (e.g., muscle group weakness, range of motion [ROM] deficits, visual skill deficits, balance disorders) may be best addressed as modifiers within functional goals. For example: "RUE shoulder flexion adequate to permit independence in UE dressing." It is not enough to establish goals and develop outcome studies that show the effectiveness of occupational therapy in improving the components of performance. We must establish goals and focus on outcome studies that demonstrate improvements in performance areas (functional outcomes).

AVOID DOUBLE-LEVEL STATUS REPORTING — In identifying a client's need for assistance within a performance area, practitioners should avoid double-level status reporting. For example, avoid the following: "Client requires min-mod [minimum-moderate] assistance with LE [lower-extremity] dressing." The double level typically means that the client inconsistently performs at the more independent level. As a rule, if there are inconsistencies in the level of performance, choose the lower baseline to permit documentation of progress as it occurs. In this example, the practitioner should rate the client as requiring moderate assistance.

ESTABLISH A FUNCTIONAL MAINTENANCE PROGRAM — If an evaluation reveals that a client does not have the potential to achieve higher levels of functional performance, the occupational therapy practitioner may design a functional maintenance program. Glickstein and Neustadt (1992) developed an elaborate program described as *functional maintenance therapy*. Although much of the authors' work was done in long-term-care settings, it can be generalized to home care. The section in the home health coverage guidelines (HCFA, 1996) entitled "General Principles Governing Reasonable and Necessary Physical Therapy, Speech–Language Pathology Services, and Occupational Therapy," states that services are skilled if they "are necessary to the establishment of a safe and effective maintenance program" (§ 205.2, A.5.c.) or are "needed to manage and periodically reevaluate the appropriateness of a maintenance program" (§ 205.2, A.2.). Although the administration of periodic reevaluations is not uniformly practiced (often to the detriment of the person who needs this type of follow-up), functional maintenance programs are commonly a part of home health care.

Functional maintenance programs are similar to what is often termed a discharge program, a *home program*, or a *home exercise program*. The basic purpose of a functional maintenance program is to assure that the client, family member, or permanent caregiver will perform activities in a health-producing manner after skilled services are terminated. If a practitioner expects the client to use adaptive equipment or orthotic devices or the family members or caregivers to perform therapeutic handling or assistance during ADL, then a functional maintenance program should be documented. An example of goals and plans designed as part of a maintenance program includes the following:

Goal: Caregiver to provide safe, return demonstration of the following:

1. Donning and doffing the hand splint.

2. Safely using and adjusting wearing schedule.

3. Identifying a need for OT reeval [occupational therapy reevaluation], reasons for professional evaluation, and need for splint modification.

4. Therapeutically handling RUE during active–assistive ROM.

5. Demonstrating the proper type, timing, and frequency of verbal cues and physical assistance for client to maintain minimal assistance level of UE and LE dressing.

Plan: Instruct caregiver in therapeutic techniques related to functional maintenance program (as outlined in goals).

Note that the goals of a functional maintenance program can identify a family member or caregiver as the person receiving instruction. Practitioners should instruct to a level that will assure that family members, caregivers, or both understand the functional maintenance goals, the benefits of doing the program, and the potential consequences if the program is not followed and that they have the skills and confidence to carry out the maintenance program. The more specific occupational therapists can be in goal setting, the easier it will be to compute and justify the number of visits needed to accomplish the goals. Additionally, specific goals will support effective follow-through by occupational therapy assistants in carrying out the program.

FOCUS ON UNDERLYING FACTORS – Skilled evaluations document the relationship between medical problems and function. More specifically, occupational therapy practitioners identify specific physical or cognitive impairments that interfere with independence or safety in performance areas. Allen et al. (1989) stated: "When reimbursement is denied or delayed, it is often due to insufficient documentation—either the documentation lacks technical accuracy or lacks *details supporting medical necessity* [italics added]" (p. 798). (Note that these experts do not say that the documentation lacks details about media or methods used in occupational therapy.) The key in this principle is to combine medical knowledge with observation and task analysis to identify the specific impairments that restrict or limit occupational function. This principle challenges practitioners to document the clinical reasoning that underlies the establishment of goals (e.g., Why should we be reimbursed for involving the client in activities to increase fine motor coordination?). For example: "Fine motor incoordination in the client's dominant right hand prevents independence in UE dressing," or "Weak mass grasp in the client's dominant right hand makes meal preparation dangerous."

The medical review guidelines related to skilled occupational therapy (HCFA, 1989) states that to be consider skilled, "The documentation must indicate that the severity of the physical/emotional/perceptual/cognitive disability requires complex and sophisticated knowledge to identify current and potential capabilities" (§ 3906.5a). Documenting the severity of the client's disability requires occupational therapy practitioners' full use of their strong medical background as well as integration of their occupational analysis skills. This principle challenges practitioners to concisely articulate the relationships that are identified and that underlie dysfunction. For example:

- Poor error awareness prevents this client from being independent in grooming and hygiene skills.

- Visual scanning and attention deficits contribute to the client's inability to feed herself independently.

- RUE arm placement deficits and awkward grasp patterns prevent independence in LE dressing.

- Client's poor standing tolerance is preventing her from returning to independence in homemaking.

- Poor postural adjustment mechanisms (fear of trunk rotation and weight bearing on LLE [left lower extremity]) contribute to unsafe functional mobility skills. Unsafe functional mobility skills contribute to a lack of independence in toileting, hygiene, bathing, and dressing skills.

In these examples, documenting the relationship supports the need for the occupational therapy practitioner to involve the client in activities to increase error awareness, improve visual scanning and attention skills, develop RUE motor control, and develop postural control in a standing position (functional mobility skills). Although the examples are not at a level of specificity typically seen in "treatment-oriented" documentation, they demonstrate statements of analysis that are important for practitioners to include in medical records in order to enable medical reviewers to agree to approve reimbursement of services.

In situations where the client is progressing slowly, application of this principle can be a strong tool for writing documentation that leads to reimbursement. Instead of focusing on the *slowness*, practitioners can document specifics about the *impairments* that are causing the functional disability. Practitioners must not become desensitized to the gravity and weight of suffering that clients are experiencing (e.g., the paralysis, the pain, the weakness and fatigue that accompanies use of compensatory methods and adaptive equipment). Their words must open the medical reviewer's eyes to the severity and complexity of the dysfunction observed during therapy. When practitioners are in the midst of an ADL retraining program, and the client is making steady, but slow, progress, it would be wise to document *underlying causes* and to avoid benign statements such as "client is progressing well." Uninformative rhetoric fills the medical records with "weeds" that the reviewer must ignore or uproot in order to discern the client's status and progress. Good documentation concisely communicates critical relationships between impairment and function.

FOCUS ON PROGRESS — A progress statement is more than that of current status; it should include a comparative analysis that informs the reader of change. The medical review guidelines (HCFA, 1989) provide clear descriptions of six levels of assistance that occupational therapy practitioners can be expected to use in evaluating progress. Although practitioners are free to use whatever scale they prefer, it is certainly an advantage to be aware of, if not use, the scale that HCFA has acknowledged. The following descriptors have been selected from this document to portray the various levels of assistance:

1. Total Assistance—initiates minimal voluntary motor actions, 100% assistance by one or more helpers

2. Maximum Assistance—75% assistance by one person, physical support needed each step, one-to-one demonstration

3. Moderate Assistance—50% assistance by one person, assistance needed every time, intermittent demonstration: occupational therapy practitioner or caregiver must be in the immediate area

4. Minimum Assistance—25% assistance by one person; requires setup; needs help to initiate or sustain an activity; needs help to review alternate procedures, sequences, and methods; needs help to correct repeated mistakes; needs periodic cognitive assistance to check safety compliance; needs assistance to solve problems posed by unexpected hazards.

5. Standby Assistance—supervision needed for safe, effective performance of adapted methods, safety precautions

6. Independent Status.

The six levels provide much room for demonstrating progress. Practitioners must accurately establish a baseline to enable progress to be demonstrated. In most cases when adaptive equipment is initially issued to a client, one-to-one demonstration is provided (i.e., maximum assistance). If on the next visit, the client requires only intermittent demonstration, he or she has progressed from maximum to moderate assistance. The client who then requires only instruction or reminders in using alternate methods has progressed from moderate to minimal assistance. A client who lacks only the confidence to perform the task without supervision (e.g., fears falling or failure) has progressed from minimal assistance to standby assistance. Clients progress from standby assistance to independent status when they do not need setup or safety supervision in performing a task.

The medical review guidelines (HCFA, 1989, § 3906.4b) also clearly inform reviewers that clients may experience progress within each level of assistance, if the occupational therapy practitioner documents a change in response to treatment, as evidenced by one of the following:

1. Decreased refusals

2. Increased consistency

3. Increased generalization.

These concepts direct practitioners to document progress when a client is not moving rapidly from maximum, to moderate, to minimal assistance. Most home care practitioners have experienced the plight of arriving at a home treatment session to find that the client has, during the practitioner's absence, attempted (or mastered) the very skill that the practitioner had planned to evaluate, adapt, or retrain. The good news is that there is no need for frustration: The practitioner has unearthed clear evidence of progress! The evaluation skills of the home care occupational therapist are a skilled service. Practitioners may document a client's progress by noting generalization of the adaptation process from one skill to another, even if the progress occurred between visits. Such progress does not indicate that recovery is occurring spontaneously (i.e., that it would occur without the occupational therapy program in place), only that it is occurring between visits. An effective occupational therapy program may facilitate progress between visits, and practitioners should document such generalization as progress.

In addition to progress being demonstrated by changes in levels of assistance and changes within an assistance level, medical review guidelines state that progress in occupational therapy is evidenced when "a new skilled functional activity is initiated" (HCFA, 1989, § 3906.4c) or "a new skilled compensatory technique is added" (§ 3906.4d). Therefore, practitioners would be wise to sequence and organize intervention plans so that visits clearly document when a new actual performance evaluation of an area is completed or when a new technique or compensatory method is attempted. Instead of providing three pieces of adaptive equipment in one visit and documenting all three during three subsequent visits, it may be clearer to focus each visit on the skilled training that occurred with one piece of equipment (or compensatory method).

FOCUS ON SAFETY – Third party payers recognize the critical importance of safety in the home. The professional skills of occupational therapy practitioners play an extremely important role in evaluating and intervening in safety issues. The medical review guidelines describe in detail occupational therapy's role in evaluating safety dependence and secondary complications (HCFA, 1989). For example, the guidelines recognize the potential for skin breakdown as a safety concern, going on to state:

> Safety dependence may be demonstrated by high probability of falling, lack of environmental safety awareness, swallowing difficulties, abnormal aggressive/destructive behavior, severe pain, loss of skin sensation, progressive joint contracture, and joint protection/preservation requiring skilled occupational therapy intervention to protect the patient from further medical complication. (§ 3906.2)

Focusing on the evaluation and treatment of these safety issues in a progress note provides a clear view of the medical necessity for occupational therapy services.

STATE EXPECTATIONS FOR PROGRESS – Occupational therapy practitioners should carefully document expectations for progress related to independence and safety. The medical review guidelines state:

> Occupational therapy services are covered only to the time that no further significant practical improvement can be expected. Progress reports or status summaries must document a continued expectation that the patient's condition will continue to improve significantly in a reasonable and generally predictable period of time [italics added]. (HCFA, 1989, § 3906.4)

The question is: *Whose* expectations? The answer cannot be "the medical reviewer who has never seen the client." The occupational therapy practitioner's professional judgment must be clearly stated: If there are expectations that the client will improve, then the progress note should include a concise statement of those expectations. Again, this is an important principle to apply if a practitioner is attempting to retrain a client in the safe, functional performance of a self-care task, and the client is not progressing quickly from one assistance level to another. The practitioner's professional judgment that the client will achieve a higher level of independence or safety is key information to be included in a progress note.

EXPLAIN SLOW PROGRESS OR LACK OF PROGRESS — The home health coverage guidelines (HCFA, 1996) use the terms *reasonable* and *necessary* to describe the amount, frequency, and duration of skilled therapy services that are covered. Although these terms may seem too vague to set clear limits, they provide the leniency needed to justify service delivery in special cases when progress is delayed by unique medical or life circumstances. The occupational therapy practitioner is responsible for documenting the aspects of the client's condition or situation that has delayed progress. In an attempt to prepare reviewers for the potential delays that occur in rehabilitation, the medical review guidelines modify the guideline calling for "significant practical improvement" by stating: "*Do not interpret* the term 'significant' so stringently that you deny a claim simply because of a temporary setback in the patient's progress" (HCFA, 1989, § 3906.4). Temporary setbacks are commonly caused by pain; medication changes; medical complications; and external circumstances, such as a death in the family. Practitioners should clearly document temporary setbacks that will delay progress toward goals. Appropriate use of the term temporary setback in the medical record could assist the medical reviewer in understanding the circumstances.

More commonly, progress may be slowed by difficulties practitioners encounter during the therapeutic process. Does Medicare cover a practice period to evaluate consistency of task performance? If a new compensatory method had been demonstrated to a client, would Medicare cover a practice session to evaluate whether the method actually improved function? The answer to both questions is yes. In a section devoted to describing skilled occupational therapy, Medicare's medical review guidelines describe the importance of granting time for effective training: "A period of practice may be approved for the patient and/or patient's caregivers to learn the steps of the task, to verify the tasks's effectiveness in improving function, and to check for safe and consistent task performance" (HCFA, 1989, § 3906.5a). The key to reimbursement in these situations is appropriate documentation. Practitioners do not "monitor performance" or simply "observe client perform" a task; the skilled evaluation purposes of the session must be clearly stated. For example:

> *Dressing:* OT [occupational therapist] evaluated the effectiveness of compensatory methods demonstrated last session. Methods were modified to increase safety. Client demonstrated inconsistence in her ability to remember the proper movement sequence needed in donning her blouse.

SUMMARIZE SKILLED SERVICES DELIVERED — The *Elements of Clinical Documentation* (AOTA, 1995) states that when writing a contact, treatment, or visit note that activities, techniques, and modalities used may be indicated by checklist or brief statement. This directs practitioners away from the "blow-by-blow" reporting of the treatment provided. Reviewers do not have the time to wade through lengthy descriptions of every action taken during each session. For reimbursement purposes, it is vital that each visit reflect the delivery of skilled services. However, this information should be a brief, summary-type statement of what occurred. Evaluations are skilled services (HCFA, 1996); therefore, any actual performance evaluation of an

ADL skill should be documented. Other skilled services can be categorized as direct intervention (e.g., ADL retraining; involvement in activities selected or adapted to challenge the development of performance components or areas; orthotic design, fabrication, fitting) or as instruction related to the maintenance program.

EVALUATIONS — Because evaluations are considered skilled services, the documentation of plans for actual performance evaluations clarifies that skilled services are still needed. Plans to evaluate a client's ability to perform an ADL skill or ability to integrate energy conservation methods (or other health-reinforcing principles) during the performance of a specific ADL skill demonstrate the continued need for occupational therapy.

DIRECT INTERVENTION — Occupational therapy practitioners spend a lot of time on ADL retraining. A simple statement informing the reviewer that ADL retraining is occurring in a specific area can be followed by statements that relate to one or more of the principles listed previously. For example:

> *Grooming:* Client was instructed in compensatory methods to overcome visual inattention problems during shaving. He has progressed from requiring moderate assistance to needing minimal assistance. He is expected to progress to independence.

Practitioners should document recommendations for adaptive equipment, regardless of the client's decision to follow the recommendation. (This can protect the practitioner from litigation directed toward the absence of equipment that could have protected a client from injury.) If equipment is issued, or if a client is trained in the safe, appropriate use of equipment, this should also be documented.

Practitioners must decide for whom they are writing. If the target audience is a supervisor concerned with service competency in a specific area, then treatment-oriented information should be included. Or, if a registered occupational therapist conducts a supervisory visit and wants to communicate more information to a certified occupational therapy assistant, then specific treatment-oriented information should be included in the medical record. However, if a practitioner is writing a visit note with the third party payer as the target audience, specifics of treatment related to media and strategies may be brief. For certified occupational therapy assistants who have already demonstrated service competency, or for registered occupational therapists who are providing continuous direct care to a client, the details of treatment may be greatly reduced in the medical record. Reducing the amount of treatment-oriented information in the medical record will enable reviewers to quickly identify important information about medical necessity and the critical role of occupational therapy in facilitating independence and safety in the home. (Practitioners should also recall that specific treatment information may be recorded in an abbreviated fashion in departmental records.)

INSTRUCTION — In the field of occupational therapy, instruction is commonly considered a part of intervention; after all, ADL retraining is often a matter of instructing clients in alternative methods. However, home care occupational therapy forms are often designed from a nursing perspective in which client instruction is separated from direct nursing. Practitioners must either accept this seemingly artificial division or develop forms that are more clearly aligned with occupational therapy models of practice. If practitioners must use forms that separate direct care from teaching and education (e.g., a checklist to indicate that instruction has been provided in a specific area), they should not feel compelled to duplicate information in the narrative section of the note.

Regardless of the format used, when occupational therapy practitioners provide any type of instruction, it is imperative that the client's (or caregiver's) response to the instruction be documented. This is especially important in cases where the learner may need more instruction than is commonly needed (e.g., because of fear, pain, memory deficits). The practitioner's expectations for the learner to understand and demonstrate the skill being addressed may also be documented, similar to expectation for progress. Any maintenance program (i.e., home exercise, discharge) should be provided in writing to the client and should be included in the medical record. In some cases, when a specific protocol is commonly followed and is on file in the departmental records, practitioners may provide a written copy to the client and state the title of the protocol or instructional material in the medical record.

Coordination with Other Disciplines — In addition to making concise statements about the skilled services provided, practitioners may also make statements about the coordination of these services with other disciplines. Some home care agencies have developed progress note forms with special sections for the documentation of interdisciplinary communication and cooperation. If no special section exists, practitioners are encouraged to write the statement in the functional section to which the communication most closely relates. For instance, if an occupational therapy practitioner discussed transfer methods with the physical therapy practitioner and was working on the development of transfer skills for bathing, then a statement about the interdisciplinary communication could be placed in the bathing section of the note. Recording interdisciplinary communication will provide the reviewer with concrete evidence of cooperation and emphasize that overlap is not occurring.

Summary: Case Example — The selection of content for documentation in the medical record is an important skill home health practitioners use after every treatment session. Although not all of the principles are expected to be applied to every progress note, they can be used to examine the "reimbursement potential" of each note. Figure 10.1 is a case example that illustrates the application, and lack of application, of the principles. The context is set with a few brief highlights. A poor example illustrates common errors found in occupational therapy records, and a good example illustrates many of the principles described in this article.

Conclusion

Home-based occupational therapy practice enables practitioners to apply the core concepts on which the discipline was founded. Therapist-designed exercises that use newly purchased materials give way to real-life activities that clients want to resume and that, echoing the essence of our profession, provide "occupation therapy." There is no time and not much reason or financial support for involving clients in exercises or drills that focus on performance com-

Figure 10.1 Poor and good case examples of progress note documentation

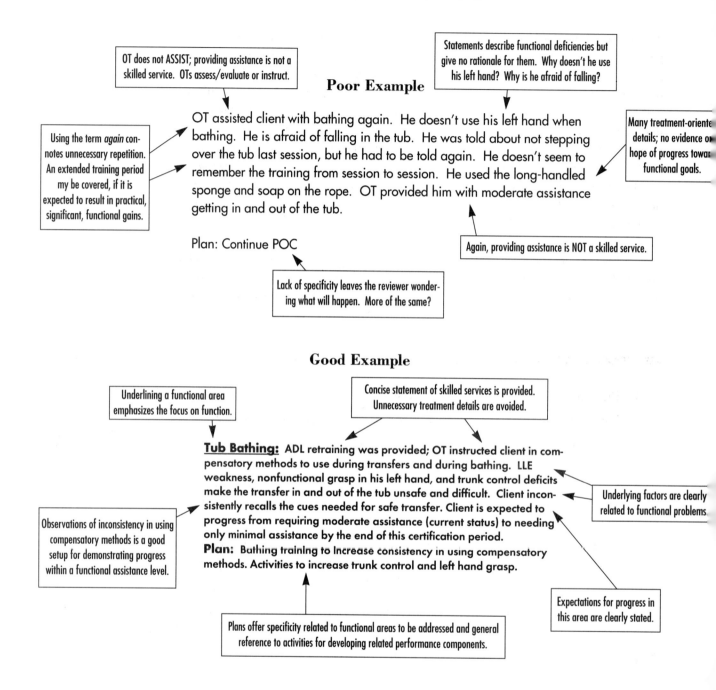

OT does not ASSIST; providing assistance is not a skilled service. OTs assess/evaluate or instruct.

Statements describe functional deficiencies but give no rationale for them. Why doesn't he use his left hand? Why is he afraid of falling?

Poor Example

Using the term *again* connotes unnecessary repetition. An extended training period my be covered, if it is expected to result in practical, significant, functional gains.

Many treatment-oriented details; no evidence or hope of progress toward functional goals.

OT assisted client with bathing again. He doesn't use his left hand when bathing. He is afraid of falling in the tub. He was told about not stepping over the tub last session, but he had to be told again. He doesn't seem to remember the training from session to session. He used the long-handled sponge and soap on the rope. OT provided him with moderate assistance getting in and out of the tub.

Plan: Continue POC

Again, providing assistance is NOT a skilled service.

Lack of specificity leaves the reviewer wondering what will happen. More of the same?

Good Example

Underlining a functional area emphasizes the focus on function.

Concise statement of skilled services is provided. Unnecessary treatment details are avoided.

Tub Bathing: ADL retraining was provided; OT instructed client in compensatory methods to use during transfers and during bathing. LLE weakness, nonfunctional grasp in his left hand, and trunk control deficits make the transfer in and out of the tub unsafe and difficult. Client inconsistently recalls the cues needed for safe transfer. Client is expected to progress from requiring moderate assistance (current status) to needing only minimal assistance by the end of this certification period.
Plan: Bathing training to increase consistency in using compensatory methods. Activities to increase trunk control and left hand grasp.

Underlying factors are clearly related to functional problems.

Observations of inconsistency in using compensatory methods is a good setup for demonstrating progress within a functional assistance level.

Expectations for progress in this area are clearly stated.

Plans offer specificity related to functional areas to be addressed and general reference to activities for developing related performance components.

In the 4th week of the certification period, a practitioner is developing safety and independence in bathing using a tub-transfer bench. The first session established that the client required maximum assistance for transfers. During the second session, the client progressed from needing maximum assistance during transfers to needing moderate assistance. During the third training session, the practitioner's note focused on performance of bathing and the performance components that interfered with safety and independence. This is the fourth bathing training session; it went much the same as the third, although the client's potential for improving became clearer. Note. ADL = activities of daily living; LLE = left lower extremity; OT = occupational therapist; POC = plan of care.

ponents that do not directly affect functional outcomes. The documentation of home care occupational therapy must stress the functional focus of our discipline. We cannot afford to have progress notes emphasize repetitive routines or small gains in the learning of home exercise programs that focus on performance components (for example upper-extremity strengthening) if there is no significant improvement expected in a meaningful performance area. The principles described in this article are meant to enable practitioners to maintain a view of the large, meaningful picture of what home care occupational therapy is about and to be able to document these services appropriately. The analysis of the third party payer as a target audience should encourage practitioners to stay focused on the essential concepts of function, safety, and underlying factors that *interfere* with function and safety, progress toward goals, and expectations of progress. This analysis also encourages a progress-oriented (or outcome-oriented) rather than a treatment-oriented approach to documentation. Occupational therapy has the potential to lead the home health team in focusing on the real needs of the client who is homebound. Occupational therapy services, and the documentation of these services, must stay true to the core values of the discipline for the sake of our clients and the future of our profession.

Appendix

ASSUMPTIONS FOR REIMBURSEMENT – Occupational therapy will be reimbursed if:

1. The client has functional limitations that can be decreased.

2. The client's physical or cognitive impairments are interfering with function or safety.

3. The client either is showing progress, has a good acute reason for not showing progress, or is expected to show progress.

4. The services delivered by the practitioner are skilled care, documented as evaluation or reevaluation; therapeutic intervention; or client, family member, caregiver instruction or training.

5. The practitioner has "skilled plans" that will significantly affect the client's level of independence or safety in performance areas or will design and implement a functional maintenance plan to be carried out by family members or caregivers.

Acknowledgments

I thank my husband, James P. McGuire, MAH, for his support and for the gift of his editorial skills. I thank the Lord for His guidance in my life: "In all your ways acknowledge Him, and He will make your paths straight" (Prov. 3:6).

References

Allen, C., Foto, M., Moon-Sperling, T., & Wilson, D. (1989). A medical review approach to Medicare outpatient documentation. *American Journal of Occupational Therapy*, 43, 793–800.

American Occupational Therapy Association. (1992). *Effective documentation in occupational therapy*. Bethesda, MD: Author.

American Occupational Therapy Association. (1994a). *Medicare guidelines for occupational therapy*. Bethesda, MD: Author.

American Occupational Therapy Association. (1994b). Uniform terminology for occupational therapy (3rd ed.). *American Journal of Occupational Therapy*, 48, 1047–1054.

American Occupational Therapy Association. (1995). Elements of clinical documentation (revision). *American Journal of Occupational Therapy*, 49, 1032–1035.

DePaoli, T. L., & Zenk-Jones, P. (1984). Medicare reimbursement in home care. *American Journal of Occupational Therapy*, 38, 739–742.

Glickstein, J. K., & Neustadt, G. K. (1992). *Reimbursable geriatric service delivery. A functional maintenance therapy system*. Gaithersburg, MD: Aspen.

Health Care Financing Administration. (1989). *Medical review (MR) of part B intermediary outpatient occupational therapy (OT) bills* (DHHS transmittal no. 1424). Washington, DC: U.S. Government Printing Office.

Health Care Financing Administration. (1996). *Medicare home health agency manual* (DHHS transmittal no. 277). Washington, DC: U.S. Government Printing Office.

Kielhofner, G. (1985). *A model of human occupation*. Baltimore, MD: Williams & Wilkins.

Kunstaetter, D. (1988). Occupational therapy treatment in home health care. *American Journal of Occupational Therapy*, 42, 513–519.

MacRae, A. (1984). Occupational therapy in a Medicare-approved home health agency. *American Journal of Occupational Therapy*, 38, 721–725.

Meyer, A. (1922). The philosophy of occupation therapy. *Archives of Occupational Therapy*, 1, 1–10.

Reed, K. (1984). *Models of practice in occupational therapy*. Baltimore, MD: Williams & Wilkins.

Robertson, S. C. (1992). Why we document. In *Effective documentation for occupational therapy*. Bethesda, MD: American Occupational Therapy Association.

Schkade, J. K., & Schultz, S. (1992). Occupational adaptation: Toward a holistic approach for contemporary practice, part 1. *American Journal of Occupational Therapy*, 46, 829–837.

Schultz, S., & Schkade, J. K. (1992). Occupational adaptation: Toward a holistic approach for contemporary practice, part 2. *American Journal of Occupational Therapy*, 46, 917–925.

Scott, S. J., & Somers, F. P. (1992). Orientation to payment. In *Effective documentation for occupational therapy*. Bethesda, MD: American Occupational Therapy Association.

Steinhauer, M. J. (1984). Nationally Speaking—Occupational therapy and home health care. *American Journal of Occupational Therapy*, 38, 715–716.

11. Special Considerations III: Mental Health

Kathleen Kannenberg, MA, OTR/L

This is the last of three chapters discussing special considerations affecting certain areas of practice. The author of this chapter focuses on special documentation issues in mental health.

Kathleen Kannenberg is an occupational therapist care manager and consultant in community mental health practice in Seattle, Washington. She is the former Mental Health Program Manager for the American Occupational Therapy Association.

The Language of Function

The results of a 3-year study by the AOTA Mental Health Special Interest Section (MHSIS) Education Task Force confirmed that the lack of clarity about the role of occupational therapy in mental health is a critical issue among students and practitioners.

Practitioners identified the need for functional outcomes, raising the concern that:

> too often, clinicians concentrate treatment interventions on components of functional skills and never reach, address, or apply these components to the actual functional performance required of the consumer (AOTA, 1995; FG01-853, FG07-159).

> what's happening again is that whole idea that people see what you do and think anyone can do it (AOTA, 1995; FG03-1240).

> there is this physical disability that doesn't come attached to a psychosocial component (AOTA, 1995; FG07-425).

A major need for students is to see that occupational therapy is effective. One student participating in a focus group said:

> 99% of our students leave their fieldwork sites not being able to see what OTs role was in mental health because they (clinicians) are not practicing OT in mental health (AOTA, 1995: FG06-1858).

Educators expressed the concern that:

> fieldwork facilities don't seem willing to incorporate psychosocial goals into traditional rehabilitation programs because of questions related to reimbursement (AOTA, 1995: FG06-829).

How can we prepare students and clinicians for practice in the next millennium if we are not able to articulate or demonstrate the role of occupational therapy interventions in providing cost-effective outcomes for individuals with mental illness?

Many occupational therapy practitioners have asked how they can demonstrate to payers and consumers the cost-effective outcomes of occupational therapy practice in mental health. Additional questions are often asked about whether psychosocial interventions for clients with nonpsychiatric conditions can be documented and receive payment. In order to survive and thrive in both current and future practice environments, occupational therapists and assistants need to focus interventions on functional outcomes, measure changes in ways meaningful and relevant to the client, and be able to articulate and document those functional changes to justify services.

This chapter will provide a brief overview of forces shaping the future of occuptional therapy practice in mental health, discuss how these trends provide a solid foundation for the use of occupational therapy services, and describe special challenges in documenting functional outcomes in mental health. AOTA's Uniform Terminology III will be presented as a tool for documenting outcomes, and the Medicare Part B Guidelines will be reviewed specific to how they relate to mental health practice. Some examples of functional, measurable, and objective goals for mental health and psychosocial goals in other practice areas are provided.

Detailed information on key elements to consider when writing functional goals as well as documenting psychosocial interventions in other practice areas can be found in this book in chapter 7 by Moorhead and Kannenberg, "Writing Functional Goals."

Directions for the Future

The health care delivery system has changed dramatically in the past decade. The advent of the Medicare prospective payment system had the first major impact on both public and privately funded health programs. In the past several years, the health care reform movement and the rapid growth of the managed care industry created additional changes in health care service delivery and in requirements for documentation. Although current health trends may appear to limit the provision of occuptional therapy services, these same trends also can serve as a rationale for using the language of function to describe and document the outcomes of occupational therapy services and as a foundation for the growth of occupational therapy practice in mental health.

The purchasers of health care, both public and private, have restructured approaches to health care delivery and finance in order to control costs. School districts, as well as state and federal governments, are experiencing severe budget constraints. Even Medicare and Medicaid, the largest public purchasers of occupational therapy services, are pursuing payment reforms and greater use of managed care (Sommers, 1996). Lines between public and private systems are blurring as funding streams merge, with the overall goal of containing costs; market forces are driving the reform that is occurring all around us, both in reimbursement forms and methods of service delivery.

Health care trends shaping the future of occupational therapy practice in mental health and other areas include:

- continued cost containment within a managed care environment
- demands for measurable, functional outcomes
- a rapidly growing consumer movement
- community based services
- multiskilled practitioners.

In making decisions about the use of health care dollars, consumers (clients, families, third-party payers, health care systems, industry, and government) are demanding services that provide good value. Because health care dollars must be stretched to cover many providers, questions must be asked about the cost-effectiveness of the treatment provided— for example, what services the client received and whether those services were necessary, what the benefit of outcome was for the client, who is the best provider of these services, and where they should be delivered (Fine, 1986).

Recently the cost of labor has come to the forefront as a major contributor to rising health care costs. Issues relating to multi-skilling and cross training have been prevalent in the occupational therapy literature. In a managed care environment, instead of occupational therapy being a revenue producing center, we are a cost center. For example, if OT is provided, managed care profits decline, whereas previously OT contributed to profits by providing services. Thus, changing the skill mix and professional level composition of the workforce has become a priority in containing costs. Cross training has forced occupational therapy to recognize that not everything we do is skilled and that we must identify nonskilled activities that can be performed by others. It becomes even more critical, then, in a mental health environment, where other professionals and paraprofessionals are providing services that look like occupational therapy, to clearly define skilled occupational therapy services and how they are unique. Occupational therapy practitioners are multiskilled and can practice in a wide variety of settings.

Despite shrinking resources and services, the consumer movement in mental health has grown rapidly, with individuals moving from being passive recipients of services to active customers. A client centered and collaborative approach is a natural for occupational therapy as we have a long history of valuing people doing for themselves. Yerxa in 1967 said "that to engage in occupation is to take control. Since self-initiated activity is our stock in trade, and since it is impossible to force any human being to initiate without his choosing to do so, choice is one of the keys to our unique therapeutic process." In a client-centered approach, the knowledge and experiences of the client are central and used in partnership with the professional's expertise. Thus, our ability to pay attention to both verbal and nonverbal expressions of what constitutes purposeful, meaningful occupational performance is an asset unique to occupational therapy (CAOT, 1993).

In addition, health care consumers, both clients and payers, are identifying the community as the locus of treatment services. The community is the least restrictive and most natural context for the development of adaptive behaviors and is often the least costly. We see validation of this trend toward community services in the development of continuums of care, with hospitals becoming part of large multisystem organizations. Managed care monitoring has significantly increased the use of outpatient services, stimulating the development of a range of ambulatory services designed to enhance the continuum of care and maintain clients in the community. These trends clearly indicate that occupational therapy practitioners must focus on service delivery emphasizing the consumer's priorities for goals and using natural settings for intervention.

Thus, market forces and external mandates for change are changing the composition of the workforce as well as influencing expansion of practice environments for occupational therapy. These trends validate the belief that occupational therapy is in a uniquely advantageous position in today's health care environment. Our services are both cost effective and can provide meaningful and relevant functional outcomes for individuals with mental illness. Our biggest challenge in mental health is to view these trends as opportunities, not barriers, and bridge the service delivery gap, moving occupational therapy services to the community where clients who need our services are living.

Psychiatry

The impact of these forces, coupled with the more limited funding available for mental health services, created a major crisis both for the field of psychiatry and for occupational therapy. The short length of inpatient stays, higher acuity, and rapid turnover of patients led to significant changes in the focus of mental health care. Inpatient treatment approaches emphasize crisis intervention, psychopharmacological approaches, rapid assessment, and early discharge planning. The bulk of mental health treatment has moved from inpatient to outpatient settings. In 1955, only 23% of patient care was in outpatient settings, but by 1990, it represented 74% of total care (Center for Mental Health Services, 1994). Both private and many public mental health systems are now controlled by managed care in an effort to contain costs. Although adequate funding resources have not yet followed the movement of clients to outpatient and community-based settings, we can be sure that services will not move back to the hospital!

What Do Payers Want?

Reimbursement and funding issues remain one of the largest obstacles to occupational therapy practice in mental health and our ability to provide needed services to our clients.

Managed care systems are designed to provide coverage at a predetermined rate, which is negotiated according to the services desired. Cost containment appears to be the primary influencing factor in the provision of health services. Peer review organizations have been established at both the federal and private levels to provide prospective and concurrent utilization review that monitors use of services in an attempt to cut costs by reducing unnecessary admissions and lengths of stay. In both systems, if the cost of care is under the predetermined rate, the setting can keep the difference. However, it must also absorb any losses if the cost is higher. This creates a powerful incentive to control costs (Fine, 1986).

Managed care goals are now the same for all payers. Both public and private reimbursement systems are looking for the following:

- expected and relevant outcomes achieved within a defined time frame, for example, the quality of life achieved through living more independently
- outcomes sustainable over time, for example, not requiring therapist intervention or a therapeutic environment
- efficient allocation and coordination of services, for example, types of staffing, equipment, and space
- defined "critical pathways," for example, a typical, expected course of treatment leading to a specific outcome for a particular diagnosis (Foto, 1994). The challenge to all health care providers, including occupational therapy, is to achieve the same or better outcomes as in the past while using fewer resources.

Functional Outcomes

Foto in 1996 defined outcome as a result of therapy or what a client is able to do after short-term and long-term goals have been met. She identifies outcome "as measured by the quality of life that a patient is able to live as a result of having achieved a certain level of independence...and the outcome measures the value of worth of that progress to the patient, the patient's family, the payer, and society in general" (p. 87).

We must be able to articulate how occupational therapy can meet consumer demands for outcomes by speaking a language with relevance to our audience. Our language is function, and our product is "productive living." Communication required that we define and document our role in a way that allows someone who is not an occupational therapy practitioner to understand the goals, methods, and outcomes of our services. This is a challenge, especially in mental health. Our practice arena in hospitals has often been a centralized "activity or adjunctive therapy" department, which lumps together similar disciplines using activity as a basis for treatment. From an administrative viewpoint, this centralization provides for cost-effective and coordinated services; the dilemma is that the uniqueness of each discipline can easily be lost. Although disciplines such as occupational, recreation, music, dance, and other creative arts therapies have distinct philosophies, there are many overlap areas, both in scope of services and treatment modalities. This creates role blurring and confusion and often leads to the concept of a generic and interchangeable staff of "activity therapists."

Community-based programs, (such as community mental health centers, day treatment centers, residential treatment programs, psychosocial clubhouses, and vocational programs) are designed to support and assist consumers in developing the social, vocational, and leisure skills necessary to successfully live in the community. Occupational therapy services are often not recognized as needed in the community because few occupational therapy practitioners work there. Program staff members from a variety of backgrounds are providing rehabilitation services, and there is little understanding of what occupational therapy does that is unique and different. Services that may look like occupational therapy, (such as budgeting, cooking, and coping skills) usually are provided by other less costly disciplines. Occupational therapy practitioners, in turn, are often unsure of what their role is in community practice. This lack of awareness of what occupational therapy has to offer and the more limited funding resources that affect salaries create a challenging environment in which to market occupational therapy services.

Regulatory bodies such as the Joint Commission on Accreditation of Healthcare Organizations (JCAHO), the Commission on Accreditation of Rehabilitation Facilities (CARF), Medicare, and state licensing agencies contributed to this dilemma by defining nonspecific standards for "activity services" that incorporate many disciplines together. For freestanding psychiatric hospitals or community mental health centers, there are no specific standards requiring that occupational therapy services be provided. Other program requirements, not specific to occupational therapy, may include a general statement regarding providing access to services the client needs. By collaborating with other disciplines toward enhancing the quality and outcomes of care as mandated by all agencies, and identifying programmatic needs, occupational therapy practitioners can communicate the role and value of occupational therapy in enhancing functional outcomes in all settings (Brinson & Kannenberg, 1996).

Payers, employers, and consumers need a clear understanding of how the goals, methods, and outcomes of occupational therapy interventions can help meet managed care demands for functional outcomes that are sustainable over time (Foto, 1994). Occupational therapy personnel shortages (especially in mental health), cost containment, and the prevalence of role blurring have all created opportunities for other disciplines to fill positions and reduced our practice to a narrow range of what we are able to do, often eliminating the unique holistic approach of occupational therapy. Unless health care administrators have a clear understanding of the role and value of occupational therapy in meeting consumer demands for functional independence and cost containment, hiring decisions may be based on available personnel, salary requirements, and reimbursement issues.

With all consumers in mental health asking why they should pay for occupational therapy services, what we do that is unique and different from other health care providers, and what is the benefit or outcome of our interventions, it becomes imperative that occupational therapy practitioners in mental health communicate their role clearly and with confidence.

Documentation

Documentation in the medical record is the primary format for communicating with both the health care team and third party payers. Reimbursement for services in mental health is an issue regardless of whether your setting includes occupational therapy in the per diem or daily rate, bills separately as a fee for service, or simply provides services. Whether you practice in an inpatient or outpatient, profit or nonprofit setting, the highest costs in the mental health delivery system are staffing costs. When administration looks at cost containment, the focus is on numbers and types of staff as well as the necessity of the services provided in meeting the financial "bottom line." The future of occupational therapy in mental health depends, in part, on our documentation skills.

Psychiatry as a field has continued to struggle with external agency reimbursements for measurable goals, documented progress, and observable outcomes. Requirements demanding a master problem list and goals developed by the multidisciplinary treatment team often lead to broadly based and generic problems and goals.

In trying to meet the requirements for an integrated and multidisciplinary treatment approach, occupational therapy practitioners have developed treatment plans that are often ambiguous, difficult to measure, and indistinguishable from other disciplines. Following are four examples of problems (in italics) followed by related goals that might have been written by occupational therapists as well as other members of the multidisciplinary treatment plan.

1. Depression: Increase mood and activity level
2. *Impaired coping skills*: List three coping strategies

3. *Impaired attention span*: Increase attention span from 10 to 20 minutes

4. *Impaired self-care*: Increase independence in activities of daily living.

In documenting progress, we have documented the process of treatment, the modality provided, what the client or therapist did, but not the outcome of our intervention and its effect on functional status. Unfortunately, third party payers and other consumers may not understand how improved self-esteem, attention span, or coping skills contribute to functional outcomes of activities of daily living, work, and leisure pursuits. If we assume this "leap of faith" by the payer, the uniqueness of occupational therapy's contribution may be lost.

Using AOTA's Uniform Terminology III

It has always been difficult for occupational therapy practitioners in mental health, as well as other psychiatric disciplines to define measurable, objective outcomes. Our colleagues in physical rehabilitation always seemed able to write more specific and measurable goals. Practitioners in mental health moved to using components of performance that seemed more measurable, for example, attention span or coping skills.

Uniform Terminology III (Appendix 8) provides a conceptual framework for documentation. It defines occupational therapy's domain of concern and the expected outcome of our service and can be used as a tool for helping practitioners identify functional outcomes. The focus of occupational therapy is always the broad categories of human performance typically part of roles in daily life, for example, activities of daily living, work and productivity, and play and leisure. Our method is to observe clients in selected functional activities critical to their desired occupational roles and integral to individual needs, goals, life stories, diagnosis, and environment. Once performance areas are identified that are meaningful and relevant to the individual, family member, or caregiver, deficits observed are usually caused by underlying factors identified in Uniform Terminology III as performance components (defined by Medicare as underlying factors). We assess and intervene with those underlying elements that contribute to or interfere with performance in the desired life area, for example, sensorimotor, cognitive, psychosocial, and psychological. Distinguishing between performance areas and performance components when writing functional goals is critical. Components in and of themselves do not necessarily correlate to competent or meaningful function in everyday life. Accordingly, if our goals are limited to component areas, although they may seem more measurable, they do not differentiate our goals from those of other disciplines, especially in mental health, and do not reflect meaningful, functional outcomes. Using the "so what" rule can be helpful in distinguishing relevant outcomes, for example, an individual can concentrate for 20 minutes, can list three coping skills, and can role play assertive behavior, but what life activities is he or she able to do as a result?

The final area of Uniform Terminology III is the most recent addition and describes situations of factors that influence an individual's behavior and engagement in desired or required performance areas. Context has been a recurring theme in occupational therapy literature but has not always been effectively used by practitioners in mental health. We have often addressed the context of the clinic setting by designing activity or environmental adaptations that have assisted the individual to function more effectively. We have rarely addressed the discharge, community, or home environment. Because adaptive responses are often facilitated by the environment, context is a critical variable in evaluation and intervention. If we have evaluated performance without considering context, we may misinterpret the behavior and plan inappropriate interventions. Occupational therapy practitioners must also consider context in determining the nature, feasibility, and appropriateness of the intervention. Understanding of the contextual aspects of performance can show the uniqueness of occupational therapy. Performance contexts as identified by Uniform Terminology III include *temporal*, for example, chronological, developmental, life cycle, and disability status; and *environmental*, for example, physical, social, and cultural.

Optimal performance is always considered to be the result of the interactive relationship among these three broad areas identified in Uniform Terminology III. Performance areas and components must always be considered within the context of performance, for example, is it the activity itself or the context that needs to be adapted for a successful outcome to occur? Interventions can be directed toward elements of any of these three areas that may allow for more cost-effective allocation of scarce resources (e.g., arranging supplies in the kitchen for easy access may make more sense than teaching new skills to an individual with decreased sequencing and organizational skills). Occupational therapy practitioners may benefit from using Uniform Terminology III as a "litmus test" of whether the functional goals they are writing include outcomes consistent with the list of performance areas. This review can eliminate using performance components as outcomes when writing goals. When the focus of intervention is on specific performance components, they can be incorporated into the goal as long as a functional (performance area) outcome is present. Performance components are often incorporated into short-term goals. Although the term *function* is commonly used by many other professionals, the way that occupational therapy practitioners conceptualize function, as described in Uniform Terminology III, is truly unique.

Medicare Part B Guidelines

Why should psychiatric occupational therapists, regardless of their practice setting and source of funding, use the Medicare Part B Guidelines for Outpatient Occupational Therapy? Because Medicare has the most stringent and specific coverage guidelines, documentation that satisfies Medicare will usually meet the requirements of other third party payers. In addition, Medicare has the only clearly defined criteria for what is considered skilled and nonskilled occupational therapy, and Medicare identifies in what circumstances it should be provided and what the outcome of the intervention must be. Although skilled has been defined by Medicare for the purpose of review, it is a helpful concept for occupational therapy practitioners.

By reviewing and understanding the Medicare guidelines for covered services, it becomes clear how we can use the guidelines to document in such a way that our role and value will be clearly delineated and reimbursement will be maximized. The new guidelines were introduced in 1989, following passage of the law that included occupational therapy in Part B, outpatient services, and these proved to be of limited value for psychiatric occupational therapists, as the following quotation from the Medicare Part A Intermediary Manual illustrates:

> Such therapy may involve the planning, implementation and supervision of individualized therapeutic activity programs as part of an overall active treatment program for a patient with a diagnosed psychiatric illness, e.g., the use of sewing activities which require following a pattern to reduce confusion and restore reality orientation in a schizophrenic patient. (HCFA, 1987 p. 3-33.5A)

The new guidelines have an historical significance since they represent the first time in the history of HCFA that AOTA was actively involved in developing standards. The advent of these guidelines presented our profession with the opportunity to revise documentation practice in all specialty areas in order to focus on the needs of the individual and the ability to function.

The specific areas in the Part B Guidelines that are of primary interest and importance to mental health are highlighted in the following selections (HCFA, 1990).

Cognition and safety are included as a functional limitation in the performance of activities of daily living. Each level of assistance identified has specific criteria for establishing baseline data and measuring progress.

§3906.4A3. MODERATE ASSISTANCE — This represents the need for 50% assistance by one person to perform physical activities or constant cognitive assistance to sustain/complete simple, repetitive activities safely. The records submitted should state how a cognitively impaired patient requires intermittent one-to-one demonstration or intermittent cueing (physical or verbal) throughout the activity. Moderate assistance is needed when the occupational therapist/caregiver needs to be in the immediate environment to progress the patient through a sequence to complete an activity. This level of assistance is required to halt continuing repetition of a task and to prevent unsafe, erratic or unpredictable actions that interfere with appropriate sequencing. (HCFA, 1990, p. 10-129)

§3906.2 SAFETY DEPENDENCE/SECONDARY COMPLICATIONS — A safety problem exists when a patient without skilled occupational therapy intervention cannot handle him/herself in a manner that is physically and/or cognitively safe. This may extend to daily living or to acquired secondary complications. Safety dependence may be demonstrated by high probability of failing, lack of environmental safety awareness, abnormal aggressive/destructive behavior, severe pain…requiring skilled occupational therapy intervention to protect the patient from further medical complication(s). (HCFA, 1990, p. 10-125)

§3906.4B. CHANGE IN RESPONSE TO TREATMENT WITHIN EACH LEVEL OF ASSISTANCE — Significant improvement must be indicated by documenting a change in one or more of the following categories of patient responses within any assistance level:

1. Refusals—The patient may respond by refusing to attempt an activity because of fear or pain. The documentation should indicate the activity refused, the reasons, and how the OT

plan addressed them. For the cognitively impaired patient, refusal to perform an activity can escalate into aggressive, destructive or verbally abusive behavior if the therapist or caregiver presses the patient to perform. In these cases, a reduction in these behaviors is considered significant progress, but must be documented, including the skilled OT provided to reduce the abnormal behavior.

For the psychiatrically impaired patient, refusals to participate in an activity frequently are symptoms of the diagnosis. The patient should not be put on a "hold" status due to refusals. If the documentation indicates that the patient is receiving OT, is contacted regularly, and is actively encouraged to participate, medically review the claim to determine if reasonable and necessary skilled care has been rendered.

2. Inconsistency—The patient may respond by inconsistently performing functional tasks from day-to-day or within a treatment session.

Approve the claim when the documentation indicates a significant progression in consistency of performance of functional tasks within the same level of assistance.

3. Generalization—The patient may respond by applying previously learned concepts for performing an activity similar to another activity. The records submitted should document a significant increase in scope of activities that the patient can perform, their type, and the skilled OT services rendered.

C. A New Skilled Functional Activity is initiated—Examples

- Adding teaching of lower body dressing to a current program of upper body dressing

- Increasing the ability to perform personal hygiene activities for health and social acceptance.

D. A New Skilled Compensatory Technique is Added—(With or without adapted equipment). Examples:

- Teaching a patient techniques such as one-handed hoe tying

- Teaching the use of a button hook for buttoning shirt buttons (HCFA, 1990, pp. 10-130-10-131).

§3906.5 *LEVEL OF COMPLEXITY OF TREATMENT* – Base decisions on the level of complexity of the services rendered by the occupational therapist and not what the patient is asked to do. Examples:

A. Skilled OT—The documentation must indicate that the severity of the physical/emotional/perceptual/cognitive disability requires complex and sophisticated knowledge to identify current and potential capabilities. In addition, consider instructions required by the patient and/or the patient's caregivers. Instructions may be required for activities that most healthy people take for granted. The special knowledge of an occupational therapist is required to decrease or eliminate limitations in functional activity performance. Occupational therapists must often address underlying factors which interfere with specific activities. These factors could be cognitive, sensory, or perceptual deficits.

Skilled services include, but are not limited to, reasonable and necessary:

- Patient evaluations

- Determination of effective goals and services with the patient and patient's caregivers and other medical professionals

- Analyzing and modifying functional tasks

- Determining that the modified task obtains optimum performance through tests and measurements

- Providing instructions of the task(s) to the patient, family/caregivers

- Periodically reevaluating the patient's status with corresponding readjustment of the OT program
(HCFA, 1990, pp. 10-131-10-132)

Uniform Terminology III and the Medicare Part B Guidelines have provided psychiatric occupational therapists and assistants with a language to identify functional problems and objective criteria to measure and document progress toward independence.

As occupational practitioners in mental health, we should not try to be all things to all people. The view of occupational therapy in psychiatry as providing generalized activities or as being interchangeable with other disciplines must be changed. This view diminishes our role as a specialty service for persons with adaptive performance problems and psychosocial rehabilitation need (Schwartz, 1988). Depending on the client population and type of setting, we must identify the services that will help our clients to achieve the highest level of function. This may involve our giving up areas that can be done by other professionals, but it will allow us to focus on those skills and interventions that only occupational therapy can provide.

Occupational therapy practitioners in outpatient or community settings will need to overcome the lack of awareness of what occupational therapy can offer in programs such as partial hospitalization, community mental health centers, mobile treatment teams, residential treatment programs, psychosocial clubhouses, drop-in centers, homeless shelters, and home health agencies. Using the language of function and demonstrating the uniqueness of occupational therapy evaluation and intervention will allow us to move into practice arenas where clients need our services.

This new format for documentation will require a different way of thinking in order to relate psychiatric problem areas of self-expression, socialization, and concentration to functional performance. However, is not that the justification for hospitalization as well as outpatient care: an inability to function effectively at a lower level of care? As we use the levels of assistance to document how progress has been achieved as a direct result of skilled intervention; as we clearly identify the underlying factors and problems that interfere with functional performance; as we establish measurable short and long-term functional goals with time frames for accomplishment, our professional boundaries will become clear. The value of occupational therapy in mental health then will be established both in our own minds and in those of our colleagues and consumers.

In 1989 Dickie stated:

> The schism between occupational therapy in mental health and those in other specialty areas narrows or disappears when we talk about reimbursement. Suddenly the language becomes function, and all of us start talking about how to document functional outcomes. Isn't it ironic that third party payers, not necessarily known for their understanding of occupational therapy, are driving this unification of language and purpose? (p. 3)

Examples of Functional Goals

Detailed information on key elements to consider when writing functional goals as well as documenting psychosocial interventions in other practice areas can be found in this book in the chapter by Moorhead and Kannenberg, "Writing Functional Goals." Although there is no perfect format for writing functional goals, the following examples may be helpful. Performance components are incorporated into some of the goals as examples of how to include them. Both goals for clients and caregivers are included.

1.   Client will improve socialization by calling a friend when feeling lonely, with prompt of a posted list of coping strategies.

2.   Client will independently prepare a can of soup for lunch, following directions on can.

3.   Client's caregiver will demonstrate independence in setting up meal preparation for client to prepare own lunch.

4.   Client will initiate and complete daily AM grooming and bathing with intermittent verbal cues from caregiver.

5.   Client will assist in meal preparation by making a salad and setting the table according to a pre-determined weekly schedule with minimal assistance.

6.   Client will independently schedule 1 hour of play time with 3-year-old son in her daily schedule of activities to improve skills in care of others.

7.   Client will complete on-site job application independently, using information pre-printed on cue card as prerequisite to job acquisition.

8.   Client will improve socialization at work, by initiating conversation with coworkers regarding daily break schedule with minimal cueing.

9.   Client will improve money management by independently getting spending money twice weekly from bank cash machine.

10. Client will improve volunteer participation by independently serving meal trays during lunch at day health program.

11. Client will improve socialization independently by asking classmate in communitycollege class to have coffee during class break.

12. Client will identify from the newspaper one interesting and free recreational activity available on the weekend and include in weekly schedule with minimal assistance.

13. Client will participate in weekly card game using adaptive devices.

14. Client will use printed cue card to fill medi-set in order to maintain medication routine.

15. Client will improve socialization by independently asking husband to eat dinner with the family twice a week.

16. Client, with minimal cueing, will follow daily schedule to complete required home management tasks.

17. Client, with moderate assistance, will ask roomate to lower the radio volume while he is doing homework.

18. Client will sustain attention to task for 15 minutes in order to prepare two sack lunches for her children.

References

American Occupational Therapy Association. (1994). Uniform terminology for occupational therapy (3rd ed.). *American Journal of Occupational Therapy, 48*, 1047-1054.

American Occupational Therapy Association. (1995). *Mental Health Special Interest Section education task force report.* Bethesda, MD: Author.

Brinson, M., & Kanneberg, K. (1996). *Mental health service delivery guidelines.* Bethesda, MD: American Occupational Therapy Association.

CAOT. (1993). Occupational therapy guidelines for client-centered mental health practice. Ministry of Supply and Services, Canada, 5.

Center for Mental Health Services. Manderscheid, & Sonnenschein (Eds.). (1994). *Mental health, United States, 1994.* Bethesda, MD: U. S. Government Printing Service.

Dickie, V. (1989). From the chair. *Mental Health Special Interest Section Newsletter, 12*(3), 3-4.

Fine, S. (1986). Trends in mental health. In S. Robertson (Ed.), *Mental health SCOPE: Strategies, concepts, and opportunities for program development and evaluation* (pp. 19-32). Bethesda, MD: American Occupational Therapy Association.

Foto, M. (1966). National speaking—outcome studies: The what, why, how, and when. *The American Journal of Occupational Therapy, 50,* 87-88.

Foto, M. (1994, November 24). California faces the future. *OT Week,* 26-27.

Health Care Financing Administration. (1987). *Medicare part A intermediary manual, part 3: Claims process.* Washington, DC: U. S. Government Printing Office.

Health Care Financing Administration. (1990). *Medicare intermediary manual, part 3*: Claims process. (DHHS Transmittal No. 1487). Washington, DC: U. S. Government Printing Office.

Schwartz, S. (1988). Prospective payment for psychiatric services: Service management strategies for occupational therapy. In S. Robertson (Ed), *Mental health FOCUS: Skills for assessment and treatment* (pp. 1-37-1-41). Bethesda, MD: American Occupational Therapy Association.

Sommers, F. (1996, July). The Demand for OT in 2005. *OT Practice.*

Yerxa, E. (1967). Authentic occupational therapy. *American Journal of Occupational Therapy, 21,* 1-9.

Fidler, G. (1994). The psychosocial core of occupational therapy. *American Journal of Occupational Therapy, 49*, 1021-1022.

Hemphill, B., Peterson, C., & Werner, P. (1991). *Rehabilitations in Mental Health: Goals and Objectives for Independent Living*. Thorofare, NJ: Slack.

Medicare Reimbursement Guidelines: Reimbursement Program, AOTA.

Stoffel, V. (1995). Psychosocial concerns with occupational therapy practice. *American Journal of Occupational Therapy, 49*, 1021-1022.

VanLeit, B. (1996). Managed mental health care: Reflections in a time of turmoil. *American Journal of Occupational Therapy, 50*, 428-433.

Additional Resources

12. Documentation for Assistive Technology

Aimee J. Luebben, EdD, OTR/L, FAOTA

Technology can make a significant difference in the lives of our patients and clients. Patients depend on the occupational therapist not only to suggest appropriate equipment but also to provide the necessary documentation for funding. Documenting the need for equipment, especially expensive high-tech equipment, is a challenge. This chapter provides clear guidance on how to accomplish such documentation, as well as sample letters written to funding sources.

Aimee J. Luebben is the Director and Associate Professor, Occupational Therapy Program, University of Southern Indiana, Evansville, Indiana.

Gaining the freedom to be productively employed, participating in recreational activities, caring for personal needs, and living life to the fullest are some of the greatest challenges faced by persons with disabilities. To meet these challenges, technology can serve as an equalizing factor, providing many of the same educational, vocational, self-help, and leisure opportunities available to persons without disabilities (Luebben, 1986).

Although occupational therapy practitioners have been involved with adaptive equipment since the beginning of the profession, assistive technology is relatively new federal terminology. According to The Technology-Related Assistance for Individuals with Disabilities Act of 1988 (PL 100-407), *assistive technology device* means any item, piece of equipment, or product system, whether acquired commercially off the shelf, modified, or customized, that is used to increase, maintain, or improve functional capabilities of individuals with disabilities. Most occupational therapy clinicians have recommended specific assistive devices to enhance the quality of life for persons with disabilities, but sometimes the equipment is not funded. The key to funding assistive technology is documentation that is thorough, appropriate, and objective.

In many ways assistive technology documentation is different from the forms of documentation discussed in other chapters. The fundamental difference is the purpose. Documenting services for reimbursement to the person or agency providing occupational therapy services is of prime importance, while documentation for assistive technology is more in the nature of advocacy. Providing funding justification for persons requiring occupational therapy services is the primary purpose for documenting assistive technology needs. Appropriate documentation can assist third party reimbursement sources in making an accurate and informed decision regarding the purchase of adaptive equipment to enhance the lives of persons who need assistive technology.

Another major difference between documenting for occupational therapy services and for assistive technology is the temporal aspect. Most reimbursement requests for occupational therapy services are sent after services have been rendered, while the majority of equipment funding must be preauthorized by the reimbursement source before any equipment can be ordered or delivered.

A third way assistive technology documentation is different from the other forms of documentation is in the variability of documentation. For the most part, when documenting occupational therapy services for reimbursement, a standard format is submitted to the third- party payers. However, there is a wide variation in the documentation needed to request financial assistance for assistive technology. The same request submitted to several funding sources may need to undergo several transformations since various funding sources have different requirements for documentation.

Siegel (1991) reported that some clinicians have taken an "ostrich" approach, prescribing equipment based only on clinical parameters and leaving the reimbursement issue to the patient. The frustration inherent in the reimbursement process, the bureaucracy, and arbitrary decisions by the reimbursement sources contribute to further clinician avoidance in becoming involved with the third party payers. If allowed, the justification paperwork for assistive technology can be time consuming and difficult.

Trefler (1989) suggests having a full-time clerical person on staff to direct the funding process; however, with some preparation and insight into the equipment approval process, documentation for assistive technology can be treated as any other type of report writing and generated by the person recommending the device. The precursors to documenting the need for assistive technology are identifying funding sources and using funding strategies. Once a payment source has been targeted and funding strategies employed, the occupational therapy practitioner can write the assistive technology documentation for the person needing the adaptive equipment. For a high degree of success in obtaining assistive technology funding, it is essential to follow the funding agency requirements.

One agency may reimburse the total price of an adaptive device, but with expensive equipment, it is becoming more common to combine financial assistance from more than one funding source ("Reimbursing Adaptive Technology," 1989). In order to find funding for specific pieces of assistive technology, it is crucial to know the local availability of funding sources. In every area there is a variety of funding sources including Medicare, Medicaid, private medical insurance, vocational rehabilitation, private and state facilities (including nursing homes, intermediate care facilities for persons with developmental disabilities, and sheltered workshops), educational agencies and schools, public fundraising, community service organizations (for example, Lions, Elks, Variety Club), health organizations (for example Muscular Dystrophy Association, United Cerebral Palsy, Easter Seals), and private foundations.

Before approaching a funding source, DeShaw (1990) recommends finding out the rules of the game (whom to contact, what information to present, and how to present the information) and also cautions that the rules for funding sources may change over time and verification of changes must be made. Knowing specific requirements of the various funding sources can reduce the amount of time spent and paperwork generated. The requirements of federally funded programs and private insurance can vary from state to state, and even missions of service organizations differ locally. Delineating the specifics for each funding group is beyond the scope of this publication; however, two sources that may be purchased are: *The Many Faces of Funding* from Phonic Ear, Inc., 250 Camino Alto, Mill Valley, CA, 94941, 800-227-0735; and *A Road Map to Funding Sources* from the Society for the Advancement of Rehabilitative and Assistive Technology (RESNA), 1101 Connecticut Avenue NW, Suite 700, Washington, DC, 20036, 202-857-1140.

To complete the information regarding available funding opportunities, two other financial options merit exploration: tax benefits and loan programs. Stating that assistive technology is virtually always tax deductible to the individual or business purchaser, Mendelsohn (1991) presents a detailed explanation of specific tax law provisions in the Internal Revenue Code that apply to the purchase of adaptive equipment. If full or partial funding of a device is denied by targeted financial assistance agencies after several appeals, private pay and use of the tax deductibility may prove useful. Planning is the key to use of the tax savings that technology offers (Mendelsohn, 1991).

Strategies

Various loan programs may provide another option in obtaining assistive technology ("Reimbursing Adaptive Technology," 1989; Rice, 1991). To offer more loan programs, partnerships are being established among combinations of governmental agencies at all levels, funding sources, community agencies, and health organizations. With partnerships sharing some of the costs and risks inherent in providing access to credit, loan programs reduce the expenses of providing financing and arrange to have the lending institution pass savings on to the person who needs financial assistance with assistive technology.

While people across the United States are receiving financial support to purchase assistive technology from a variety of funding agencies, other persons with similar disabilities are being denied funding from the same sources for the same adaptive equipment (Pressman, 1987). A theme that is evident from the funding literature is the need for an adviser or advocate, one person who has been designated as the team leader in the pursuit of funding dollars (DeShaw, 1990; Pressman, 1987). Other members of the assistive technology assessment and funding-seeking team are important, but for the most efficient continuity of efforts, one person (a clinician, durable medical equipment dealer, caregiver, or person who is seeking funding for the device) should be named by the team to coordinate each funding search. The advocate becomes the contact person for all involved, compiling information, coordinating communications to funding agencies, and directing necessary cooperative efforts for the team.

In addition to selecting one person to coordinate funding efforts, there are other ways of increasing the likelihood of obtaining funding for assistive technology. Enders (1988) has proposed 10 strategies to assist in receiving financial support to purchase adaptive equipment:

1. Learn the specifics of local service delivery systems that provide funding.
2. Be aware that the entrances to all systems are controlled by gatekeepers.
3. Remember that all funding systems operate within a bureaucratic environment.
4. Request funding in terms consistent with the purpose or mission of the system whose financial assistance is being sought.
5. Be professional in conduct.
6. Educate the funding system on the efficacy of the agency requesting funding.
7. Remember that systems work because of the efforts of the people within them.
8. Remember that all systems have an appeals process.
9. Use external systems to approach the funding systems if needed.
10. Be persistently patient.

Learning the specifics of local service delivery systems that provide funding is the first strategy. Although some funding sources require a large amount of objective documentation, these agencies are not the norm. Many sources prefer a simple justification discussing the equipment and the person. Before wasting needless time and energy on paperwork, the practitioner should talk to a person within the organization to determine the exact needs of the funding agency.

The second strategy is being aware that the entrance to all systems is controlled by gatekeepers. Each agency has specific rules, regulations, and protocols. It is important to take the time to investigate the procedures required to request funding for assistive technology.

To remember that all funding systems operate within a bureaucratic environment is the third strategy. While a bureaucracy can be viewed as an obstacle, this system can work to the advantage of the persons requiring and requesting funding for assistive technology. A bureaucratic hierarchy can be used as a self-contained appeals process if a denial is made at a lower level.

The fourth strategy is to request funding in terms consistent with the purpose or mission of the system from which financial assistance is being sought. The terminology used may make the difference between whether a device receives funding or not.

Hofmann (1990) and DeShaw (1990) have compiled a list of words and phrases used in funding assistive technology with previous success. *Medically necessary, reasonable and necessary, durable medical equipment*, and *prosthetic device* are key phrases for Medicare. Terminology for potential Medicaid and private medical insurance reimbursement includes

- *achieving and maintaining self-support to prevent, reduce, or eliminate dependency*
- *self-sufficiency*
- *preserving, rehabilitating, or reuniting families*
- *health related*
- *prosthetic appliance*
- *physician-prescribed equipment*
- *part of the client's medical treatment plan*
- *restoration of the patient to his or her best functional level.*

For vocational rehabilitation services, successful phrases are

- *services, training, and equipment used to enhance the employability of the person with a disability*
- *vocational potential*
- *promoting independent living*
- *vocationally enabling.*

The reauthorization of PL 94-142, the Education for the Handicapped Act, as the Individuals with Disabilities Education Act (IDEA) has served to increase special education funding of assistive technology if the multidisciplinary team determines the device to be

- *educationally relevant*
- *needed in order to receive a free appropriate public education*

- *utilized to facilitate a child's education in the least restrictive environment*
- *providing related services* (Golinker, 1991).

Being professional in conduct is the fifth strategy. Often funding agency personnel never meet the occupational therapy practitioner making the adaptive device recommendation. With many pieces of assistive technology becoming more costly, agencies are cautious about the level of professionalism exhibited by the clinician. Well-written, professional-looking documentation can assist in obtaining funding for adaptive equipment.

The sixth strategy is educating the funding system on the efficacy of the agency requesting funding. Because most funding sources are large bureaucracies, individual staff members often relish the continuity of working with the same clinicians. With a high success rate of determining the most appropriate equipment to meet the needs of the person requiring the device combined with the funding source's conception of purchasing a piece of adaptive equipment that provides value for the money, that funding agency staff person and the clinician are likely to continue having more successes. On the other hand, a clinician without a track record with the reimbursement source may take some time to establish credibility. If literature on the agency requesting funding exists, the clinician should be sure to send it to the funding source.

Meetings prior to requests for funds are also a good way to present the clinician or group of clinicians who will make equipment recommendations. Putting a face to a name often helps the funding agency personnel later when funding is requested. An invitation to provide input to the assessment procedure is always welcomed by the funding agency staff member, though scheduling conflicts often preclude attendance.

To remember that systems work because of the efforts of the people within them is the seventh strategy. To improve the likelihood of receiving funding for adaptive equipment, Pin Dot News ("ABCs of Funding," 1990) gives this advice: Write for the reader. Writing for the reader is probably the most important aspect of documenting the need for funding a piece of assistive technology. The person who reads the request may not have an allied health background and may need a more complete explanation of both the device and aspects of the person's disability that warrant recommendation of the piece of adaptive equipment.

The eighth strategy is to remember that all systems have an appeals process. DeShaw (1990) reminds assistive technology funding seekers that denials should not be taken personally but rather as an indication that a particular funding system is unable to respond to requests at this time. For reimbursement denials, taking a reasoned approach was recommended in an *OT Week* article ("Claims Denials," 1991), and several tips were given. First, for the recommendation that was denied funding, check the documentation. Perhaps there were written aspects that either were unclear or did not receive the emphasis needed for the funding source. After clarifying the language and strengthening the weak points, the practitioner should resubmit the recommendation to the same source. Any communication, including telephone calls, with the funding source should be documented in written form. The record may be used later to show compliance with protocol. If there are repeated denials, the clinician should use the professional network to talk to clinicians who have had similar recommendations funded by the same reimbursement source. Clinicians with funding success may have some insight into the process with that particular agency.

Using external systems to approach the funding systems if needed is the ninth strategy. According to Beck (1991) funds for assistive technology have become increasingly more accessible than in the past, and two ways of solving the funding problem are consumer advocacy and educational efforts. The person for whom the funding is being requested and the family are often key players in the acquisition of funding. If objective documentation justifying the need for equipment fails, often snapshots, videotapes, and letters supporting professional recommendations can change the decision of the funding source in favor of reimbursing for the device.

The tenth strategy is to remain patient and persistent. This is a key factor. Funding of assistive technology is often a process that is long and filled with obstacles. The practitioner must always remember the person for whom funding is requested. The needs of that person and the improvement in that person's quality of life should supersede the time and effort involved in the process.

Proving the need is essential to the acquisition of assistive technology. According to Hofmann (1990) funding requests should contain the following information:

- a cover letter
- the appropriate agency forms
- the physician's prescription for the equipment
- therapy evaluation(s)
- diagnostic reports.

When appropriate, pertinent literature describing the device may also be sent.

Often the occupational therapy practitioner has not been designated as the funding advocate but is responsible only for the justification of equipment. To begin writing the justification, clinicians should remember several points. For the most part, the funding agency staff person reading the documentation and also making the decision regarding the disposition of the equipment may never have met the person with the disability and may be lacking in the background of the disability in functional terms. Appropriate assistive technology justification becomes the link between the current functional picture of the person needing equipment described by the justification writer and the ramifications of the proposed adaptive device and changes in the user's life made by the equipment. In addition, the decision maker is often unfamiliar with the specific pieces of equipment, and since there is ongoing change in technology, adaptive device unfamiliarity will continue. Consider the justification an educational process for the reader; describe the device in easily understandable terms, and discuss how the equipment will affect the life of the user.

Assistive Technology Justification

While many therapists once sent lengthy evaluation reports, some clinicians found that a well-written justification in the form of a letter is a welcome substitute for the funding agency. Ideally, the justification should be no longer than two pages and kept to one if possible. Even a lengthy justification can be shaped into a two-page document using a new printer that has the ability to select different sizes and shapes of fonts as well as spacing for printing.

To make the best impression on the reader, the justification should be clear, attractive, and free from therapeutic jargon. In a way this piece of documentation is somewhat akin to a sales promotion as the clinician is trying to "sell" the funding source not only on providing financial assistance on the recommended equipment but also on the credibility of the recommendations. A justification written in a professional manner, using correct English, punctuation, and spelling, has a better chance of receiving proper attention by funding agencies.

Since the justification is written in the form of a letter, the salutation is important. For the greatest impact on the prospective funding source, the salutation should greet the reader by name. For the reader, a salutation of "To whom it may concern" may show the need for assistive technology, but it may also be an indication of inadequate follow-through of the team requesting funding assistance. It may take some work to find the exact name of the person in charge of determining funding and to obtain the correct spelling, but the payoff in terms of receiving funding is worth the time and energy expended.

Following the salutation, the justification should contain identifying information (name and birthdate at the minimum) about the person for whom the equipment is being recommended, a statement of the person's diagnosis with a description of the nature of the disability stated in functional terms, a statement regarding the person's abilities, and a prognostic statement regarding the improved ability to function with the device. The prognostic statement can contain information on potential changes in life functioning, including potential maximization, environmental control, independence enhancement, and self-sufficiency improvement.

The next sections should describe the device (model number and company, with address) and discuss the benefits for the person for whom funding is being sought. If there are optional components requested for the device, each piece should have a brief description with a short statement of justification. These individual justification statements for each adaptation, seemingly tedious at the time of writing, may provide necessary information to the decision makers. Unjustified components often result in funding denials that require lengthy appeals.

Several other areas may warrant inclusion in justification documents. Sometimes the funding agency requests that costs be listed in the justification, but often the prices come from another source, the durable medical equipment dealer who was involved in the assistive technology team. Communication with the funding source prior to writing the justification can clarify this issue. Another area that may be included in the justification is a description of the persons comprising the team that evaluated and made the recommendations for the person needing assistive technology. Most funding agencies laud a multidisciplinary evaluation effort with evidence of consumer involvement. Borin (1990) writes that if other pieces of equipment have been tried without success, specific information regarding those devices and the reason for failure should be cited in the justification. This aspect may anticipate questions from funding sources about other equipment available. If equipment had been leased for a trial period, the person's performance with the assistive technology should be documented for the agency making a decision about financial assistance.

A successful formula for the justification is the identification of the person, diagnosis, functional statement, and evaluation team in the first paragraph, with the name of the assistive technology device being requested in the last sentence. The middle paragraphs should contain the individual justification statements for each component of assistive technology being requested. The last paragraph should start by thanking the agency for consideration and assistance, followed by a statement describing some possible consequences for the person needing assistive technology if the device is not funded, and end with a name and telephone number to contact if the agency has any questions. The practitioner should complete the justification with a signature and the complete name and credentials (nonabbreviated versions) of the occupational therapy practitioner requesting funding. The clinician should remember to use terminology that is consistent with the funding agency from which financial assistance is being sought.

Conclusion

Following the text in this chapter, several letters are shown that have been successful in obtaining funding for assistive technology. Since funding requirements change from state to state and locale to locale, these documents should be read as guidelines, not copied and used verbatim. Computer technology has assisted in automating justification writing to the point that portions of many of the carefully worded justification documents used in the past may be saved and reused for persons with similar assistive technology recommendations.

An alternative to the justification letter, the Seating/Wheeled Mobility Payment Review Summary, is a form developed by the Specialized Product/Equipment Council through RESNA, an interdisciplinary association for the advancement of rehabilitation and assistive technologies. The form, designed to serve as a communication link between the clinical team and the funding source, summarizes information and organizes evaluation materials and methods (Borin, 1990). Developed to improve the efficiency and effectiveness of the prior authorization system for assistive technology, this form provides a consistent format for concise and complete information regarding the person needing equipment and the adaptive device being recommended by the team. While the Seating/Wheeled Mobility Payment Review Summary deals with only one aspect of adaptive equipment, similar forms using the same format could be developed for other areas of assistive technology. Before using this form or any other formal format, the clinician should check with the funding agency to determine whether the decision makers will accept the form and whether other information will be required.

Two advocacy purposes are accomplished by documentation that is successful in receiving assistive technology financial assistance. First, for the person who needs the adaptive device, the equipment purchased with the requested funds will produce a marked change in his or her quality of life. The second aspect of advocacy is more global in nature. While adaptive devices seem expensive at the onset, assistive technology is proving to be cost saving. Occupational therapy practitioners should not stop communicating with the funding agency after equipment has been approved for funding. Rather clinicians should thank the agency for the needed financial assistance and keep staff members apprised of the user's ongoing progress with the device. This will keep doors open with the funding agency for future requests and also present a current picture of the use of assistive technology. System change occurs more easily at a local level, but clinicians can influence the funding system at the legislative level by showing evidence of successful equipment funding in case studies that have been well-documented to show cost benefits.

References

ABCs of funding. (1990, Spring). *Pin Dot News, 3*(1), 1-2.

Beck, J. (1991). Consumer advocacy: The key to funding. *Communication Outlook, 12*(4), 7-9.

Borin, L. (1990). Documentation for specialized adaptive equipment. *AOTA Developmental Disabilities Special Interest Section Newsletter, 13*(1), 1-2.

Claims denials: Tips on keeping your cool and getting paid. (1991). *OT Week, 5*(7), 9.

DeShaw, D. (1990). Funding issues. *Assistive Technology Information Network, 4*(4), 1-2.

Enders, A. (1988). *The bottom line: Finding funding for technology*. Seminar conducted at the International Conference of the Association for the Advancement of Rehabilitation Technology, Montreal, Canada.

Golinker, L. (1991). *You want us to fund what?* Ithaca, NY: United Cerebral Palsy Associations.

Hofmann, A. C. (1990). The many faces of funding. In B. M. Reid (Ed.), *Branching out in the 90s.* Denver, CO: Colorado Department of Education.

Luebben, A. J. (1986). Low cost high tech: People, equipment, and money resources. In H. J. Murphy (Ed.), *Proceedings of the Second Annual Computer Technology/Special Education/Rehabilitation Conference, 2*, 225-239.

Mendelsohn, S. (1991). Tax deductibility of assistive technology: A hidden federal subsidy. In H. J. Murphy (Ed.), *Proceedings of the Sixth Annual Conference on Technology and Persons with Disabilities, 6*, 639-648.

Pressman, H. (1987). Funding technology devices. *Exceptional Parent, 17*(7), 48-52.

Reimbursing adaptive technology. (1989, Winter). *NARIC Quarterly, 2*(4), 1, 7-11, 13-15, 17.

Rice, S. R. (1991). Funding assistive technology: Charting the waters of loan programs. In Siegel, J. D. (1991). Strategies for reimbursement. *Proceedings of the Seventh International Seating Symposium: Seating the Disabled, 7*, 263-265.

The Technology-Related Assistance for Individuals with Disabilities Act of 1988, 29 U.S.C. §2201 (1988).

Trefler, E. (1989). The funding challenge for pediatric technology. In *The AOTA practice symposium 1989: Program guide* (pp. 38-42). Bethesda, MD: American Occupational Therapy Association.

Figure 12.1 Initial letter requesting adaptive equipment

PL
Crippled Children's Services
Extant, IL

Dear PL,

During school annual reviews this year LP, the mother of EP (DOB: 1982), a student with a diagnosis of cerebral palsy resulting in spastic quadriplegia, indicated that the family was having difficulty placing EP in the bathtub and supporting her during her bath. Mrs. Powers asked about the availability of bath chairs. After sending her information with specific measurements, the family decided [on] the Ortho-Kinetics (W220 N507 Springdale Road, P.O. Box 436, Waukesha, WI 53187, 800-558-7786) 52-inch TLC bath chair (#6741) with waterproof headrest (#6701-01). In addition to utilizing the device for its intended purpose, the family will also use the bath chair for an extra positioning device both in the house and in the yard during nice weather.

Mrs. P also inquired about the adaptive toilet chair utilized in the classroom. As part of her classroom programming, EP uses a stand-alone child-sized potty chair for toilet training and has been most successful. To ensure continuity and also decrease the need to buy expensive diapers, I recommend that she have the same system at home. The chair is a wooden and metal chair manufactured by Rifton, Route 313, Rifton, NY, 12471, 914-658-3141. Recommended are E82, Large Child's Potty Chair; E822, Backpad; E817, Footrest with seven inch sandals; and E861, tray. All components may be found on page four of the 1990/91 Rifton catalog.

Thank you for your assistance in this matter. The bath chair and potty chair will afford safety and optimal positioning during bathroom tasks. If you have any questions, please contact me at the above number.

Sincerely yours,

Aimee J. Luebben
Licensed Occupational Therapist
Certified Educator

Figure 12.2 Initial letter requesting augmentative communication device

KB
Community Club
King Road
St. Louis, MO

Dear KB,

In the course of speaking with you in the last few years, I have mentioned that I will be coming to you sometime in the future to ask for funding on a speech prosthesis for a very deserving person. CA (DOB: 1973) is the young man I have been speaking about and he is now ready to have his own RealVoice augmentative communication device.

CA has a diagnosis of cerebral palsy resulting in spastic quadriparesis. So motorically involved that he is unable to speak and has little reliable, voluntary movement, CA makes laughing noises at jokes so we know that intelligence is locked inside his body. One day, when we first got the computer at school and provided access for CA, we found that he knew his colors, shapes, letters, and numbers, all of which had been untestable in the past. For the last two years CA has been using my RealVoice two days a week when I am scheduled to be in his facility and a flashlight when the RealVoice is unavailable. In the classroom he now makes requests by utilizing the RealVoice.

There is excellent followup at home. CA's mother is a teaching assistant in an early childhood classroom and his sister, TA, is working while going to school to become an early childhood teacher. They report CA is much more relaxed at home than at school and is able to accomplish some complex motor movements. With the consistent success we have had at school, we had a team meeting of teacher, teaching assistants, speech pathologist, and therapists and decided CA was ready for his own device. After consultation with the speech pathologist, we recommend that CA have a similar system for his own use. Available from Adaptive Communication Systems (800-247-3433) and recommended are a RealVoice (male) with the light board placed in a pan that fits over the keyboard, a light pointer, and a Quick and Easy Mount to attach the system to his wheelchair. His wheelchair is new and was funded through CHAMPUS, but this insurance does not fund communication devices.

His mother, LA, is aware there is an application process for Community Club funding process and eagerly awaits your information. Thank you for your assistance in this matter. With a speech prosthesis, CA will not only gain a "voice," but also will be more independent and have some control over one aspect of his life. If you have any questions, please contact me at the above number.

Sincerely yours,

Aimee J. Luebben
Licensed Occupational Therapist
Certified Educator

Figure 12.3 Initial letter requesting custom positioning after trying other systems

JR
Crippled Children's Services
Extant, IL

Dear JR,

JF of Rehab Medical; JO, Physical Therapist; BT, Physical Therapist Assistant; and I evaluated CH (DOB: 1974) for a seating and mobility system. CH has a diagnosis of cerebral palsy resulting in right spastic hemiparesis and, because of her physical limitations, requires assistance for all activities.

Her current system consists of an Everest and Jennings standard manual wheelchair with Otto Bock lateral supports, heel loops, lap belt, and lap tray. Since the Pin Dot prefabricated contour seat did not provide adequate positioning, it was removed and she is now sitting on a piece of egg crate foam, but assumes a windswept posture with her hips twisted and trunk flexed laterally to the other side. At the last clinic her physician prescribed that CH wear her body jacket all day. Although she wears it at school, compliance with the wearing of the orthosis at home is inconsistent. Because CH has the functional use of one arm, independent propulsion for mobility of a standard wheelchair is difficult and slow.

Recently CH had a trial use of a Meyra one hand drive (left) mobility system. As soon as she was placed in the chair, she was able to propel herself independently and was learning to fine tune maneuvers such as turning and backing up. This same Meyra system we recommend for mobility.

The seating system is more easily assessed by separating the back from the seat component. We recommend a Jay Back with deep lateral supports that will accommodate CH during the times when she is wearing the orthosis and when she is not. A Danmar chest harness will assist in providing circumferential type pressure at the trunk when the orthosis is removed. She has been positioned in just about every other type of planar, hybrid, and prefabricated contour seat available; positioning was unsatisfactory in each case. For this reason we recommend a contour seat, custom fabricated for CH.

Since her feet move around in the standard foot plate with figure eight straps, a more aggressive system, shoe positioners/channels, is recommended for CH. We recommend a laptray for anterior upper extremity support and a surface for fine motor activities, and a hip strap mounted at 45 degrees of the hip angle to position her correctly in the chair.

Thank you for your assistance in this matter. With a one arm drive mobility system CH will gain more independence and control of her life; the seating system will provide support for postural integrity and decrease the potential for surgical procedures. If you have any questions, please contact me at the above number.

Sincerely yours,

Aimee J. Luebben
Licensed Occupational Therapist
Certified Educator

Figure 12.4 Initial letter requesting customized seating and wheeled mobility system

LS
Medical Social Consultant
Crippled Children's Services
High Street, Nemo, IL

Dear LS,

JF of Rehab Medical and I evaluated JC (DOB: 1971) on July 23, 1990 with JC's mother, a caregiver, and two people from UCP present during the assessment. JC is currently not using a wheelchair. He has been unable to tolerate his current planar type manual push wheelchair and was placed on homebound status in his school district since he screamed when placed into his old wheelchair. JC has a diagnosis of cerebral palsy resulting in spastic quadriplegia. He currently has no method of positioning and desperately needs a new wheelchair.

JC's muscle tone is increased and a strong asymmetrical tonic neck reflex interferes with positioning. Secondary to hypertonia JC's range of motion is limited; he has fixed deformities of the hips, shoulders, knees, and elbows and tightness in other joints. Little voluntary movement was observed; however, it was noted that when the seating system was completed, JC relaxed his fisted hands.

Because of his severe deformities and physical limitations, a standard, planar seating system is not reasonable or appropriate and a contour seating system custom molded to his body is needed for proper support. He was fitted in a molding frame adjusted to accommodate the few degrees of trunk flexion he has. The Comfi back and seat cushions are Contour U components which will be fabricated from soft supportive material from the molds made of JC on site.

While the molds of the seating system were custom molded during the assessment, the mobility unit was researched and carefully selected since the seating system approximates a full reclining position. A Motion Designs Zippie Tilt wheelchair was chosen, and the 14 inch wide seating system will fit between the bars of the 16 inch frame. The tilt mechanism is recommended because, with the presence of primitive reflexes, it is necessary to angle JC in space to provide position changes and shifts in weight-bearing areas. The standard Zippie seating system was deleted and trunion and pan components will be used to attach the seating system to the mobility unit.

Thank you for assistance in this matter. A new wheelchair will provide necessary support to assist in maintaining JC's remaining postural integrity. If you have any questions, please contact me at the above number.

Sincerely yours,

Aimee J. Luebben
Licensed Occupational Therapist
Certified Educator

Figure 12.5 Initial letter requesting van modifications

PL
Crippled Children's Services
Extant, IL

Dear PL,

CC (DOB: 1987) has recently been fitted with a standard type wheelchair in a child's size. As you recall, CC has a diagnosis of cerebral palsy resulting in spastic diplegia and is dependent on others for her self care needs. The family has purchased a minivan, but needs financial assistance in obtaining a lift for the van. To promote safety in moving CC into and out of the family's transportation system as well as during travel, I recommend the van be modified by professionals to include a lift and the appropriate wheelchair tiedowns.

Thank you for your assistance in this matter. If you have any questions, please contact me at the above number.

Sincerely yours,

Aimee J. Luebben
Licensed Occupational Therapist
Certified Educator

Figure 12.6 Initial letter requesting expensive seating and wheeled mobility system

BJ
Nursing Consultant
Crippled Children's Services
High Street
Nemo, IL

Dear BJ,

LY, Physical Therapist, JF of Rehab Medical, and I evaluated HE (DOB: 1975) for a new seating and power mobility system. As you know he has a diagnosis of high-level spinal cord injury and is outgrowing his present system which has not proven reliable in terms of mobility.

Because HE is unable to manually operate a wheelchair, we recommend another powerdrive wheelchair, a narrow adult model with an 18 inch seat depth. He must recline at various times during the day to shift his weight and prevent costly skin breakdown; for this a tilt and zeroshear recline mechanism is recommended for HE.

To access the mobility and recline mechanisms, recommended are the following: a joystick mount, a short throw chin joystick with appropriate hardware and electronics, and a dual function recline interface. The interface mounting kit will be mounted on a bib and will not swing out of HE's range as his current system does. HE needs a ventilator and battery tray with adaptor mounts to support his various supportive apparatus and two batteries for his use.

For the seating system HE is positioned well in an extra long Jay cushion with adductor pads, hip guides, and an abductor. The Jay is a hybrid cushion which provides the proper support while assuring skin integrity via flotation gel. An Otto Bock headrest with multiaxis offset hardware and headrest adaptor mount will provide support for his head and two large scoliosis pads with left and right support hardware will align his body within the narrow adult wheelchair.

A buckle seat belt mounted at 45 degrees to the angle of his hips will keep HE back in the wheelchair, and an acrylic tray will provide necessary anterior upper extremity support. To position his feet properly, angling footplates and velcro straps are needed.

Thank you for your assistance in this matter. If you have any questions, please contact me at the above number.

Sincerely yours,

Aimee J. Luebben
Licensed Occupational Therapist
Certified Educator

Figure 12.7 Appeals letter requesting additional funds for adaptations to seating and wheeled mobility system

JR
Crippled Children's Services
Extant, IL

Dear JR,

I understand Illinois Medicaid has placed a ceiling dollar amount on specific seating adaptations. In a letter dated April 22, 1991 I outlined specific recommendations for a seating system for MS (DOB: 1986) who has outgrown his Orthokinetic travelchair. According to the dealer, Rehab Medical, Medicaid has allowed limited funding for three specific pieces of equipment: a biangular back, trunk laterals, and Danmar harness. This letter is written to clarify why these specific wheelchair adaptations were recommended and to reiterate the medical necessity of these particular devices.

MS has a diagnosis of cerebral palsy resulting in spastic diplegia and he prefers sitting in his current wheelchair with his back in a rounded position. This is causing a reversal of the normal curves of his back and is also promoting scoliosis. If this process is not retarded, MS will require costly surgical procedures for correction. The biangular back is designed to assist MS in sitting up straight and to discourage leaning over. The laterals recommended for his trunk are more expensive as they are curved. The curved devices are stronger and decrease the potential for skin breakdown. Since we have already tried the harness that meets the Medicaid dollar amount without success as the straps move off his shoulders during bus transportation, the Danmar chest harness, a one piece design that can be bent to fit MS's chest shape, was recommended.

Thank you for your assistance in this matter. In all of our recommendations we try to provide the optimal positioning for the best value, and as Illinois taxpayers, we are mindful of the costs involved. The three specific pieces of equipment are the ones that are needed to provide support for postural integrity, decrease the potential for surgical procedures, and allow safety during transportation. If you have any questions, please contact me at the above number.

Sincerely yours,

Aimee J. Luebben
Licensed Occupational Therapist
Certified Educator

13. Documentation Review

Cathy Crispen Pinson, MA, OTR/L

It is usually difficult to review your own notes and look for omissions. This author presents a form for chart review based on the Medicare Part B guidelines, the most stringent reimbursement guidelines. It is therefore an excellent tool to review your own notes or to conduct peer review of documentation. It offers a valuable tool for improving documentation.

Cathy Crispen Pinson was formerly Payment Program Manager for the American Occupational Therapy Association and is currently Assistant Professor in the Occupational Therapy Program at Shenandoah University, Winchester, Virginia. She is an experienced medical reviewer of Medicare and third party payer claims.

After a patient has received occupational therapy services and the appropriate documentation has been completed, the service provider then sends the payer of record the bill for those services performed. The payer may elect to complete a medical review of the claim to ensure that the occupational therapy services billed were actually covered by the patient's policy or the payer's coverage guidelines. In many instances, to complete the medical review, the payer requests the documentation from the provider of the services. This documentation is then reviewed for two purposes: technical accuracy and medical necessity. Claims are paid or denied based upon both the accuracy and the appropriateness of the therapist's documentation.

When reimbursement is denied or delayed, it is frequently due to insufficient documentation or technical errors. It is recommended that the therapist take time to review the documentation and claim form before they are sent to the payment source to screen the material for errors or incomplete documentation. It is now a requirement of Joint Commission on Accreditation of Healthcare Organizations (JCAHO) that periodic review of claims and documentation occurs on an ongoing basis in accredited facilities.

The Documentation Review Form

The guidelines and sample forms presented in this chapter are to assist therapists in providing the proper documentation and patient information necessary for a fair review of their claims to any payment source. Figure 1 shows a typical patient information sheet. Figure 2 shows a sample documentation review form.

Payers such as Medicare, Medicaid, worker's compensation, and private insurance companies have personnel that perform the review of therapy claims. A majority of the reviewers are not occupational therapists; they are nurses or other health care professionals. Payers have varied criteria or guidelines for reviewing their respective claims.

Since the Health Care Financing Administration (HCFA) Medicare, Part B Medical Review Guidelines are the most stringent of all payers, using the elements in these guidelines to review documentation will ensure that it meets or exceeds the standards of all payers.

Technical Aspects

The first step in a payer medical review and in a peer review is to check the claim for the correct patient information (technical requirements). A review of the technical requirements (a Level 1 Review for Medicare purposes) typically includes verifying the ICD-9-CM (*International Classification of Diseases-9th Revision*) diagnosis code(s) that correlate with the diagnosis that is directly related to the occupational therapy service rendered. The ICD-9-CM diagnosis codes are frequently found on the patient's medical chart or can be found in the ICD-9-CM code manual (U.S. Department of Health and Human Services, 1996). The first or primary code that is listed on the therapy claim should be for the primary functional problem for which occupational therapy services are provided. You may list a secondary code if there is an additional problem that relates to occupational therapy treatment. If a diagnosis code is listed that pertains to the medical treatment of the patient, such as ICD-9-CM code 599.0 (Urinary Tract Infection), and not the problem necessitating therapy, such as ICD-9-CM code 342.1 (spastic

Figure 13.1 Medicare Outpatient Part B, therapy billing information (OT,SP,IT,PR,CR)

Item 10-Patient's Name:		Smith, Margaret	
Item 22-Billing Period:		08/13--9/13	
Item 28-Occurence Code:	11	Onset Date:	06/21
Item 33-Occurence Code:	35	Start of Care Date:	07/13
Item 51-Revenue Code:	430	(OT-430, SP-440, IT-412, PR-949, CR-943)	
Item 52-Visits:		11	

Actual number of visits this billing period

Item 68-HIC: 123   45   6789A

Patient's Health Insurance Claim Number

Item 77-Primary Diagnosis: Multiple Sclerosis

Diag. must substantiate why therapy is being given

ICD-9 CODE: 340

Therapist: OTR   Date: 10/18

hemiplegia), the claim may be denied because the patient does not require skilled occupational therapy for that particular primary code.

The technical review also includes verifying the onset date for the occupational therapy treatment diagnosis and the date of the start or the occupational therapy care. Only in rare instances should these dates be the same. The onset date should precede the start of care date (see Figure 13.1).

The number of treatment visits should also be listed on the bill. If the initial evaluation visit(s) fall within that billing period, those should appear in the visit total. Frequently, the number of procedures given during the visit (session) is mistaken for the number of actual visits. This error causes the number of visits to appear excessive for that billing period (see Figure 13.1).

This information corresponds to the patient information sheet. Often billing or medical record clerks complete the above technical information on patient claims. They may misunderstand the therapist's documentation or have a lack of experience in therapy coding. If you are having difficulty with excessive Level 1 reviews of your claims, it is important to train billing personnel to interpret the therapist's documentation. If the technical requirements are met on the claim, the payer may or may not elect to further review the actual documentation to determine the "medical necessity" of the claim. The documentation may be provided to the payer in an attachment to the bill or sent in separately upon the payer's written request.

Medical Necessity Aspect

A review of the documentation for occupational therapy services typically includes the following:

- a physician's referral when required

- a physician's certification on the HCFA 700/701 form when required (see Appendix 2)

- an initial evaluation that includes a summary of the patient's medical history

- daily notations of the therapy visits

- monthly and/or weekly progress notes

- an itemized statement of the daily therapy charges.

If you use a peer review form to analyze your documentation for appropriate content and completeness of information, you may avoid the submission of deficient documentation, resulting in a claim denial.

Physician's Order

Therapy records should include a written physician's order if it is required by the payment source. The complete order should include the occupational therapy treatment diagnosis, the onset date of the diagnosis, the request for evaluation and/or specific treatment orders, an estimation of frequency and duration, the date and the physician's signature. If the physician makes a referral for services, the therapist should establish a treatment plan outlining the type of activity or procedure(s) and the frequency and duration of that treatment with the therapist's signature and the date, at the time of the initial evaluation. The physician's order can be in the form of a signed and dated HCFA 700 form. Any changes or additions to this plan by the therapist or physician must be in writing, should be signed and dated, and should appear in the record. If the physician writes specific treatment orders, they must be followed unless the therapist receives a written change in orders signed by the physician (see Figure 13.2).

Frequency and Duration

Frequency and duration of therapy are estimated by the therapist about the patient's potential to successfully attain the therapy goals within the prescribed time. The *frequency* (number of treatment sessions per week) and *duration* (length of the course of occupational therapy treatment) must be specific rather than a span of time, e.g., 5 times per week for 6 weeks (see Figure 13.2). If the initial estimate of either the frequency or duration proves to be inappropriate during the course of therapy, an adjustment can be made by documenting the change in either the progress notes or the monthly plan of care (physician's certification or HCFA 701 form).

Physician Certification

Payers such as Medicare, Part B and Medicaid require *certification* for therapy services. This is a statement written by the therapist and agreed to by the physician, indicating that the patient needs occupational therapy services. This certification is valid for 30 days from the initial evaluation/plan of care date or for 30 days from the previous certification. Many payers accept the initial written physician's order as the first certification. Most payers require that the signature is in writing, not a stamp or computer generated. The physician must also date the certification.

Certification or recertification may be placed on a form provided by the payer or one developed by the therapist, but it should contain the following elements:

Figure 13.2

DEPARTMENT OF HEALTH AND HUMAN SERVICES
HEALTH CARE FINANCING ADMINISTRATION

FORM APPROVED
OMB NO. 0938-0227

PLAN OF TREATMENT FOR OUTPATIENT REHABILITATION *(COMPLETE FOR INITIAL CLAIMS ONLY)*

1. PATIENT'S LAST NAME	FIRST NAME	M.I.	2. PROVIDER NO.	3. HICN

4. PROVIDER NAME	5. MEDICAL RECORD NO. *(Optional)*	6. ONSET DATE	7. SOC. DATE

8. TYPE: ☐ PT ☐ OT ☐ SLP ☐ CR ☐ RT ☐ PS ☐ SN ☐ SW

9. PRIMARY DIAGNOSIS *(Pertinent Medical D.X.)*	10. TREATMENT DIAGNOSIS	11. VISITS FROM SOC.

12. PLAN OF TREATMENT FUNCTIONAL GOALS

GOALS *(Short Term)*

OUTCOME *(Long Term)*

PLAN

13. SIGNATURE *(professional establishing POC including prof. designation)*

14. FREQ/DURATION *(e.g., 3/Wk x 4 Wk.)*

I CERTIFY THE NEED FOR THESE SERVICES FURNISHED UNDER THIS PLAN OF TREATMENT AND WHILE UNDER MY CARE ☐ N/A

15. PHYSICIAN SIGNATURE

16. DATE

17. CERTIFICATION FROM   THROUGH   ☐ N/A

18. ON FILE *(Print/type physician's name)* ☐

20. INITIAL ASSESSMENT *(History, medical complications, level of function at start of care. Reason for referral)*

19. PRIOR HOSPITIALIZATION FROM   TO   ☐ N/A

21. FUNCTIONAL LEVEL *(End of billing period)* **PROGRESS REPORT**   ☐ CONTINUE SERVICES *OR* ☐ DC SERVICES

22. SERVICE DATES FROM   THROUGH

FORM HCFA-700 (11-91)

*U.S. Government Printing Office: 1993 — 771-5

- a statement that is written or checked off indicating that the physician has seen the patient during the 30-day certification period (if required by the payer)

- a statement of need for continuing therapy services

- a statement of the specific frequency and duration of treatment

- a statement that the physician will review the plan every 30 days (if required by the payer)

- the physician's signature and date

- the therapist's signature and date.

Initial Evaluation

Documentation should include *an initial evaluation*. Within this record should be information to substantiate the need for skilled occupational therapy intervention. The patient's medical history should be detailed, with an emphasis on the patient's prior level of function. The record should also contain baseline functional data, in both subjective and objective form, that relate to the medical necessity for occupational therapy services. The data can be obtained in various ways and should be specific to the patient's diagnosis and functional problems and needs.

The trend of many payers is to follow Medicare's lead in stressing client-centered care. They want verification that the patient and/or caregiver(s) participated in selecting the therapy goals and activities that they feel are important to accomplish during the course of therapy. Payers also want evidence that the therapist observed the patient perform specific functional activities and determined the baseline functional level (see Figure 13.3). If the therapist notes a possible need for adaptive equipment, environmental adaptation, or instruction in compensatory techniques, there should be a correlation with the identification of factors that are interfering with the performance of the task, such as decreased ability to perform activities of daily living tasks, cognitive deficits, and/or inability to access areas of the home due to confinement to a wheelchair for mobility, etc.

Long-term goals should be listed. They should be goals that the patient is expected to have accomplished at the end of the occupational therapy treatment course (see Figure 13.3). Short-term goals that are related to the accomplishment of each long-term goal should also be outlined. The short-term goals need to be broken down into activities that can be accomplished within that monthly billing period.

Goal statements should contain two parts: the *functional outcome statement* and the *enabling intent*. A functional outcome statement identifies the desired patient performance resulting from therapy. Enabling intent identifies the method by which a therapist enables a patient to accomplish the stated goal.

Notations and Progress Notes

Many payers, such as Medicare, require that each patient visit be documented with a *notation*. At a minimum, this documentation should include the date of treatment, the length of the session, the activities or procedures, and any changes that occur in the patient's progress towards the goals.

Figure 13.3

WINCHESTER REHABILITATION CENTER
OUTPATIENT/DAY PROGRAM
PEER REVIEW

THERAPIST _____   REVIEW DATE _____

PATIENT NAME _____   REVIEWER'S INITIALS_____

INITIAL EVALUATION:	YES	NO	NA
1. OT order written clearly?			
2. Date of doctor's certification documented?			
3. Onset date included?			
4. Precautions listed?			
5. Past medical history recorded?			
6. Is there a subjective statement?			
7. Social History			
a) Prior level of function listed including self-care, home management and work responsibilities?			
b) If appropriate, is previous rehabilitation experience documented?			
c) Is specific home environment described?			
8. Are all areas addressed? (Cognition, visual/perceptual, communication, sensation, VE function, balance/endurance, driving)?			
9. Functional Status			
a) Is grid completed in full?			
b) Is type of home management indicated? If not, is reason documented for TBE?			
10. Assessment Plan			
a) Are functional limitations listed?			
b) Are there at least two strengths and two limitations identified?			
c) Is rehab potential documented?			
d) Are the expectations for improvement documented?			
11. Goals			
a) Are there at least 3 functional/measurable STG's stated?			
b) Are there at least 2 functional/measurable LTG's stated?			
c) Is patient's willingness or ability to learn documented?			
d) Treatment plan documented			
PROGRESS NOTES:			
1) Subjective information from patient.			
2) Objective information includes: c) Number of visits this claim (if documentation is at time of recertification) (NA if daily outpatient note).			
a) Treatment received (including frequency & duration)			

b) Patient's response to treatment described in measurable terms?			
c) Number of visits this claim (if documentation is at time of recertification) (NA if daily outpatient note).			
3) Assessment includes:			
a) Patient progress			
b) Reference to goals (every two weeks)			
c) Statement of remaining functional deficits?			
d) Rehab potential documented?			
4) Plan includes:			
a) Treatment type			
b) Frequency and duration in weekly terms			
c) New goals (every two weeks)			
DISCHARGE SUMMARY			
1. Reason for referral or OT order clearly written?			
2. Date of doctor's most recent recertification?			
3. Onset date included?			
4. Precautions listed?			
5. PMH recorded to include significant past medical history?			
6. Is there a subjective statement?			
7. Are the discharge plans clearly stated?			
8. Social History a. Patients prior level of function (including self-care, home management, and work responsibilities)?			
b. Is specific home environment described?			
c. Are driving recommendations listed?			
9. Are all areas addressed: (Cognition, Visual/Perception, Communication, UE function, Sensation, Balance/Endurance)			
10. Functional Status a. Is the grid completed in full?			
b. Is type of home management indicated?			
11. ASSESSMENT:			
a. Are there at least two strengths and two limitations identified?			
b. Are at least 1-2 functional outcomes from therapy documented?			
c. Has the achievement of STG's/LTG's by the patient been documented?			
d. If a goal has not been met, is a reason stated?			
e. Is the type of equipment and home exercise program we recommended documented?			
f. Is there a statement reflecting patient/family response to therapy, equipment, home program, etc.?			

Total				

Total # Applicable   _____   Total LTG # Applicable   _____
Total # YES Applicable   _____   Total LTG YES Applicable _____
Total % YES Applicable   _____   Total % Goals Applicable   _____

General Comments/Praises/Recommendations _____

_____

_____

_____

Is charge sheet present?_____

_____   _____

Signature of Participants (Reviewer):

OT\PEERREV.DAY

These daily notations are then used to write the required weekly and monthly *progress notes* (see Figure 13.3). The progress note should document changes in the patient's performance of the stated goals from the beginning of the notation period to the end. Relevant underlying factors such as pain, a change in the patient's medication, or a change in behavior or cognitive status should be related to the activity performance and noted in the documentation. If a patient accomplishes a goal, it should be noted and that goal deleted from the list. If a goal is not reached, an explanation should be provided. It may be necessary to modify the non-accomplished goals due to inappropriateness, lack of patient relevance, or the exacerbation of underlying factors (see Figure 13.3).

Discharge Summary

Upon discharge from therapy, a *discharge summary* becomes a final progress note. It should summarize progress on goals throughout the course of treatment and include any training given to caregivers, home program instruction, and equipment issued to the patient. Further need for occupational therapy services should be described as well as any follow-up that will occur.

Other Reports

Often therapists are required to supply a *report* on their patients to attorneys, worker's compensation boards, employers, schools, physicians, and other health care settings. These reports provide a means of making decisions regarding the patient by persons who are not occupational therapists or perhaps, not even health care professionals. Reports should be written with the specific audience in mind and the reason(s) for which the report was requested. The audience for whom the report is written is often not familiar with occupational therapy terminology and abbreviations, and these should be avoided. Common definitions of words should be used as well as simplified descriptions. The report contents are organized into three or four sections: introduction/ history, findings, interpretations, and recommendations/summary.

To partially fulfill the requirements of some federal and state regulations that there be a demonstration of adequate supervision of certified occupational therapy assistants (COTAs), it is recommended that notes written by COTAs be cosigned by an occupational therapist or that the therapist writes a note detailing supervision received by the COTA for that specific patient after every fifth treatment session. This is a requirement of Medicare's Conditions of Participation as well as of many state occupational therapy licensure regulations. It is wise to confirm the requirements for your particular setting.

The most frequent cause of denial is the policy, plan, or guidelines does not cover the service(s) the therapist performed. There could be several reasons why the services given by the therapist are deemed noncovered by the payer, including the following examples.

Reasons for Denial of Claims

1. *The documentation does not demonstrate that a skilled occupational therapy service was provided.* The treatment must have a certain level of complexity that can only be performed safely and effectively by an occupational therapist or COTA under the supervision of a therapist. If the patient or a caregiver could provide the documented care (e.g., daily feeding program, repetitive range of motion exercises, endurance activities, daily practice in an activity of daily living skill) or another service could provide the same care, then the skills of an occupational therapist may be unnecessary.

2. *The documentation does not show that there was significant practical improvement and progress on the patient's goals in a reasonable amount of time.* If the patient has not sustained gains, the therapy is considered to be at maintenance level or not reasonable for the expectations set. Therapists need to document movement in levels of assistance and/or improved patient response to assistance given).

3. *The documentation fails to establish that the patient with a specific diagnosis would not improve naturally without the intervention by occupational therapy.* At times, the typical progression of the medical condition would spontaneously return the patient to normal function. Occupational therapy may be necessary when there are extenuating circumstances that would hinder that spontaneous recovery. That information must appear in the documentation for consideration; otherwise the payer will assume that the treatment was not "medically necessary" for that particular diagnosis.

4. *Some payers, due to restrictions in their policies or guidelines, only pay for certain types of occupational therapy services in certain therapy settings.* Your documentation may be excellent, but the patient might not be covered in their policy for your services. It is recommended that insurance policies and payer guidelines be reviewed on an ongoing basis for restrictions or changes in coverage. Medicare coverage remains stable for long periods, but the remaining payers change coverage guidelines frequently. Private insurance policies vary from individual to individual and are the most difficult to track.

5. *A majority of payers will only pay for direct service provision.* They usually do not pay separately for the therapist to attend case conferences, staffing, or inservices. They also will not accept billing for separate documentation time by the therapist. The expectation is that these activities will be built into the cost of the treatment time.

Conclusion

It is the therapist's responsibility to demonstrate that the occupational therapy service provision is reasonable and necessary for that particular patient. The payers cannot make interpretations or suppositions based on information not present in the record. Again, it is recommended that the therapist screen the claim forms for accuracy and take time to review documentation prior to its being sent to the payer. Provision of inservices to billing clerks and medical records personnel may be useful in decreasing billing (technical) errors for occupational therapy claims. By following the documentation review guidelines, therapists should be able to provide documentation to the payer that includes all of the elements necessary to establish medical necessity for that occupational therapy service.

The documentation following this chapter is provided to gain practice using the *Documentation Review Form* (Figure 13.3) with actual occupational therapy documentation. Case A is from a psychiatric facility. Case B is from a skilled nursing home, and Case C is from an inpatient rehabilitation facility. This particular review form can be used with all occupational therapy documentation and is patterned after Medicare requirements.

References

American Occupational Therapy Association. (1994). *Uniform terminology for occupational therapy* (3rd ed.). Bethesda, MD: Author.

U.S. Department of Health and Human Services. (1989). *International classification of diseases, 9th revision, clinical modification* (3rd ed.). (DHHS Publication No. PHS 89-1260). Washington, DC: U.S. Government Printing Office.

Case A

GENERAL OBSERVATIONS

	Intact	Impaired	Comments
Grooming		✓	bizarre dress – sunhat
Affect		✓	flat
Reality Orientation		✓	x2; confused
Memory		✓	unreliable historian
Activity Level		✓	hyperactive
Thought Process/Content of Speech		✓	paranoid
Self-Concept		✓	low

INTERPERSONAL BEHAVIOR

	Intact	Impaired	Comments
Independence		✓	
Cooperation	✓		
Socialization		✓	seclusive, lacks skills
Expression of Anger		✓	
Expression of Feelings		✓	internalizes

TASK PERFORMANCE

	Intact	Impaired	Comments
Attn. Span/Concentration (30 min.)		✓	10 min, pre-occupied
Fine Motor Coordination	✓		
Decision-Making	✓		
Ability to Follow Directions		✓	1 step, requires refocusing
Attention to Detail		✓	
Organizational Skills		✓	requires external structure
Impulse Control	✓		
Frustration Tolerance	✓		
Problem-Solving		✓	requires assistance
Interest in Activity		✓	engages, lacks interest

FUNCTIONAL SKILLS

Activities of Daily Living (age appropriate)	Intact	Impaired	Comments
Self-Care		✓	has skills, does not initiate
Money Management		✓	
Transportation		✓	
Meal Planning & Preparation		✓	
Home Management		✓	
Safety & Health		✓	poor judgement

COPY

Ingleside Hospital
Rosemead, California

**REHABILITATION SERVICES
OCCUPATIONAL THERAPY
EVALUATION SUMMARY AND TREATMENT PLAN**

Patient # 00300

FUNCTIONAL SKILLS (cont).

	Intact	Impaired	Comments
Time Management:			
Ability to Structure Productively		✓	lacks self gratification
Balance of Work and Leisure		✓	imbalance
Identifies Interests/Aptitude		✓	isolative
Awareness of Community Resources	✓		
Ability to Utilize/Follow Through		✓	

Occupational Role: __unemployed__

   Ability to Function __Unable to secure or maintain employment (chronic)__

Precautions/Contraindications __none indicated__

Diagnosis (Axis 1) __Major Depression w/ Psychotic features R/o Bipolar, mixed__

Patient Goals __refused to Identify__

Referral Recommendations __none__

Comments __Patient was cooperative w/interview, but guarded in disclosing personal information.__

OCCUPATIONAL THERAPY RECOMMENDATIONS/TREATMENT PLAN

It is felt that _____ __patient name__ _____ is appropriate for and would benefit from the Occupational Therapy treatment program. The patient will be seen in occupational therapy for __1-2__ hour(s), __5-6__ time per week, or as tolerated, in small groups/individual treatment sessions. Treatment will continue for the duration of hospitalization, unless otherwise indicated by a physician order.

PROBLEM	GOAL
① PAranoia	① increase frequency + length of interactions with others
② Psychotic thought + behavior	② improve ability to sustain attention to task + conversation
③ Dysphoric Mood	③ increase spontaneous expression of affect

METHOD

___ one to one	✓ communication/self expression
✓ living skills	___ health education
✓ task skills	✓ sensory motor
___ prevocational/vocational	Other: _____

Date of Evaluation __December 8,__ _____ Therapist _____ _____ __MA, OTR__

Treatment Program Approved _____

                                 Physician

Ingleside Hospital
Rosemead, California

REHABILITATION SERVICES
OCCUPATIONAL THERAPY
EVALUATION SUMMARY AND TREATMENT PLAN

Patient #00300

ATTENDANCE CODE

✓ = Attended
E = Excused

R = Refused
O = Did not attend

Attendance from _December 8_ to _December 14_

OCCUPATIONAL THERAPY TREATMENT	MON	TUES	WED	THURS	FRI	SAT	SUN
Evaluation				comp KRK ✓	✓	✓	
Task skills							
Living skills				O	✓		
Communication/self expression							
Prevocational/vocational							
Health education							
Sensory motor							
One to one							✓/R
Other							

DATE _Dec. 14_   OT Weekly Progress Note

Patient is consistent in group attendance, responding to a kind firm approach, despite her paranoia. She is a passive group participant, observing from the periphery of the group. Problems:

1) Paranoia — Patient displays a decrease in paranoia, as demonstrated by improved eye contact and ability to respond briefly to approach. She is reluctant to engage in process, but has made the first step of attendance.

2) Psychotic thought + behavior — She continues to demonstrate psychotic thought process, as seen by her apparent responses to internal stimuli and continued difficulty sustaining attention. She does respond to refocusing and is able to work for brief periods on simple tasks.

3) Depressive Mood — She continues to appear depressed, as seen by her flat affect and seclusiveness. It is difficult to determine progress in depressed mood ⟶

Patient # 00300

12/14   because of her paranoia.

Plan

Continue to implement current OT treatment plan, with special emphasis on developing a rapport & providing structure that supports reality.

                                     JTR

ingleside hospital

Rosemead, California

UNIFIED PROGRESS NOTES

PAtient # 00300

ATTENDANCE CODE

✓ = Attended   R = Refused
E = Excused   O = Did not attend

Attendance from _Dec 15_ to _Dec 22_

OCCUPATIONAL THERAPY TREATMENT	MON	TUES	WED	THURS	FRI	SAT	SUN
Evaluation	✓		✓	✓	✓		
Task skills					✓		
Living skills							
Communication/self expression		✓		✓			
Prevocational/vocational							
Health education							
Sensory motor		✓				✓	
One to one							✓
Other							

DATE _12/22_   OT Weekly Progress Summary —

Patient is attending groups regularly and requires only minimal reminders to participate.

1) Paranoia — Although she continues guarded and is minimally self-disclosive, she has/has increased trust and is able to respond to longer interactions with both peers and staff. Posture continues rigid.

2) Psychotic thought & behavior — Her behavior is increasingly reality oriented ie although she continues to wear summer clothes in winter, she will take off her sunhat while in group. She is occasionally distractible and pre-occupied, but is no longer responding to hallucinations. She is oriented x3 now.

3) Dysphoric mood — Her mood continues depressed. Affect remains flat and when in unit milieu, she remains withdrawn from peers. She does not verbalize any feelings, needs, although she will respond to task oriented questions. ———→

PATIENT #00300

12/22 | cont.

Plan continue current OT plan. Focus on
depressed mood, by initiating one to ones to
support verbalization of feelings. ————————
X ————— —OTR

ingleside hospital

Rosemead, California

UNIFIED PROGRESS NOTES

#0030d

ATTENDANCE CODE

✓ = Attended
E = Excused
R = Refused
O = Did not attend

Attendance from 12/22 to 12/24

OCCUPATIONAL THERAPY TREATMENT	MON	TUES	WED	THURS	FRI	SAT	SUN
Evaluation	✓						
Task skills							
Living skills							
Communication/self expression		✓					
Prevocational/vocational							
Health education							
Sensory motor		O					
One to one		D/C					
Other							

DATE 12/24 OT Discharge Summary

Patient participated regularly in groups during her hospitalization. Participation within group process continued passive & required facilitation.

Initial OT goals –

1) increase frequency & length of interactions
2) improve ability to sustain attention to task & conversation
3) increase spontaneous expression of affect

Goals 1 & 2 were met; goal 3 unmet due to patients' chronic paranoia and limited length of stay. She demonstrated increased trust + ability to engage w/others. Only minimal reminders were required to elicit group attendance and she was able to dress appropriately at time of discharge.

Her speech, although minimal in content and length, was goal directed and she was able to request needs in an appropriate manner. She continued to appear depressed. Affect brightened minimally in

#00300

response to group involvement. She was not able to spontaneously interact, but was responsive to approach. Interest level in activities improved only slightly, although she was able to verbalize positive feelings related to accomplishments. Self esteem continued low.

Master Treatment Plan Problems:
Problems 1, 2, and 5 were addressed in the OT treatment plan & progress is indicated above.
Functional Abilities & Deficits:
Patient requires external structure and support to organize & follow-through on basic activities of daily living. Within this structure, she is able to carry out self care, but requires assistance in all other areas. She would benefit from a structured living environment which would provide the support required for her to maintain in the community.

K. _____ OTR

ingleside hospital

Rosemead, California

UNIFIED PROGRESS NOTES

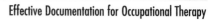

Case B

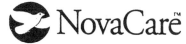

Patient's Name	Birth Date	Sex F	Eval Date: 1/3
Facility Boulder Manor Room	Medicare #		Co-Insurance #
Diagnosis IT Fx Neck of Femur (L)	Onset Date 12/20		Physician

Previous OT None

Medical Hx osteoarthritis (B) shoulders
obesity

UPPER EXTREMITY   (R) Hand dominant

STRENGTH

RT	LT	AREA	ACTION		ROM RT	LT		RT INTACT	IMPAIRED	LT INTACT	IMPAIRED
3	2+	shoulder	flex	extend	120/30	90/10	Coordination	X		X	
2+	2	shoulder	abd	add	110/90	100/90	Muscle Tone	X		X	
2+	2+	shoulder	int rot	ext rot	50/60	50/55					
3	3-	elbow	flex	extend	WNL	WNL					
3	3	forearm	sup	pro			Contracture None				
3	3	wrist	flex	extend			Tremor None				
3+	3	hand			↓	↓	Pain 4o (L) Hip pain ; (B) shoulder				
16#	14#	grip					pain upon movement				

COGNITION	INTACT	IMPAIRED	SENSORIMOTOR	INTACT	IMPAIRED
Orientation	X		Vision	X c̄ glasses	
ST Memory		X mildly	Visual Tracking	X	
LT Memory	X		Hearing		X HOH
1 Step Command	X		Body Scheme	X	
2 Step Command	X		Motor Planning	X	
Judgement		X safety	R/L Discrimination	X	
Attention Span	X		Spatial Relations	X	
Problem Solving		X	Sequencing	X	
Receptive Language	X				
Expressive Language	X			RT	LT

ORAL MOTOR			SENSATION	int	imp	int	imp
Tongue Movements	X		Lt Touch	X		X	
Chewing	X		Temperature	X		X	
Swallowing	X		Proprioception	X		X	
			Stereognosis	X		X	

ACTIVITIES OF DAILY LIVING (IND – independent; SUP – supervised; VQ – verbal cueing; MIN – minimum physical assist; MOD – moderate physical assist; MAX – maximum physical assist; U – unable; NT – not tested).

Feeding IND	Grooming MOD	Oral Care MIN	Toileting MAX x 2
U/E Dress MOD	L/E Dress U	Fasteners IND	Bathing NT
Bed Mobility MAX x 2	Sitting Balance 4-/5	Transfers MAX x 2	Ambulation NT
W/C Mobility U	Endurance 2/5		

Equipment W/C   Ted hose

Precautions NWB (L) L/E ; SOB upon exertion

Prior level of function Lived alone in Sr. Apt. complex ; (I) in self-care, functional

Add Comments mobility. 3 meals/day provided along c̄ housekeeping
& laundry services

    - Supportive family ; pt & family motivated for d/c home

REHAB POTENTIAL Good for stated goals

GOALS 1) ↑ grooming/oral care to (I) 2) ↑ U/E dressing to min, L/E dressing to mod (A)
3) ↑ func. xfers to max x 1 4) ↑ w/c mobility to mod (A) 5) ↑ (B) U/E strength, ROM
to 3+/5   LTG: (I) self-care ; d/c home

RX PLAN Self-care trng., functional mobility trng., assess for & train in use of
adaptive equipment ; (B) U/E therapeutic exercise.

FREQ OF RX 5x/wk x 6 wks AMT 45-50 DUR up to 2 months   THERAPIST'S SIG _____ OTR
then 3x/wk

FORM APPROVED
OMB NO. 0938-0233

Medicare Rx For Prescription Therapy Only
Initial - Part A

PHYSICIAN USE THIS FORM TO PRESCRIBE: ☐ PHYSICAL THERAPY (P.T.) ☒ OCCUPATIONAL THERAPY (O.T.)
☐ SPEECH PATHOLOGY (S.P.)

COMPLETE THE FOLLOWING TO ASSURE PROPER MEDICARE REIMBURSEMENT

BENEFICIARY NAME

AGE **84**

BENEFICIARY ADDRESS (Street, City, State, Zip Code)

HEALTH INSURANCE CLAIM NO.

PRIMARY DIAGNOSIS (conditions for which therapy is prescribed)
IT Fx Neck of (L) Femur 820.21

DATE OF ONSET OF PRESENT CONDITION
Month **12** Day **20** Yr

SECONDARY DIAGNOSIS (bearing on condition therapy)
osteoarthritis (B) shoulders 715.01

DATE PATIENT FIRST RECEIVED THERAPY FOR CURRENT CONDITION
Mo. **01** Day **03** Yr

WAS SURGERY PERFORMED FOR PRIMARY DIAGNOSIS? ☒ YES ☐ NO (If "Yes," indicate nature of surgery and date)
ORIF

Mo. **12** Day **21** Yr

ASSESSMENT OF REHABILITATION POTENTIAL
Good for stated goals

GOALS OF TREATMENT PLAN
1) ↑ grooming/oral care to (I) 2) ↑ U/E dressing to min, 4E to mod (A) 3) ↑ functional xfers to max (A) x 1 4) ↑ w/c mobil. to mod (A) 5) ↑ (B) U/E strength, ROM to 3⁺/5 LTG: (I) self-care a/c home

PRESCRIPTION (agents and techniques ordered — indicate changes or variations)
Eval
self-care trng., functional mobil. trng., assess for a/ train in use of adapt. equip. (B) U/E therapeutic exercise

ORDERED FREQUENCY OF TREATMENT
5x/wk

NUMBER OF TREATMENTS ORDERED
20-25

DURATION OF TREATMENT PROGRAM
1 month, renewable

HAS PATIENT RECEIVED PRIOR ☐ P.T. ☒ O.T. ☐ S.P. FOR SAME CONDITION? ☐ YES ☒ NO (If "Yes," give location and date)

LOCATION

DATE

PROGRESS SUMMARY INCLUDING PERTINENT MEDICAL INFORMATION AND SIGNIFICANT CHANGES
Pt. was living alone in apt. in Sr. complex, (I) in basic ADL's, when she fell a/ fractured hip. Eval. results indicate pt. requires mod (A) grooming a/ U/E dressing (unable to participate in 4E dressing 2° pain), max (A) x 2 functional mobility. (B) U/E function ranges from 2-3⁺/5. Pt. is currently NWB (L) 4E. Judgement/problem solving skills are mildly impaired. Skilled O.T. indicated to ↑ pt.'s functional (I) for d/c home.

*See attached eval

COMPLETED BY

TITLE
OTR

DATE
1/3

PHYSICIAN NAME

PHYSICIAN SIGNATURE (required only when used as prescription)

PHYSICIAN ADDRESS (Street, City, State, Zip Code)

DATE

Documentation Review

171

Attn. Nursing:

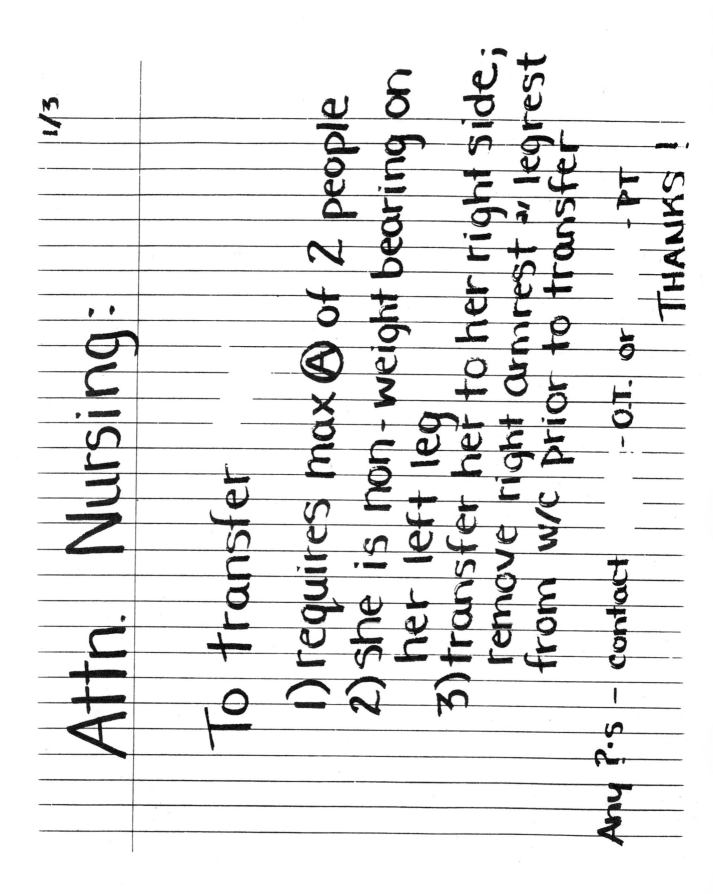

1/3

To transfer

1) requires max Ⓐ of 2 people
2) she is non-weight bearing on
   her left leg
3) transfer her to her right side;
   remove right armrest & legrest
   from w/c prior to transfer

Any ?·s — contact _____ -OT- or _____ -PT
THANKS !

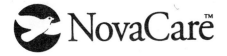
NovaCare™

FOURTEEN DAY PROGRESS REPORT

PT (OT) ST

Patient: _____ Physician_____

Initial Tx. Date: _1/3_____ Facility: **Boulder Manor**

Today's Date: __1/17_____ Tx. to Date _Eval + 10_

Diagnosis: IT Fx Neck of (L) Femur
osteoarthritis (B) shoulders

Goals: 1)↑ grooming /oral care to (I)
2)↑ U/E dressing to min, 4E to mod (A)
3)↑ func. xfers to max (A) x1
4)↑ w/c mobility to mod (A)
5)↑ (B) U/E strength. ROM to 3⁺/5

Progress:
Grooming /oral care has ↑ from min/mod (A) to (I). U/E
dressing has imp. from mod to min (A) ; 4E from unable
to mod/max (A) + use of adapt. equip. Func. xfers have
imp. from max (A) x 2 to mod max (A) x 2. w/c mobility
skills have imp. from una..e to min/mod (A) up to
50! (B) U/E grip strength ↑ from 16# to 19#, (L) from 14# to
16# Pt. voicing fewer c/o (B) shoulder pain during ADL
tasks.

Plan: Cont tx 5x /wk. Goals: 1)↑ dressing to min (A) 2)↑ func.
xfers to min/mod (A) 3)↑ w/c mobility to (I) 4)↑ (B) U/E strength/.
ROM to 3⁺/5

☒ Please sign and return

_____   ~~~~~~~~~~~   _____OTR____
         Physician   Therapist

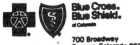

FORM APPROVED
OMB NO. 0938-0233

Medicare Rx For Prescription Therapy Only

PHYSICIAN USE THIS FORM TO PRESCRIBE: ☐ PHYSICAL THERAPY (P.T.) ☒ OCCUPATIONAL THERAPY (O.T.)
☐ SPEECH PATHOLOGY (S.P.)

COMPLETE THE FOLLOWING TO ASSURE PROPER MEDICARE REIMBURSEMENT

BENEFICIARY NAME | AGE **84**

BENEFICIARY ADDRESS (Street, City, State, Zip Code) | HEALTH INSURANCE CLAIM NO.

PRIMARY DIAGNOSIS (conditions for which therapy is prescribed)
IT Fx Neck of (L) Femur   820.21

DATE OF ONSET OF PRESENT CONDITION
Month **12** Day **20** Year

SECONDARY DIAGNOSIS (bearing on condition therapy)
osteoarthritis (B) shoulders   715.01

DATE PATIENT FIRST RECEIVED THERAPY FOR CURRENT CONDITION
Mo. **01** Day **03** Yr.

WAS SURGERY PERFORMED FOR PRIMARY DIAGNOSIS? ☒ YES ☐ NO (If "Yes," indicate nature of surgery and date)
ORIF

Mo. **12** Day **21** Yr.

ASSESSMENT OF REHABILITATION POTENTIAL
Good for stated goals

GOALS OF TREATMENT PLAN
1)↑dressing to (I) c̄ adapt. equip. 2)↑ functional mobility to (I) 3)↑ u/e strength ROM to 3⁺/5 4)↑ toileting to (I) 5) D/C home

PRESCRIPTION (agents and techniques ordered — indicate changes or variations)
Self-care trng (dressing, toileting, bathing), functional mobility trng; trng. in use of adapt. equip., therapeutic exercise, home assessment / d/c planning

ORDERED FREQUENCY OF TREATMENT
5x/wk 2 wks, then 3x/wk 2 wks

NUMBER OF TREATMENTS ORDERED
18

DURATION OF TREATMENT PROGRAM
1 month

HAS PATIENT RECEIVED PRIOR ☐ P.T. ☒ O.T. ☐ S.P. FOR SAME CONDITION? ☐ YES ☒ NO (If "Yes," give location and date)

LOCATION | DATE

PROGRESS SUMMARY INCLUDING PERTINENT MEDICAL INFORMATION AND SIGNIFICANT CHANGES
Pt. has made significant gains in tx. u/e dressing imp. from mod (A) to (I), u/e from unable to min/mod (A), toileting from max (A) x 2 to mod (A) x 1, w/c mobility from unable to (I) 150'. Pt. is now PWB (L) u/e (as of 2/1) (B) u/e shoulder ROM has imp. an average of 10° each movement; grip strength has ↑'d from 16# to 20# on the (R); from 14# to 17# on the (L). Skilled O.T. necessary to further ↑ functional (I) for d/c home.

COMPLETED BY | TITLE **OTR** | DATE **2/2**

PHYSICIAN NAME | PHYSICIAN SIGNATURE (required only when used as prescription)

PHYSICIAN ADDRESS (Street, City, State, Zip Code) | DATE

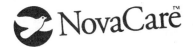
NovaCare™

DISCHARGE SUMMARY

Physical Therapy/(Occupational Therapy)/Speech Therapy

Name:

Physician:

Facility: Boulder Manor

Diagnosis: IT Fx Neck
of (L) Femur

Treatment:
self-care training
func. mobility trng.
therapeutic exercise

Date of Initial
Treatment: 1/3

Number of Treatments:
Eval: 1
Part A 28
Part B 7

History, Prior Level of Function:
Prior to hip fx pt. lived alone in Sr. Apt. complex. She was Ⓘ
in self-care, functional mobility. Three meals/day, laundry
a/ housekeeping services were provided. Pt. has supportive
family living close-by.

Therapy Goals	Initial Status	Final Status (Highest Level Reached)

1) ↑Ⓘ self-care
   grooming
   oral care
   dressing
   toileting
   bathing

   mod Ⓐ
   min Ⓐ
   mod Ⓐ u/e; unable l/e
   max Ⓐ x 2
   not tested

   Ⓘ
   Ⓘ
   Ⓘ
   Ⓘ
   min Ⓐ

2) ↑ Ⓘ functional mobility
   bed mobility
   transfers
   w/c mobility

   max Ⓐ x 2
   max Ⓐ x 2
   unable

   Ⓘ
   Ⓘ
   Ⓘ

3) ↑ Ⓑ u/e strength;
   ROM (shoulders)

   Grip strength Ⓡ 16# Ⓛ 14#
   60% active function

   Ⓡ 20# Ⓛ 18#
   75% active function

Comments: Home visit/assessment completed 2/27.   Pt. d/c'd home
c̄ following adapt. equip: raised toilet seat c̄ arms, tub grab bar,
tub safety bench, extended arm reacher, dressing stick, sock aid,
longhandled shoehorn, longhandled sponge.

Goals Met? Yes ✓   Partial_____ No_____

Reason for Discharge:
   Goals met; pt d/c'd home 3/3

Recommended Follow-up Care
   1) Aide to Ⓐ c̄ bathing 3x/wk
   2) Pt. to follow u/e exercise program as per instructions

3/3
Date of Discharge

O.T.
Type of Therapy

_____, OTR
Therapist Signature

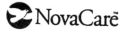

PHYSICAL/OCCUPATIONAL/SPEECH THERAPY PROGRESS NOTES

NAME OF PATIENT _____   NAME OF FACILITY _Boulder Manor_

DATES	
1/3	O.T. eval completed as per physician's order. See data sheet for details. Medicare Rx completed a̅ sent to MD. Requested a̅ received telephone order for specific tx. Worked c̅ P.T. to present inservice to Nrsg. staff on transferring pt. bed ⇄ w/c. Pt. pleasant a̅ cooperative. Plan to begin tx 1/4/89. ⌐⌐⌐⌐⌐⌐⌐, OTR
1/4	Pt. seen in AM for self-care a̅ func. mobil. trng.; B u/e therapeutic exercise. Instructed in grooming/ oral care following set-up at sink; pt. required mod A to comb hair, min A to clean dentures, able to wash face/hands c̅ Ø A. Following instruction in overhead technique, pt. able to doff blouse min A; don mod A. B u/e therapeutic exercise: AROM x 10 (AAROM shoulders), cone stacking (11 on R, 8 on L). xfer w/c → bed c̅ max A x 2, toward R, NWB L u/e. Plan to cont tx 5x/wk as per eval goals. ⌐⌐⌐⌐⌐⌐, OTR
1/5	Pt. in bed; c/o L hip pain. Instructed in bed mobility skills: rolled R a̅ L c̅ mod A, scooted c̅ max A. xfer supine → sit max A → w/c max A x 2. Groomed following set-up at sink + min A. Dressed u/e c̅ mod A utilizing overhead tech. Xfer w/c ⇄ commode c̅ max A x 2. B u/e ther ex: AROM, AAROM x 10, cone stacking, balloon toss. Pt. tolerated tx well. Cont 5x/wk. ⌐⌐⌐⌐⌐⌐, OTR
1/6	Pt. seen for self-care a̅ func. mobil. trng., ther. ex. Instructed in functional xfers for ADL's (w/c ⇄ commode; w/c ⇄ bed) c̅ pt. requiring mod/max A x 2. Rolling in bed to ↑ ease in u/e dressing (L min A; R mod A). Undressed/dressed u/e c̅ min A. B u/e AROM + AAROM (shoulders) x 10. Pt. c/o fatigue, no additional ex. attempted. Attended weekly rehab. mtg. to discuss eval results, plan of tx. c̅ rehab team. Will schedule O.T. sessions in AM, as PT plans to see pt. in P.M. ⌐⌐⌐⌐⌐⌐, OTR

MONTH	1	2	3	4	5	6	7	8	9	10	11	12	13	14	15	16	17	18	19	20	21	22	23	24	25	26	27	28	29	30	31
JAN			E	X	X	X																									

P.T. _____ O.T. _X_ S.T. _____

NAME OF PATIENT _____   NAME OF FACILITY _Boulder Manor_

DATES	
WEEKLY SUMMARY	Pt. seen for eval + 3 tx sessions. Responding well to tx a/ beginning to show progress. Plan to cont tx 5x/wk as per eval goals. ⌒_____ , OTR
1/9	Pt. seen for AM care trng; therap. ex. xfer supine→sit max Ⓐ → w/c mod/max Ⓐ x2. Performed grooming/oral care c̄ min Ⓐ. Undressed/dressed ᵁ∕ᴇ c̄ min Ⓐ + v. cues for technique. Began teaching pt. w/c mgmt. a/ w/c propulsion skills; following instructions + demonstration pt. required mod Ⓐ to propel 15'. v'd problem solving skills noted. ⌒_____ OTR
1/10	Pt. seen in AM. ᵁ∕ᴇ dressing while supine in bed; required max Ⓐ. Pt. able to roll, but unable to bridge 2° obesity, weakness. xfer bed ↔ w/c mod/max Ⓐ x2. Dressed ᵁ∕ᴇ c̄ min Ⓐ. Pt. required max Ⓐ to reposition self in w/c. Instructed in w/c mobility; propelled self 15' min/mod Ⓐ. Ⓑ ᵁ∕ᴇ ther. ex: w/c push-ups x10 (unable to lift buttocks), dowel ex: 2 sets x11. Pt. motivated to be more Ⓘ; however expresses fear of pain upon any movement. ⌒_____ OTR
1/11	Pt. seen for self-care, func. mobil. trng, ther. ex. Instructed in wt. shifts in w/c, trunk anterior flexion ex x10 to ↑ sit→stand xfers. xfer w/c ↔ commode c̄ max Ⓐ x2. Pt. demonstrated v'd fear given ample time + opportunity to Ⓐ more in her xfer: "I feel more in control." Undressed/dressed ᵁ∕ᴇ min Ⓐ. Ⓑ ᵁ∕ᴇ dowel ex: 2 sets x11. Pt. requested pain pill 2° Ⓛ hip pain: Nurse informed. ⌒_____ ; OTR
1/12	Pt. seen for self-care a/ func. mobil. trng., ther. ex. Undressed/dressed ᵁ∕ᴇ min Ⓐ. Introduced use of adaptive equip. for ᵁ∕ᴇ dressing. Instructed in techniques to don/doff shoes using extended arm reacher to open/close velcro tabs, long handled shoe horn. After 3 reps, pt. required

MONTH	1	2	3	4	5	6	7	8	9	10	11	12	13	14	15	16	17	18	19	20	21	22	23	24	25	26	27	28	29	30	31
JAN									X	X	X	X																			

page 2

P. T. _____	O. T. _X_	S. T. _____

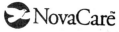
NAME OF PATIENT _____ NAME OF FACILITY _Boulder Manor_

DATES	
1/12 cont.	max Ⓐ Ⓛ shoe, mod Ⓐ Ⓡ. Instructed in w/c mobility; pt. propelled self 25' c̄ min Ⓐ (in straight line). Plan to begin to work on maneuvering w/c about in room. ; OTR
1/13	Pt. seen for self-care ā func. mobility trng, u/e ther ex. xfer bed → w/c mod/max Ⓐ x1. Undressed/ dressed u/e occas. min Ⓐ; groomed c̄ set-up, occas. min Ⓐ. Instructed in w/c mgmt. skills (locking brakes, raising ā swinging away legrests). Played "Balloon Volleyball" to ↑ active shoulder mvmt. No c/o ↑'d shoulder pain. Grip strength measured: 19 lbs Ⓡ 16 lbs Ⓛ. Attended weekly rehab mtg to discuss progress, goals c̄ rehab team. Pt. also c/o hip pain Ⓛ to P.T. ┌ ┐; OTR
WEEKLY SUMMARY	Pt. progressing in all tx areas: u/e dressing from mod Ⓐ to min Ⓐ, w/c mobility from 11 to mod Ⓐ, func. xfers max Ⓐ x2 to mod/max Ⓐ x2. Beginning to work on u/e dressing skills. Cont tx 5x/wk. ┌ ┐ OTR
1/16	Pt. seen in AM. Instructed 2 Nrsg. aides in w/c ⇆ commode xfers as pt. cont. to verbalize fear if a different person is involved in xfer. Anterior flexion ex x10, wt. shifts in w/c prior to xfer. xfer w/c ⇆ commode c̄ max Ⓐ x1 + Ⓐ of another to pull pants up/down. Pt. performed grooming/oral care following set-up at sink. Don/doff shoes c̄ adapt. equip. + max Ⓐ Ⓛ, min/mod Ⓐ Ⓡ. Propelled w/c 50' c̄ min Ⓐ. ; OTR
1/17 *14 day progress report sent to MD	Pt. seen for self-care trng c̄ instruction in use of adapt. equip, func. mobil. trng. ā ther ex. Performed grooming/oral care Ⓘ at sink. Don/doff blouse occas. min Ⓐ. Following 3 reps + constant v. cues pt. able to don/doff Ⓡ shoe min Ⓐ; Ⓛ mod. Demonstrate use of dressing stick ā dressing tape for donning pants.

MONTH	1	2	3	4	5	6	7	8	9	10	11	12	13	14	15	16	17	18	19	20	21	22	23	24	25	26	27	28	29	30	31
JAN													X			X	X														

P. T. _____ O. T. __X__ S. T. _____

page 2

NAME OF FACILITY __Boulder Manor__

NAME OF PATIENT _____

DATES	
1/17 Cont.	but pt. stated she was too fatigued to try today. Anterior flexion, w/c push-ups × 10 to imp. sit → stand xfer. Ⓑ U/E AROM × 10, cone stacking (13 on Ⓡ, 10 on Ⓛ). Cont tx. ⌐_____ OTR
1/18	Pt. seen in AM, cheerful ⱥ cooperative. Dressed U/E c̄ v. cues + Ⓐ to hook bra. Recommended velcro closure on bras; pt will ask daughter to sew them on. Don/doff shoes c̄ use of adapt. equip: mod Ⓐ Ⓛ, Ⓘ Ⓡ. Instructed new nurse's aide in w/c ⇄ commoc xfer. Required max Ⓐ of 1 + Ⓐ of another to pull pants up/down. xfer w/c → bed max Ⓐ of 1 + SBA of 1. Instructed in rolling, scooting, bridging skills to pull pants up/down: required mod Ⓐ. Ⓑ U/E AROM exercises c̄ dowel (each joint × 10) while supine in bed, no c/o pain in shoulders. Pt. displayinc ↓'d fear, ↑'d active participation in functional mobility. Cont tx 5×/wk. ⌐_____ OTR
1/19	Pt. seen in A.M. In good spirits; daughter present to observe session. Introduced use of dressing stick for L/E dressing ⱥ demonstrated its use. Pt. required mod/max Ⓐ to get slacks over feet, then remove them. Instructed in sit ⇄ stand xfers to ↑ ease for L/E dressing (× 5) c̄ pt. requiring v. cues for correct position ⱥ NWB status Ⓛ L/E + mod Ⓐ. Don/doff blouse c̄ v. cues + Ⓐ to hook bra. Daughter will bring bras c̄ velcro closures next week. Ⓑ U/E AROM × 10, cone stacking (14 on Ⓡ, 11 on Ⓛ), balloor toss. No c/o shoulder pain. Cont tx. ⌐_____ OTR
1/20	Pt seen for self-care ⱥ func. mobil. trng. ↓ther ex. Instructed in use of adapt. equip for L/E dressing. Using dressing stick. pt able to don/doff panties min/mod Ⓐ. slacks mod Ⓐ (excluding standing to pull them up). Don/doff Ⓡ shoe Ⓘ Ⓛ shoe min/mod Ⓐ

MONTH	1	2	3	4	5	6	7	8	9	10	11	12	13	14	15	16	17	18	19	20	21	22	23	24	25	26	27	28	29	30	31
JAN																		X	X	X											

P. T. _____ O. T. __X__ S. T. _____

page 2

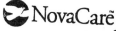
NAME OF PATIENT _____   NAME OF FACILITY <u>Boulder Manor</u>

DATES	
1/20 cont.	Undressed/dressed U/E c̄ (A) to hook bra. Pt. propelled w/c 100' c̄ min (A). Sit ⇄ stand xfers x 5 c̄ mod (A). (B) U/E ther ex AROM x 10, bean bag toss. Pt. stated she enjoyed bean bag toss. Pt. is displaying mild problem solving skills in all ADL skills a/ needs frequent verbal cueing. Attended weekly rehab mtg. to discuss pt's case c̄ Rehab team. r_____, OTR
WEEKLY SUMMARY	Pt. cont. to make progress in all tx areas: U/E dressing from min (A) to (A) to hook bra only, U/E from max to mod (A), grooming/oral care from set-up, occas. min (A) to (I), func. xfers from mod/max (A) x 2 to max (A) x 1 + SBA of 1. w/c mobility skills ↑ from mod (A) to min (A) 100'. Plan to cont tx 5x/wk as per stated goals. r_____, OTR
1/23	Pt. seen in AM for self-care a/ func. mobil. trng, ther ex. Pt's daughter had brought in bras c̄ velcro closures. Instructed in donning/doffing bra x 3; on 3rd attempt pt was (I). U/E dressing c̄ use of adapt. equip. Min/mod (A) to don/doff panties a/ slacks (s̄ standing to pull them up). Don/doff shoes x 2 c̄ adapt equip + min (A) (L). Pt. refused any further tx "I feel like I'm coming down c̄ something." Nrsg. informed. r_____, OTR
1/24	Attempted to see pt in AM. Stated she wasn't feeling well. Checked c̄ Nrsg; pt had temp. of 100.7°, "flu-like" symptoms. No tx. r_____, OTR
1/25	Pt. ill. No tx r_____, OTR
1/26	Pt. ill No tx. r_____, OTR
1/27	Pt. seen in AM. Stated she was feeling better a/ ready to resume tx. Cleared c̄ Nrsg. Instructed in dressing skills c̄ use of adapt. equip. Undressed/dressed U/E c̄ v. cues. Don/doff U/E clothing (s̄ coming to stand)

MONTH	1	2	3	4	5	6	7	8	9	10	11	12	13	14	15	16	17	18	19	20	21	22	23	24	25	26	27	28	29	30	31
																							X	I	I	I	X				

P.T. _____	O.T. X_____	S.T. _____

page 2

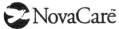 NovaCare

PHYSICAL/OCCUPATIONAL/SPEECH THERAPY PROGRESS NOTES

NAME OF PATIENT _____   NAME OF FACILITY _Boulder Manor_____

DATES	
1/27 cont.	c̄ min Ⓐ. Worked on sit⇄stand xfers in preparation for standing to pull pants up. Required min/mod Ⓐ; able to let go c̄ 1 hand. Expressed ↓'d fear, no c/o Ⓛ hip pain. Ⓑ U/E AROM x 10, cone stacking (13 on Ⓡ 11 on Ⓛ). Pt. fatigued easily, but no notable func. loss following bout c̄ "flu." Attended weekly rehab. mtg. to discuss pt's case c̄ rehab team. P.T. reports pt. to have x-ray 2/1/89 c̄ possible change in weight-bearing status on that date. ⌃_____, OTR
WEEKLY SUMMARY	Pt. ill 3 days this week. Progressed from mod Ⓐ to min/mod Ⓐ sit⇄stand xfers. Expressing ↓'d fear when standing, & now able to let go of walker c̄ 1 hand. Pt. now Ⓘ in U/E dressing c̄ use of Velcro-closure bras. Cont tx 5x/wk. ⌃_____, OTR
1/30	Pt. seen for self-care & func. mobil. trng, ther ex. Dressed U/E Ⓘ. Dressed L/E c̄ instruction in use of adapt equip + min Ⓐ. Sit⇄stand xfers x5 c̄ min Ⓐ (NWB Ⓛ L/E). Pt. able to adjust her position in chair c̄ min Ⓐ when uncomfortable. Propelled w/c 100' Ⓘ incl. maneuvering doorway; demonstrating imp. problem-solving skills. Ⓑ U/E ex incl. dowel ex. 2 sets x 10 + bean bag toss. Plan to begin working on pulling pants up/down. ⌃_____, OTR
1/31	Pt. seen in AM. Instructed in L/E dressing c̄ use of adapt. equip. Dressed L/E (excl. Ted hose) c̄ min Ⓐ + mod/max Ⓐ to pull pants up/down. xfer w/c⇄ commode mod/max Ⓐ x 1. Pt. propelled w/c 150' Ⓘ today (distance to dining room). Ⓑ U/E ther ex incl. Balloon volleyball, bean bag toss, dowel ex x 12. Informed Nrsg. of pt's ability to propel w/c to d.r. They will encourage her to propel herself at least 2 meals/day. ⌃_____, OTR

MONTH	1	2	3	4	5	6	7	8	9	10	11	12	13	14	15	16	17	18	19	20	21	22	23	24	25	26	27	28	29	30	31
																															X	X

P. T. _____	O. T. _X_	S. T. _____

page 2

Documentation Review

181

NAME OF PATIENT _____ NAME OF FACILITY __Boulder Manor__

DATES	
2/1	Pt. at Dr's Appt. this AM, so seen by O.T. in early P.M. X-ray reveals fx healing well; pt now PWB Ⓛ U/E. Instructed in U/E dressing skills: pt. required occas. min Ⓐ Ⓛ shoe, min/SBA to come to stand, mod Ⓐ to pull pants up/down. Xfer w/c ⇄ commode c̄ mod Ⓐ. Pt. refused U/E ther ex as she still had to go to PT a/ didn't want to be too tired. Plan to observe pt's ambulation skills c̄ P.T. 2/2. _____, OTR
2/2 *Medicare re-cert sent to MD	Pt. seen in AM for self-care a/ func. mobil. trng, U/E ther ex. Undressed/dressed U/E Ⓘ; U/E c̄ mod Ⓐ to pull pants up/down (PWB Ⓛ U/E). M.D. d/c'd order for Ted hose, so demonstrated use of sock aid to pt. for donning socks. Ⓑ U/E ther ex AROM x 11 (each joint), cone stacking (14 on Ⓡ, 12 on Ⓛ). Grip strength measured: 20#'s Ⓡ, 17# Ⓛ. Observed ambulation skills c̄ PT; requires walker + min/mod Ⓐ. Plan to begin ambulating pt. to bathroom for toilet xfers. _____, OTR
2/3	Pt. seen for self-care a/ func. mobil. trng, U/E ther ex. Undressed/dressed c̄ adapt. equip + mod Ⓐ to pull pants up/down. Instructed in use of sock aid. Following 3 reps, pt was able to don socks c̄ occas. min Ⓐ; doff socks using dressing stick Ⓘ Ⓡ, min Ⓐ Ⓛ. Ambulated 18' via walker (PWB Ⓛ U/E) a/ toileted (incl. xfer; pulling pants up/down) c̄ min/mod Ⓐ. Ⓑ U/E ther ex: dowel ex: 2 sets x 12, balloon volleyball. Attended weekly rehab mtg. to discuss pt's progress c̄ Rehab team. Nsg. reports pt. is propelling self to dining room 2 meals/day. _____, OTR
WEEKLY SUMMARY	Pt. has made significant progress this week. U/E dressing imp. from mod Ⓐ to min Ⓐ. Pt is now able to ambulat

MONTH	1	2	3	4	5	6	7	8	9	10	11	12	13	14	15	16	17	18	19	20	21	22	23	24	25	26	27	28	29	30	31
FEB	X	X	X																												

P. T. _____	O. T. __X__	S. T. _____

NAME OF FACILITY __Boulder Manor__

NAME OF PATIENT _____

DATES	
WEEKLY SUMMARY, cont.	to bathroom via walker (PWB Ⓑ UE) ⩗ toilet c̄ min/mod Ⓐ (imp. from mod Ⓐ.). W/C mobility has imp. from min Ⓐ to Ⓘ ⩗ pt. now propels self to meals. Cont. tx 5x/wk. ⌒ _____ , OTR
2/6	Pt seen in AM. Pt. lying in bed. c̄/o stiffness Ⓑ shoulders. U/E AROM (each joint x 12). Xfer supine→sit mod A → w/c min/mod Ⓐ. Dressed U/E Ⓘ; L/E c̄ occas. min Ⓐ + mod Ⓐ for standing balance while pulling up pants. Ambulated to bathroom ⩗ toileted c̄ min/mod Ⓐ. Raised toilet seat in place, but grab bar appears to strain shoulder. Will request raised seat c̄ arms to ↑ ease of xfer, ↓ strain on shoulder. Pt. stated "I finally feel like I'll be able to get well enough to go home." Cont tx 5x/wk. ⌒ _____ , OTR
2/7	Pt seen in AM. Ⓑ U/E AROM x 12. Goniometric measurements taken Ⓑ shoulders. Ⓡ: flexion 130°, abduction 125°, adduction 110°, IR 60°, ER 60°. Ⓛ flexion 110°, abduction 110°, adduction 100°, IR 60°, ER 65°. Measurements show an average ↑ of 10° each movement. No c̄/o shoulder pain. Instructed in L/E dressing techniques c̄ use of adaptive equipment (sock aid, dressing stick, reacher, longhandled shoehorn). Pt. required v. cues, occas. min Ⓐ to manipulate equip. + mod Ⓐ for standing balance/pulling pants up. Raised toilet seat c̄ arms in place; pt xferred to/from toilet c̄ min Ⓐ. Pt stated new seat was much easier. ⌒ _____ OTR
2/8	Pt. seen in AM for self-care ⩗ func. mobil. trng. ther. ex. xfer supine→sit → w/c min/mod Ⓐ. Dressed c̄ occas. min Ⓐ + adapt. equip. + min/mod Ⓐ standing/pulling pants up. Pt. has difficulty

MONTH	1	2	3	4	5	6	7	8	9	10	11	12	13	14	15	16	17	18	19	20	21	22	23	24	25	26	27	28	29	30	31
FEB							X	X	X																						

P. T. _____	O. T. X	S. T. _____

page 2

NAME OF PATIENT _____ NAME OF FACILITY _Boulder Manor_

DATES	
2/8 cont.	pulling pants up in back 2° obesity. Ambulated to b.r. via walker & toileted c̄ min/mod Ⓐ. Ⓑ u/e ex: cone stacking (15 on Ⓡ, 12 on Ⓛ), bean bag toss. Cont tx 5x/wk. ∧ _____, OTR
2/9	Pt. seen in AM for self-care, func. mobil trng, ther ex. Undressed/dressed c̄ v. cues + Ⓐ for standing balance. Quizzed pt. re sequence for dressing & stressed its importance r/t energy conservation & safety factors. Ambulated to b.r. & toileted c̄ min Ⓐ. Ⓑ u/e dowel ex: 2 sets x 13. Plan to cont tx toward ↑ing func. Ⓘ. ∧ _____, OTR
2/10	Pt. seen in AM. Worked on ↑ing standing endurance. Pt. stood c̄ walker at sink & completed grooming, oral care, hygiene tasks. Pt needed to stop x 2 to sit & rest. Undressed/ dressed c̄ occas min Ⓐ using adapt. equip + min Ⓐ for standing balance. Ⓑ u/e ex: bean bag toss, dowel ex x 13. Attended weekly rehab. mtg to discuss case c̄ Rehab team. U.R. Subcommittee denial given. Plan to cont. tx 5x/wk for 1 wk, then 3x/wk (Part B) for 2 wks. ∧ _____, OTR
WEEKLY SUMMARY	Pt. cont. to progress in all tx areas: u/e dressing from min Ⓐ to occas. min Ⓐ; toileting from min/mod Ⓐ to min Ⓐ. Ⓑ u/e shoulder movements have ↑'d approx 10° each movement. ∧ _____ c
2/13	Pt. seen in AM. Undressed/dressed c̄ adapt equip + min Ⓐ to stand & pull up pants. Pt. demonstrating imp. standing balance; no longer voices fear of falling. Quizzed pt x 3 re dressing sequence; 75% accurate. Instructed in func. mobil. skills: standing at

MONTH	1	2	3	4	5	6	7	8	9	10	11	12	13	14	15	16	17	18	19	20	21	22	23	24	25	26	27	28	29	30	31
FEB									X	X			X																		

P. T. _____ O. T. __X__ S. T. _____

page 2

NAME OF FACILITY __Boulder Manor__

NAME OF PATIENT _____

DATES	
	walker a/ opening a/ closing door, closet, drawers. Pt. required v. cues r/t safety. Ⓑ U/E ex: wall pulleys ½# wt : 2 sets x 12. ⌒ _____, OTR
2/14	Pt. seen in AM. xfer supine → sit → w/c min Ⓐ. Dressed c̄ 80% accuracy for sequencing skills (energy conservation, safety); required min Ⓐ to stand a/ pull up pants. Ambulated via walker to bathroom (PWB Ⓛ U/E) a/ toileted c̄ contact guard Ⓐ for xfer, min Ⓐ to pull pants up. Ⓑ U/E ex: wall pulleys ½# wt: 2 sets x 12. Cont tx. ⌒ _____, OTR
2/15	Pt. refused tx 2° diarrhea. ⌒ _____, OTR
2/16	Pt. seen in AM. xfer supine → sit min Ⓐ → w/c contact guard Ⓐ. Dressed c̄ 80% accuracy for sequencing; min Ⓐ to stand a/ pull up pants. Stood at sink to perform grooming/ hygiene tasks c̄ contact guard Ⓐ. Ⓑ U/E ex: cone stacking (16 on Ⓡ, 14 on Ⓛ). Grip strength measured: 20# Ⓡ, 18# Ⓛ. Plan to begin seeing pt. 3x/wk (Part B benefits). Phone conf. c̄ daughter to discuss new tx schedule, set up appt. for home assessment. ⌒ _____, OTR
2/17	Pt. seen for self-care a/ func. mobil. trng.; ther ex. Undressed/dressed using adapt equip + min Ⓐ to stand a/ pull up pants. Groomed while standing at sink c̄ contact guard Ⓐ. *rest break. Ambulated to b.r. a/ toileted c̄ contact guard/min Ⓐ. Ⓑ U/E ex: balloon volleyball, dowel ex: 2 sets x 13. Attended weekly rehab mtg. to discuss pt's case c̄ rehab team. Plan to begin working on tub xfer trng. ⌒ _____, OTR
WEEKLY SUMMARY	Progress this week as follows: U/E dressing from occas. min Ⓐ to Ⓐ for standing balance only while

MONTH	1	2	3	4	5	6	7	8	9	10	11	12	13	14	15	16	17	18	19	20	21	22	23	24	25	26	27	28	29	30	31
FEB														X	I	X	X														

P.T. _____	O.T. _X_	S.T. _____

page 2

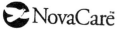

PHYSICAL/OCCUPATIONAL/SPEECH THERAPY PROGRESS NOTES

NAME OF PATIENT _____ NAME OF FACILITY <u>Boulder Manor</u>

DATES	
WEEKLY SUMMARY, cont.	pulling up pants. Toilet xfer imp. from min Ⓐ to contact guard Ⓐ. Pt. now able to stand at sink for grooming tasks demonstrating ↑'d endurance + balance. Plan to cont. tx 3x/wk for 2 wks to further ↑ Ⓘ for d/c home.
2/20	Pt. seen for tub xfer / bathing trng. Demonstrated safe tub xfer x 2 using tub grab bar + tub safety bench. Pt xfer to/from tub c̄ mod Ⓐ to lift Ⓛ leg. Bathed using long handled sponge c̄ occas. min Ⓐ. Phone conf. c̄ daughter to recommend getting raised toilet seat c̄ arms, tub grab bar, & tub safety bench. Home visit planned for 2/27. Received t.o. from M.D. for home assessment. _____ OTR
2/22	Pt. lying in bed. xfer supine → sit occas. min Ⓐ → w/c SBA. Dressed c̄ SBA + v. cues for sequencing. Pt. given written instructions for correct sequence during undressing/dressing. Copy placed in chart. When pt. gets out of sequence she has poor problem solving skills & becomes nervous. Pt. amb. via walker to b.r. & toilet c̄ SBA. Adheres to PWB status Ⓛ UE. Ⓑ UE ther ex: cone stacking (17 on Ⓡ, 15 on Ⓛ), bean bag toss. _____ OTR
2/24	Pt. seen for dressing / bathing trng. Undressed (using written sequence instructions) c̄ SBA & use of adapt. equip. Pt. xfer in/out of tub c̄ min/mod Ⓐ to lift Ⓛ leg (using tub bench, grab bar). Bathed, dried self c̄ occas. min Ⓐ + use of long handled sponge. Dressed c̄ SBA. Attended weekly rehab. mtg. to discuss pt. c̄ team. Recommend pt. have aide to help her c̄ bathing at home. Social worker will contact daughter to make arrangements. _____ OTR

MONTH	1	2	3	4	5	6	7	8	9	10	11	12	13	14	15	16	17	18	19	20	21	22	23	24	25	26	27	28	29	30	31
FEB																				X		X		X							

P. T. _____	O. T. X	S. T. _____

page 2

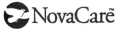

PHYSICAL/OCCUPATIONAL/SPEECH THERAPY PROGRESS NOTES

NAME OF FACILITY __Boulder Manor__

NAME OF PATIENT _____

DATES	
WEEKLY SUMMARY	Pt. cont. to make progress toward d/c home. 4̄ dressing has imp. from (A) for standing balance + v. cues to SBA; toileting from contact guard to SBA. Began working on bathing skills; pt. requires min (A) a̅ will need aide to (A) her at home for safety reasons. Plan to cont. tx 3x/wk for 1 wk c̄ home assessment scheduled 2/27. _____, OTR
2/27	Pt. seen for home visit/assessment. Pt's daughter present. Pt. xfer into car c̄ min (A) (L)4̄. Amb. up sidewalk at home c̄ SBA. Ø stairs at home. Throw rugs removed from floors for safety reasons. Bedroom: pt xfer in/out of bed c̄ v. cues. Able to manage doors a̅ drawers s̄ difficulty. Arranged clothes in top drawers. Living area: furniture re-arranged slightly to ↑ ease of maneuvering walker. Pt. able to get into/out of all chairs a̅ on/off sofa (I). Bathroom: tub grab bar + tub safety bench in place. Bath aide services set up for 3x/wk. Raised toilet seat c̄ arms in place. Pt. xfer c̄ supervision. Kitchen: sm refrigerator, sink only. Pt. receives 3 meals/day in common dining room. Pt amb. c̄ supervision only to d.r. Saw several friends a̅ informed them of return home at end of week. Returned to SNF a̅ held conf. c̄ Nrsg, PT, soc. worker re results of home visit. Plan to cont. tx 2 more sessions to further ↑ (I) for d/c home. _____, OTR

MONTH	1	2	3	4	5	6	7	8	9	10	11	12	13	14	15	16	17	18	19	20	21	22	23	24	25	26	27	28	29	30	31
FEB																											X				

page 2

P.T. _____	O.T. __X__	S.T. _____

PHYSICAL/OCCUPATIONAL/SPEECH THERAPY PROGRESS NOTES

NAME OF PATIENT _____ NAME OF FACILITY Boulder Manor

DATES	
3/1	Pt. seen in AM for self-care a/ func. mobil. tng., ther.ex. xfer supine in bed → chair c̄ supervision. Amb. via walker to sink a/ performed grooming /oral care while standing at sink.; did not require any rest periods. Pt dressed c̄ supervision + adapt equip. Referred to dressing sequence instructions x 2, but did not require V. cues. Toileted c̄ supervision. (B)u/e AROM ex x12. Goniometric measurements taken (R) shoulders. (R): flexion 130°, abduction 130°, adduction 110°, IR 60°, ER 70°. (L): flexion 120°, abduction 115°, adduction 110°, IR 60°, ER 70°. Measurements show an average ↑ of 15° each movement. Plan to see pt. for final tx session 3/3/89. _____, OTR
3/3	Pt. seen for final tx session. Able to complete AM care routine (I) c̄ use of adapt. equip (bed mobility, xfers, dressing, grooming, toileting). Daughter present to (A) c̄ d/c. Pt. provided c̄ following adaptive equip: reacher, dressing stick, sock aid, long handled shoe horn, long handled sponge. Also given written instructions for dressing sequence, u/e AROM exercises, bathtub xfers. Grip strength measurements taken: 20# (R), 18# (L). Pt. to be d/c'd home to apt. this date c̄ (A) for bathing 3x/wk. D/C summary completed a/ sent to MD. _____, OTR

MONTH	1	2	3	4	5	6	7	8	9	10	11	12	13	14	15	16	17	18	19	20	21	22	23	24	25	26	27	28	29	30	31
MARCH	X		X	DC																											

| P.T. _____ | O.T. X | S.T. _____ |

page 2

Case C

PATIENT DATA SHEET

FUNCTIONAL DIAGNOSIS: ℗ CVA, ℗ HEMI, global aphasia

REFERRING PHYSICIAN (NRH): OZER
REASON FOR REFERRAL: Comprehensive Rehab.

HISTORY:
Date of onset: 9-5
Description of Condition: Admitted to N. Va Dr's Hosp 9/5 c̄ sudden HA ℗ sided weakness, unresponsive - admitted to NORH 9/28 - recieve PT, OT, SLP. CT reveals intracerebral hemmonhage ℗ fronto-parietal c̄ compression of lateral ventrical
Previous Therapy/Surgery/Dates: ∅

Other PMHX: HYPOTENSION, HX DEPRESSION c̄ HYPOTHYROID CONDITION. Orthostatic hypotension, hypokalcemia

FAMILY/ENVIRONMENTAL HISTORY: S Ⓜ W D LIVES c̄ WIFE, SON + DTR. IN-LAW, GRAND CHILD IN HOUSE - HOUSE IS ONE LEVEL c̄ 5 STEPS TO ENTER

ORIENTATION: UNABLE TO ASSESS 2' TO GLOBAL APHASIA.

OCCUPATION: RETIRED REAL ESTATE BROKER / ENGINEER, enjoyed gardening Carpentry, mechanical tasks, music, reading, game shows, homemaking tasks
DOMINANCE: Left (Right) Ambidextrous
SUBJECTIVE INFORMATION:
Complaints: Pt expresses frustration over inability to communicate + to complete simple tasks.

Priorities: FAMILY GOALS: "HELP HIMSELF MORE, BE AMBULATORY, CONTINENT"

Activity Level: prior to 1987 - very active, employed, since 1987 - depressed, unemployed, inactive

Assistive devices used: has rental wc, glasses

PROBABLE DISCHARGE DISPOSITION: HOME c̄ FAMILY IF POSSIBLE.

Therapist(s):   Date: 10/27

NAME   INITIAL

NRH
NATIONAL
REHABILITATION
HOSPITAL

THERAPY SERVICES

FORM 200/210-008   10/85

PATIENT DATA SHEET

ADDITIONAL OBJECTIVE DATA

Address appropriate categories(s) from the following: Skin status, Respiratory Status, Muscle Tone, Balance, Coordination, Endurance, Posture/Body Mechanics, Gait, Reflex Testing, Reflex Integration, Prosthetics/Orthotics, Musculoskeletal Assessment, Cognitive/Behavioral Status.

10/27 (R) scapula demonstrates "winging" from chest wall. (R) Scapula is elevated and abducted on chest wall. (R) UE appears "ro" to have no active, however this is difficult to assess 2° pt's ↓ ability to follow commands. PROM WFL c Mod ↑'d tone at shoulder, elbow, wrist + hand. Mild edema present in (R) hand. There is 1½ finger subluxation at (R) shoulder.

10/30/91 In gravity eliminated position, pt demonstrates active elbow flexion + extension + horizontal abduction within synergy. Severe tightness noted upon PROM of pecs + forearm pronators. Moderate tightness noted in upper traps + wrist/finger flexors. Active movement is limited by tone and by pt's inability to follow commands.

11/2   Physical Therapy

Gait: Ambulation c WBQC attempted. Pt. required mod (A) → max (A) to ambulate × 5'. Gait deviations include: ① inconsistent c ability to advance (R) LE in sequence c v. cues ② ↓ isolated movement c swing (i.e. leg advanced c hip & knee flexion / abduction synergy. Pt. able to shift ^wt (To 20%) (R) in stance. Pt. requiring manual (A) to advance cane in sequence, Stairs not tested.

Balance: maintains sitting unsupported through mod. excursion maintains standing × ▓▓▓▓▓▓▓▓ requires min → mod (A) to achieve symmetry & (R) LE extension

DATE 11/1/9/

DIAGNOSIS (L) CVA, global aphasia

SENSORY EVALUATION

PAIN: SHARP/DULL

COMMENTS: *Unable to assess 2°*
aphasia - pt appears to experience
(B)UE pain at shoulder, forearm &
wrist during PROM exercises cm
Unable to assess 2° un-
reliability of pt. responses

VIBRATION: (256 cps)

Indicate most intact distal bony prominence. Test distal to proximal in the following order:

UE	LE
DIP INDEX FINGER	GREAT TOE
WRIST	ANKLE
ELBOW	KNEE
CLAVICLE	ILIAC CREST

COMMENTS: *Unable to assess 2° aphas*
NT in LE 2° cognitive
deficits

NRH
NATIONAL REHABILITATION HOSPITAL

THERAPY SERVICES

KEY:

NORMAL:	☐
ABSENT:	■
DECREASED:	↓
HYPERSENSITIVE:	↑
NOT TESTED	NT

DOUBLE SIMULTANEOUS STIMULATION

HANDS	KEY: (CHECK)	FEET
NT	NORMAL: EXTINGUISHES NEITHER	NT
	EXTINGUISHES R (WHEN BOTH TOUCHED)	
↓	EXTINGUISHES L (WHEN BOTH TOUCHED)	↓

STEREOGNOSIS

Occlude patient's vision. Manipulate objects in hand if patient is unable to do so. + = correct response; − = incorrect (explain)

R	OBJECT	L
NT	SAFETY PIN	NT
	COIN	
	SCREW	
	NAIL	
	BUTTON	
↓	KEY	↓

R	SHAPE	L
NT	CIRCLE	NT
	TRIANGLE	
↓	SQUARE	↓

PROPRIOCEPTION: Position Sense

a. Motion: Difference between up and down by passively moving upper extremity, holding at bony prominences.

RUE		LUE
NT	SHOULDER	NT
	ELBOW	
	WRIST	
	THUMB	
	INDEX FINGER	
↓	LITTLE FINGER	↓

RLE		LLE
NT	HIP	NT
	KNEE	
	ANKLE	
↓	TOES	↓

b. Position: Patient duplicates position of moved side with other side.

RUE		LUE
NT	SHOULDER	NT
	ELBOW	
	WRIST	
	THUMB	
	INDEX FINGER	
↓	LITTLE FINGER	↓

RLE		LLE
NT	HIP	NT
	KNEE	
	ANKLE	
↓	TOES	↓

KEY: NORMAL: N
     IMPAIRED: I
     ABSENT: O
     NOT TESTED: NT

NT = Not tested as results are unreliable 2° communication deficits (CM)

DLS / FUNCTIONAL PERFORMANCE

Dx: ① CVA, global aphasia   Dominance: Ⓡ

KEY:
1—Independent without equipment   4—Supervision
2—Independent with equipment   5—Assistance
3—Independent with set-up   6—Dependent

OT ☒   PT ☐

EATING	Date	11-2		
	Initials	CM		
open containers		6		
cut meat		NT		
butter bread		NT		
eat with fork		4		
eat with spoon		4		
drink from glass		4		
finger feed		4		
maneuver utensils		4		
oral motor function		4		

comments: Required cues for proper use of utensils, use of straw & rate of eating (CM)

HYGIENE & GROOMING	Date	10-31		
	Initials	CM		
wash hands cues for Ⓡ hand		4		
wash face		4		
brush teeth		NT		
clean dentures		NT		
comb hair cues for proper use of comb		4		
wash hair		NT		
set hair		NA		
apply make-up		NA		
shave—elec. & safety		NT		
deodorant		NT		
trim & clean nails		NT		
manage wig/toupe		NA		
manage glasses/contacts		NT		

comments:

BATHING	Date	10-31		
	Initials	CM		
shower c̄ shower chair Mod		5		
tub		NT		
sponge bath		NT		

comments: (equipment) Required demonstration, Mod physical assist + cues to attend to Ⓑ LE/Ⓡ LE (CM)

DRESSING (on/off)	Date	10-31					
	Initials	CM					
		O	F	O	F	O	F
hospital clothing	Max		5				
bra/male support		N	A				
undershirt, T-shirt	Max	5	S				
button front blouse/shirt	Max	5					
panties/shorts		N	A				
slacks	Max	5					
skirt/slip		N	A				
dress		N	A				
socks, hose	Mod/Max	5	5				
shoes	Mod/Max	5					
braces		N	A				
sweater		N	T				
coat							
boots							
gloves/mittens							
scarf							
tie							
other							

comments: Pt required much cueing + demonstr. s̄ difficulty following commands. Pt demonstrated neglect of ⒷLE/ⓇLE & difficulty distinguishing Ⓡ from Ⓛ extremities. Misuse of objects noted (CM)

TOILETING	Date	10-31		
	Initials	CM		
bath use appro. reg. or adapted		NT		
total bath care				
bed pan				
urinal				
empty catheter				
apply int. catheter				
skin inspection				
sterilization				
tampax				
suppository				
dig stim.				

comments:

FASTENING DEVICES	Date 10-31		
	Initials CM		
lace shoes			
fastening shows			
buttons—large/small *c̄ difficulty*	3		
zippers—side, front, back			
snaps			
hooks			
suspenders			

comments: Pt demonstrated low frustration tolerance during fine coord activities

ORTHOTICS/PROSTHETICS	Date 10/31		
	Initials CM		
splints	NA		
brace	NA		
armrest	6		
seat cushion	6		

comments:

COMMUNICATION	Date 10/30		
	Initials CM		
write name	6		
handle telephone (hold call, hold book, turn pages)	6		
typewriter	NT		
tape recorder	NT		

comments:

MISCELLANEOUS	Date 11/1		
	Initials CM		
light and hold cigarette	NA		
wind watch and set	NT		
handle money	NT		
pick up object from floor	5		
reach and remove object from tabletop	3		
operate faucets	NT		
operate doors and pass through			
operate elevator			
light switches			
open and close drawer			
use scissors			
electrical outlets			
bed controls			

comments:

BALANCE	Date 11/2		
	Initials CMS		
sitting—unsupported	*		
supported			
standing—unsupported	↓		
supported			

comments: * see obj. data sheet

BED MOBILITY	Date 10/30		
	Initials CMS		
roll to left	SBA	1/5	
roll to right		1	
supine to prone		NT	
prone to supine		NT	
sit to supine	to L/R	5 LT	
supine to sit	L/R	5 NT	
bridging		5	

comments: bridging requires min A for R LE placement; sit → supine c̄ min A → mod A & v. cues for technique

TRANSFERS	Date 10/31		
	Initials KL		
bed to chair	SBA c̄ min/mod	5	
chair to bed		5	
chair to toilet	Min/Mod	5	
toilet to chair	Min/Mod	5	
bathtub – shower chair	Min/Mod	5	
to floor		NT	
from floor		NT	

comments: Pt attempted ax c̄ tub bench transfer Mod A. Requires demonstration cues to complete. Demonstrates impulsivity CM

WHEELCHAIR MOBILITY	Date 10/31		
	Initials KL		
straight-aways	4		
corners	4		
doors	NT		
inclines			
uneven terrain			
elevators	↓		

comments:

AMBULATION	Date 11/2		
	Initials CMS		
level surfaces	*		
stairs			
inclines			
uneven terrain			
curbs			

comments (gait deviation, device, etc.): * see obj. data sheet

SUMMARY STATEMENT

THERAPIST(S):

**THERAPY SERVICES
EVALUATION SUMMARY**

PROBLEM	GOAL(S)	TREATMENT PLAN
#1 Self Care Ⓐ Feeding	S: Complete TFT as per Dr's orders L: To be determined	Eval. swallowing + self-feeding skills & provide tx as indicated ē possit referral to SSG.
Ⓑ Dressing	S: Pt will don pullover shirt ē Mod Ⓐ + cues L: Pt will complete dressing from wc ē Min Ⓐ + Min cues overall.	DLS training 2-3 x/wk ē equipment as indicated
Ⓒ Groom/Hygiene	S: Pt will demonstrate proper use of comb ē Min cues + setup L: Completion of bathing + grooming tasks ē Min Ⓐ + cues ē equipment as needed.	
#2 Functional Mobility Ⓐ Bed	S: Pt will move supine → sit in bed ē Mod Ⓐ L: Bed mob. ē Min cues	
Ⓑ WC	S: Pt will apply breaks for transfers ē reminders L: wc Mob ē Ⓢ to complete DLS & move about the home	wc mob during functional activities
Ⓒ transfers	S: Pt will complete transfer to/from toilet ē Min Ⓐ + cues.	
#3 Work/Leisure	S: Investigate premorbid interests L: Resume activity in premorbid work/leisure tasks ē Ⓢ + cues.	
#4 Sensory Motor Ⓐ AROM/PROM	S: Pt to participate in PROM exercises L: Pt to complete AROM exercises ē Ⓢ + cues.	

MR 200 / 210-009 Rev. 3/88

Effective Documentation for Occupational Therapy

**THERAPY SERVICES
EVALUATION SUMMARY**

PROBLEM	GOAL(S)	TREATMENT PLAN
® Tone	S: Evaluate need for splint to ↓ tone in Ⓡhand. L: Pt to assist in maintaining tone-inhibiting positioning of Ⓡ LE.	Splint eval + fabrication as indicated Train pt in tone-inhibition technique c̄ equipment
© Coordination	S: Pt to participate in Ⓛ LE coord activities & functional tasks L: Use of Ⓛ hand as dominant extremity for functional tasks	fine Coord + functional tasks
Ⓓ Sensory awareness - Ⓡ neglect	S: Pt to attend to Ⓡ side of tray during meals c̄ Min cueing L: Pt to attend to Ⓡ LE/Ⓡ LE, Ⓡ environment c̄ occasional cues.	SSG,
#5 Equipment	S: Equipment eval to be initiated L: DME & small equipment recommendations + train pt in use.	Equipment eval + recs
#7 Cognition	S: Continue eval using functional tasks L: Adequate cognition to complete daily tasks c̄ min/mod cueing overall.	Functional Activities Co Tx c̄ SLP
#9 Psychosocial	S/L: Provide support throughout Rehab process. S: Provide tasks to insure small success & thereby ↓ pt frustration level L: Pt will tolerate therapy c̄ minimal frustration	

THERAPIST(S):

_____ 11/3
                   Date

_____ _____ _____
Name   Service   Date

NRH
NATIONAL REHABILITATION HOSPITAL

THERAPY SERVICES

PROGRESS NOTE
Occupational Therapy ☑

Physical Therapy ☐

Treatment Period: From ___11/3___ To ___11/9___

REASON FOR REFERRAL
Primary Medical Diagnosis: _Ⓡ CVA Ⓛ hemipareas, global aphasia_
Therapy/Treatment Diagnosis: _Ⓛ hemiparesis, cognitive +
perceptual deficits_

S: _Pt is easily frustrated when completing tasks._

O: For summary of goal accomplishment and status see reverse.

A: Summary statement of functional status including underlying
factors and significant issues that impact treatment or attainment
of goals: _Pt making small gains in DLS tasks,
however cognitive/perceptual deficits and inability
to follow verbal commands has limited progress.
It is felt that he will continue to progress
in continued tx. Further, O is also necessary
to complete positioning adaptations +
splint to maintain tone inhibiting postures.
Family conference scheduled for 11/14/89_

Long term goals met or revised. ☐ No Revisions
_New LTGs stated upon completion of
therapeutic Feeding Team Eval
#1A Proper use of utensils, attention to Ⓡ
side of tray + maintain normal pace of
eating c̄ occasional cues_

Goals reviewed with and agreed upon by patient and/or caregiver
Y _✓_ N ___

Plan: _Continue toward LTG's as stated in
eval summary. Begin family training in
equipment needs at time of family
conference._

For summary of goal accomplishment, see reverse side.

Therapist: _____ Date _11/9_

Occupational/Physical Therapy Progress Note

Problem #/Title — Last Short Term Goal	Goal Met Y/N	Objective tests/measurements (accompanying forms) as well as Current Status/Comments/Why Goal Not Met	New Short Term Goal
#1A Feeding - Complete TFT	Yes	TFT completed - per results in next portion	Pt will attend to Ⓔ pels ç tray ç min cues during meal
#1B Dressing - Don pull-over shirt ç Mod Ⓐ + cues	Yes		
#1C Grooming - Demonstrate proper use of comb ç min cues + set up	No	Pt requires Mod cues + setup for proper use of comb 2° apraxia	Pt will demonstrate proper use of comb ç Min cues + setup
#2B Pt will apply ç brakes ç reminders for transfers	No	(partially met) Pt requires reminders + cues to locate/apply brakes; requires verbal contact guard / min Ⓐ	Pt will apply brakes ç reminders before transfers
#2 Pt Bed Mob - Pt will move supine → sit ç mod Ⓐ	Yes		
#3A Will review - not addressed this week	—	Pt able to perform range exercises ç demonstration + cues	
#4A Sensory Motor - Pt to participate in PROM exercises	Yes	Currently fabricating resting hand splint to maintain tone/wrist positioning	Pt will tolerate resting hand splint for 4 hour periods daily
#4B Tone - Evaluate need for splint to ↓ tone in Ⓡ hand	Yes		
#4C Coordination - Participate in Ⓔ/ⓔ coordination activities	Yes	Pt demonstrate ↑ use Ⓡ hand during functional tasks (dressing)	
#4D Sensory Awareness - Pt to attend to Ⓔ edge of tray during meal ç min cues	No	requires minimal cues 2° Ⓔ field cut	Pt will attend to Ⓔ ve/ce ç mod cues during dressing

NRH
NATIONAL
REHABILITATION
HOSPITAL

THERAPY SERVICES

PROGRESS NOTE
Occupational Therapy ☑

Physical Therapy ☐

Treatment Period: From ⁱⁱ|9 _____ To ___ ¹¹|16.
REASON FOR REFERRAL
Primary Medical Diagnosis: ⓇCVA c̄ Ⓛhemiparisis, globalaphasia
Therapy/Treatment Diagnosis: Ⓛhemiparisis, severe cognitive
& perceptual deficits.

S: _____
_____

O: For summary of goal accomplishment and status see reverse.

A: Summary statement of functional status including underlying
factors and significant issues that impact treatment or attainment
of goals: Improvement noted in attention to Ⓛextremite
which has improved patients skill in dressing and
bathing tasks. Pts frustration level during
treatment sessions has ↓'d, allowing him greater
participation in treatment with improved ability
to follow commands. Further treatment is warranted
to order equipment and complete family training
and ↑ Ⓛ in DLS and complete home evaluation.
Family conference held ¹¹/14 and wife & son
surviture. They are scheduled to participate in
treatment ¹¹/20/91. Home eval scheduled ¹¹/21/91

Long term goals met or revised. ☐ No Revisions
_____
_____
_____
_____
_____
_____
_____
_____
_____

Goals reviewed with and agreed upon by patient and/or caregiver
Y ✗ N___ _____

Plan: Continue toward LTG's as stated in
eval summary. Complete home eval. Begin
family training.
_____

For summary of goal accomplishment, see reverse side.

Therapist: _____ Date ¹¹|16.

Occupational/Physical Therapy Progress Note

Problem #/Title	Goal Met Y/N	Objective tests/measurements (accomplishing forms) as well as	New Short Term Goal
Last Short Term Goal		Current Status/Comments/Why Goal Not Met	

1A. Pt will attend to Ⓡ side ç min cues during meals — **No** — Pt requires min/mod cues. It is felt that pt. will attain this goal ç ↑ time. — Attend to Ⓡ side ç tray ç min cues during meals

1B Dressing - no STG stated — Requires mod Ⓐ + cues to don clothing

1C Grooming/Hygiene - Proper use ç comb ç min cues + petup — **No** — Partially attained- required min/mod cues + petup — Pt will insert Ⓡ UE through sleeve ç Min Ⓐ + cues. Proper use ç comb ç min cues + petup

2A Bed Mobility no STG — Requires CG/Min Ⓐ for supine→ sit during DCS routine — Supine → sit ç CG Ⓢ for DCS completion

2B WC Mobility - Pt will apply ç ç brakes ç reminders before transfer — **No** — Partially attained· requires cues to locate brake — Apply ç brakes ç reminders

2C' Transfers - no STG — Overall requires Min Ⓐ for bed, tub + toilet transfer ç equipment — W/c ⟷ tub bench transfer ç CG/Min Ⓐ + cues

4a Sensory Motor - no STG — Pt able to perf 10% shoulder ç max cues + Ⓢ — ↑ shoulder ROM ç min cues to attend to Ⓡ pole

4b Splint Pt will tolerate resting hand splint for 5 hours period — **Yes** — Resting hand splint is effectively worn. Hand-Splint completed ç wearing schedule provided to nursing — Pt will tolerate splint nightly

NRH
NATIONAL
REHABILITATION
HOSPITAL

THERAPY SERVICES

PROGRESS NOTE
Occupational Therapy ☑

Physical Therapy ☐

Treatment Period: From _11/16_ To _11/22_

REASON FOR REFERRAL

Primary Medical Diagnosis: _⊘ CVA ® hemiparesis, global aphasia_

Therapy/Treatment Diagnosis: _® weakness severe cognitive + perceptual deficits_

S: _Pt appears less agitated during treatment sessions_

O: For summary of goal accomplishment and status see reverse.

A: Summary statement of functional status including underlying factors and significant issues that impact treatment or attainment of goals: _Pt making progress in ® side awareness + DLS. Wife has participated in DLS sessions and in equipment ordering. Further training is recommended to increase comfort level c patient. Apraxia + perceptual deficits are limiting progress to a slow pace. Home eval completed 11/21/9- — see report in evaluation section of chart._

Long term goals met or revised.   ☒ No Revisions

Goals reviewed with and agreed upon by patient and/or caregiver
Y___ N___ _____

Plan: _Complete DME prescriptions._

For summary of goal accomplishment, see reverse side.

Therapist: _____ Date _____

Problem #/Title	Goal Met Y/N	Objective tests/measurements (accomp- aning forms) as well as Current Status/Comments/Why Goal Not Met	New Short Term Goal
Last Short Term Goal			
1A Feeding Pt will attend to ® plate ſ stay c min c cues	Ⓨ	Pt requires min / mod A/cue	no new goal
1B Dressing Pt will inper ®UE through sleeve c min A + cue	Ⓨ		
1C Grooming/Hygiene Pt opin use ſ comb c min cues + pick up	No	Unable to attain 2° apraxia STG revised	Pt will brush teeth c mod A + cue
2A Bed Mob Supine → Sit c Cↆ + cue	Ⓨ	Pt requires Ⓢ + occasional cↆ to move Supine → sit vertbal	Pt will move Supine → Sit c Ⓢ for DLS completion
2B W/c Mob - Pt will apply w/c brakes c reminders	No	Partially attained Pt applies brake c reminders + cues to locate	Pt will apply w/c brakes c reminders
2C Transfers - W/c → tub bench c cↆ + min A	Ⓨ	Pt's wife able to perform/assist c transfer	Transfer w/c → tub/w/c c Ⓢ using w/c program
4A Sensory Motor - Pt will progress to ® hand mapping	Ⓨ		Pt will position ®UE in/out of bed activities
4B Tone Pt will tolerate splint nightly	Ⓨ	Pt effective in edema reduction + tone inhibition Pt tolerate splint for 8 hours at night	Pt will position ®UE in weight bearing activities in sitting
4D Sensory Awareness Pt will attend to ® side c reminders in dressing	Ⓨ		Pt will incorp ®UE through sleeve c min A + cue

NRH
NATIONAL
REHABILITATION
HOSPITAL

THERAPY SERVICES

PROGRESS NOTE
Occupational Therapy ☒

Physical Therapy ☐

Treatment Period: From 11/22 To 11/29
REASON FOR REFERRAL
Primary Medical Diagnosis: ○ CVA ® hemiparesis
Therapy/Treatment Diagnosis: ® side weakness, global
aphasia, cognitive/perceptual deficits

S: Ø

O: For summary of goal accomplishment and status see reverse.

A: Summary statement of functional status including underlying
factors and significant issues that impact treatment or attainment
of goals: Pt continues to make slow steady
progress in PLS + awareness of ® side during
functional tasks, ↓ impulsivity, + ↑ frustration
tolerance. Further training is necessary to
↑ ○ c̄ PLS, further family training + complete
equipment training

Long term goals met or revised.   ☐ No Revisions

#2A Bed Mobility c̄ min cues attained

Goals reviewed with and agreed upon by patient and/or caregiver
Y ✓ N ___

Plan: Work on LTG's as stated in last
summary.

For summary of goal accomplishment, see reverse side.

Therapist: _____ Date _____

Problem #/Title Last Short Term Goal	Goal Met Y/N	Objective tests/measurements (accompanying forms) as well as Current Status/Comments/Why Goal Not Met	New Short Term Goal
#1A →7 Feeding/Cognition Attend to ⓛ side → tray	yes	Reg. min Ⓐ + cue to don shirt over Ⓛ UE	Progress w/utensils c occasional cues Pt will stand + amb parts c CG + cues
1B Dressing/UE pullor dress Ⓛ UE through sleeve	yes		
1C Grooming Brush teeth	yes	Requires set up to clearing task STG attained	
c min/mod Ⓐ + cues	yes		
2A Bed Mob-supine→sit c supervision	yes		
2B w/c Mob-apply brakes c reminders	yes		
2C Transfers w/c ↔ toilet c CG using UN frame	yes		
3 Wash/dress w/o STG		Pt refuses to participate will attempt again Now tolerating weight bearing c ↑ ability to follow through	Pt will progress up to attain D/S stand c verbal cues
4A ROM - Position Ⓛ UE in w/b activities in sitting	NO		routine c started STG
4B Sensory Awareness Ⓛ UE through sleeve c min Ⓐ + cues	yes		
5 Equipment - Complete DME prescription	yes		

14. Computerized Documentation

John Austin, OTR/L, CHT

"Render unto man the things which are man's and unto the computer the things which are the computer's. This would seem the intelligent policy to adopt when we employ men and computers together in common undertakings. It is a policy as far removed from that of the gadget worshipper as it is from the man who sees only blasphemy and the degradation of man in the use of any mechanical adjuvants whatever to thoughts. What we need now is an independent study of systems involving both human and mechanical elements."

Norbert Weiner, God and Golem, Inc. (1964)

John Austin is a graduate of the Medical University of South Carolina and Clinical Administrator of the Chattanooga Hand Rehabilitation Center. For the past 5 years, he has spoken nationally on the topic of computerization and health care documentation and has worked to help the UENet® outcomes database become a reality.

The quotation neatly summarizes the current state of healthcare informatics. The electronic health record (EHR), defined as "a computer-stored collection of health information about one person linked by a person identifier" (Medical Records Institute, 1995a) is a grand vision of computerized documentation that is moving healthcare informatics into the electronic realm. For now, it remains an elusive, but enticing, goal for vendors and clinicians alike.

Although most clinicians continue to accomplish clinical documentation by manual means, computers are slowly beginning to permeate the healthcare environment as they have infiltrated many other aspects of our lives. As devices specifically useful for the management and communication of information, nothing yet invented has approached the abilities of the computer. Ideally, computerized documentation offers an efficient and practicable means of gathering, standardizing, and disseminating clinical information to those individuals who require the different types of information clinicians can provide.

The previous chapters have described the multiple components and procedures that can make up appropriate clinical documentation. This chapter will attempt to provide background concerning the larger environment of healthcare informatics, the current state of computer technology, and insight into some of the software packages particularly useful to occupational therapists.

A Brief Historical Perspective

The traditional paper-based patient record suffers from several significant deficiencies: size, duplication of information, lack of transferability, unavailability to multiple users, and lost or misplaced information. The Institute of Medicine has reported that "11% of laboratory tests must be reordered because of lost results and that 30% of treatment orders are not documented at all." (Council on Competitiveness, 1996a). Of importance to note is the financial effects of these deficiencies. Estimates indicate that "between 20% and 30% of our national healthcare expenditures are associated with informational paperwork for the hundreds of millions of transactions that take place every month."(Council on Competitiveness). These issues are moving the healthcare industry to provide more efficient, complete and standardized information systems.

Efforts to produce computer-based patient records (CPR) or electronic patient records (EPR) have been occurring since the early 1960s. However, the challenges facing the development of the CPR are many and varied. There are technical difficulties presented by fragmentation of information from multiple medical services; the lack of standardization in inter/intra-departmental terminology; and the limited access environment produced from issues of privacy, and legal and ethical concerns. The differing media utilized to record information, the exorbitant cost, and logistical difficulties presented in hardware acquisition and installation are contributing factors. Although computers have been used in medical clinics and hospitals for several decades, they were implemented mostly for accounting and materials management purposes. These "mainframe" computers were quite large and often required specialized environments. They also required specialized training to operate and were difficult for the average individual to understand. During the early 1980s, the evolution of computer technology produced the personal computer (PC) as the Apple Computer and later the IBM PC. These smaller units began to appear in many environments, including business offices, but for purposes of creating electronic medical records, they were used primarily as glorified typewriters. They were limited in ability and continued to require specialized training in order to operate.

The early efforts to create CPRs were hampered by high cost, lack of appropriate computer technology, limited permanent information storage systems, and the unfriendly nature of early computer interfaces. Even with the advent of smaller, more powerful systems, efforts to produce CPRs today result in "computerized zones," as each department interacts with equipment and software designed only for their specific needs. They continue to be unable to access other important clinical information and test results.

During the last decade, computers have become smaller, more powerful and much easier to use. Although they continue to be utilized to create documents, spreadsheets, and database records, their ability to store, manipulate, and communicate the information these activities produce has become much more "user-friendly." In addition, they are able to gather, store, and communicate much more complex information such as photographs, sound, and video.

Because of the increased capabilities these personal computers (PC) now offer, the feasibility of using them for producing a true electronic patient record is greatly enhanced. Currently, applications directly written for medical documentation are becoming available and implemented in larger hospitals and corporate rehabilitation centers. Unfortunately, these efforts do not truly represent the grand vision of the EHR, but is a step toward that goal.

Because of the early efforts at creating EHRs, the need for developing a standardization structure became apparent. The American National Standards Institute (ANSI), a nonprofit accrediting body for standards development in the United States, formed the Healthcare Informatics Standards Board (HISB) to coordinate the efforts of system vendors, professional organizations, standards and developing organizations, and other users of standards. The resultant Joint Working Group for a Common Data Model (JWG-CDM) supports and promotes the development of a common data model that can be shared by developers of healthcare informatics standards. Working with over 1300 national and international companies; 30 governmental agencies; 20 institutional members; and 250 professional, technical, trade, labor and consumer organizations, ANSI will produce and accredit the final standard for the collection, storage, and distribution of healthcare information (Council on Competitiveness, 1996b).

A Current Perspective

The current environment concerning computerized documentation is best summarized by the Medical Records Institute's five levels of computerization (Medical Records Institute, 1995b).

LEVEL 1: AUTOMATED MEDICAL RECORDS – This involves computerization that automates functions around the paper-based record. Much of the information is computer-generated and stored as computer printouts within the medical record. Examples of automating functions include:

- admission/registration

- digital dictation systems
- accounting and its linkage to clinical information
- departmental systems (such as in an occupational therapy clinic)
- order entry/results reporting.

These systems work in parallel with the paper-based record, but the paper-based record is essentially unchanged by these systems. Information continues to be organized and displayed in a typical paper-based entity in computer printout forms.

LEVEL 2: COMPUTERIZED MEDICAL RECORD SYSTEM – This includes computerization that places the paper-based documents into a computer medical record through direct document imaging or other digitizing method. Imaging requires optical storage technology (typically a scanner, a device that converts an image on paper into digital form or "copies" the page into the computer). Documents are created on paper, then routinely indexed and scanned into a computerized system that allows multiple users to view the information much like you would in a paper-based record. However, the need to have a physical paper-based record is eliminated, and the computerized medical record can be more easily stored and transmitted.

Level 2 computerization brings to the forefront security issues not experienced with paper-based records. Of importance is that the paper-based record must be imaged as a single document. Optical Character Recognition (OCR) or Intelligent Character Recognition (ICR) technologies that digitize text in a form that can be altered are unacceptable due to the ability to modify the information. The clinician, patient ,and medical institution must be assured that the recorded information cannot be altered by others using advanced software.

LEVEL 3: ELECTRONIC MEDICAL RECORDS – This includes computerization that converts all of the processes and attributes (including legal attributes such as signatures and dates) of a paper-based record directly to computer information. The information collected is typical of paper-based records, but is rearranged for computer processes.

Several criteria are required to establish an electronic medical record.

1. An infrastructure is required for appropriate capture, processing, and storage of information.
2. A structure must be defined by computer processes rather than time-sequenced encounter information.
3. The paper-based record must be active within the computer-based records system (which can provide interactive aiding of the decision making processes by knowledge coupling, providing decision support, and other functions)
4. The record must seamlessly encompass and link financial and management functions.

The electronic medical record has the advantage of simultaneously making patient information available to multiple caregivers and standardizing terminology. Other advantages will be the ease of long-term storage of patient information, *information mining for outcomes* (a term to describe the process of producing data sets of differing types from a large database or spreadsheet), and the ability to link information to larger networks such as Community Health Information Networks (CHINs) or Public Health Information Networks (PHINs).

Security issues become paramount with the development of the electronic medical record. Of importance are:

Access Control is a method of linking abilities to a caregiver's classification within the medical community (e.g., only a physician can order medications)

Electronic Signature is a method of affixing a caregiver's electronic signature to an entry in the electronic record. (This technology already exists as evidenced by anyone who has used a credit card at many nationally-based stores, i.e., Circuit City, Service Merchandise)

Information Integrity is a method of assuring that information entered into the record cannot be altered. Changes/corrections to the information are accomplished through amendments

Auditing is a method of reviewing when and whom has accessed the electronic medical record

Availability means the system must be designed to be available at all times.

For all practical purposes, current technology has allowed only a partial realization of Level 3. The lack of full integration with financial information, continuing difficulties with standardizing terminology across diverse disciplines, and security issues remain problematic areas for full computerization.

LEVEL 4: ELECTRONIC PATIENT RECORD SYSTEMS – The electronic patient record differs significantly from the computerized information structures discussed above. Information is based on the patient rather than the entity collecting the information (i.e., hospital, HMO, physician's office, or outpatient rehabilitation facility). Before implementation of the electronic patient record can proceed, several issues have to be resolved:

- A national (or international) system of identifying all patient information within the larger network must be developed.
- Patient information conformity and standardization of terminology must be developed.
- A consensus on security issues must be created.
- Public health information systems must be developed.

LEVEL 5: THE ELECTRONIC HEALTH RECORD – The electronic patient record will include all of the health information for a patient regardless of the source (e.g., hospital, HMO, physician's office, outpatient rehabilitation facility, dentist, and wellness information). "It differs from the electronic patient record in the unlimited amount of health information captured by caregivers regarding a person. It includes wellness information and other health-related information that is not part of the traditional care delivery process" (Medical Records Institue, 1995).

Computers   Before we begin discussing the specifics of computerized documentation within the framework of occupational therapy, we need to understand the basics of computer jargon. Just as in our own medical environment, a specialized language has developed concerning computers.

First is the distinction between hardware and software. Hardware is the actual physical components that make up a computer. Software is the description used to distinguish the operating system and applications used by the computer.

HARDWARE – Although a computer may have many different types of devices within its framework or attached to various ports, it is important to understand the basic components and their functions. A port is a description of any connector for an internal or external computer device. Typically, a computer will have a communication port, a video port, an input/output port, a keyboard port, and a serial port. The following sections describe some of the more important computer components.

PROCESSOR – One of the most important computer components is the processor, since it is the true work area of the computer. Several different types are available from different manufacturers (including Pentium, Pentium Pro, Pentium II, PowerPC), but all are generally rated by the speed at which they can manipulate information given in megahertz (MHz). Typically the larger the MHz number, the more information (bytes) that can be processed in a given time frame.

MEMORY – The second most important area is memory. Memory (typically referred to as RAM for random access memory) is physically a small set of computer chips in which the information being worked on is stored. Memory is like the top of a desk. The more space you have, the more items you can place on your desktop. The larger the memory, the more items you can have working at one time. Unlike other types of storage, RAM is temporary. The information is stored only for the time you are actually working. Once you have turned your computer off, RAM is cleared of all information.

STORAGE – Third in this hierarchy is storage. If RAM is the desktop, then storage forms the filing cabinet of your computer. Storage can come in many forms, but all allow the information to be permanent in the sense that it remains in place after the computer is turned off. Some examples are 3.5-inch floppy disk, Zip, Jaz, Ditto, SuperDrives, DynaMo, hard drives, CD-R, and CD-RW. The primary difference between differing storage devices is the cost of the equipment and the media. The table below shows the differing types of media in order of increasing cost. (See Table 14.1).

Table 14.1 Examples of Storage Media

Media	Capacity	Removable
3.5" Floppy	1.44-2 megabytes	Yes
Zip, Jaz, Ditto, SuperDrive, DynaMo,	Varies. Up to 2 gigabytes	Yes
Hard Drives	Varies. Generally in the gigabyte range	No
CD-R (Recordable CDs)	Varies. Up to 750 megabytes	Yes
CD-RW (Re-recordable CDs)	Varies. Up to 1.5 gigabytes	Yes

INTERFACE – The interface describes any method used to provide information, commands, and instructions to the computer. Keyboards are the most common type of interface; however, other devices such as the mouse, touch screens, digital pens, and voice input are all examples.

OUTPUT – Output is the method used to display, print, or communicate the information on which the computer has completed work. Regardless of the method used, a printer, displaying the information on a monitor, playing an educational CD or communicating by modem output allows the user to visually see, hear, or transmit the information.

ACCESSORY EQUIPMENT – Some other interesting and important aspects of computers pertain to the accessory equipment used with many systems. Modems, scanners, CD-ROM drives, and sound cards are other devices that can be very useful.

Modems are devices that allow a computer to communicate over telephone lines. Two distinctive types are available.

- Analog modems use regular phone lines to send or receive information. Speed is limited, but they are less costly of the two types.

- ISDN (Integrated Service Digital Network) modems use special phone lines that can handle more information and different kinds of information better than regular analog phone lines. They require installation of a special phone line and are typically more expensive than analog modems. Both of these types use different speeds and have models with differing features. Information concerning ISDN lines and modems can be obtained from your local telephone company.

Scanners are devices that allow pictures and text to be digitized and input into the computer. Once the information is digitized, manipulation of the photograph or text can be accomplished with specialized applications designed to perform such task.

CD (Compact Disc) drives are devices that run CD disc to either allow the computer to use the information stored on the disc or with newer models, write information to the disc. CDs store large amounts of information compared to floppy disk. CDs come in several different forms with differing abilities. CD-ROM (CD-Read Only Memory) is a type of CD that can only be played. CD-R CD-Recordable) is a one- time recordable type of CD that can be used as a storage device. CD-RW (CD-Re-recordable) is a type of CD that can have information written, erased, and rewritten many times. A new and emerging technology is Digital Versatile Disk (DVD). DVD is similar to CD-ROM but with much higher storage capacity. A DVD-ROM Disc can store a maximum of 4.7 GB (gigabyte; a gigabyte equals 1 billion bytes) compared to the 650 MB (megabyte; a megabyte equals 1 million bytes) maximum capacity of CD-ROM. For now, they cannot have information written to them.

Lastly, sound cards are computer boards that allow the computer to play sounds, music, video sound tracks, and take input from a microphone for such activities as voice input or sound recordings.

SOFTWARE — Software is a term used to distinguish applications from the computer that runs them. Software uses specialized "languages" to instruct and command the computer. These languages are what allow the computer to "do" the activities it performs. Software can be broken down into two specialized categories: operating systems and applications.

Operating systems are used to translate commands from other types of software into instructions the computer can understand and act on. Operating systems tell the computer how to use the "drivers" that run the monitor, the printer, modem, etc. They regulate how items are stored and how the information is compressed. The most common operating systems today are DOS, OS/2, Unix, Windows 95, Windows NT, and Macintosh GUI (graphical user interface) System 8.x.

Applications are groups of programs that allow you to actually perform work. Many different types of applications exist in the market today: databases, word processors, spreadsheets, desktop publishers, and communications are some examples.

Databases store information in highly organized groups of files. Unlike many other types of applications, databases allow for easy sorting, retrieval, and mining of information. Most databases currently utilize the Open Database Communications (ODBC) standard to allow easy exchange of information with other programs. The importance of two types of databases is of particular interest to computerized documentation.

> **Interrelational databases** manage information in "tables" (user-defined groups of information) that allow multiple records to access the information without the need to duplicate the related information in each record.
>
> **Federated databases** collect information from multiple information sources. Federated databases are particularly useful for research (such as outcome studies) since multiple sites can compile large amounts of information.

Word Processors are applications that create and store documents such as letters, memos, or reports. These applications can reduce the time required to produce forms, letters, or contracts and provide many useful subprograms that can ease typing duties. For computerized documentation, two types of subprograms are very useful: macros and templates. (These are also found in many spreadsheets and databases.)

> **Macros** are a subprogram that stores user-defined phrases. Phrases that are used to describe particular situations or special endings for letters can be easily retrieved with a single command.
>
> **Templates** are a subprogram that creates and stores user-defined documents. By pre-defining the bulk of a document and entering only the information that changes, a significant reduction in typing time can be achieved when producing routine types of documents.

Spreadsheets are powerful number managers. They are used to track, sort, manipulate, and compile information in numerical format. Although often used for tracking financial information, many have the capability of performing calculations for research such as ANOVA, t-test, means, and medians.

Desktop Publishers are sophisticated word processors that easily combine graphics and text to create forms, manuals, and advertisements.

Communications software provides the method for a computer to transfer information between locations using a modem. Many different types are available, but they may have functions to manage telephone operations, fax, and email, as well as data packages containing information from databases and spreadsheets.

There are many different configurations and ways to apply some or all of this technology for use in the typical occupational therapy clinic. It may be difficult for anyone not familiar with some of the equipment and hardware mentioned thus far to imagine how all of this can fit into the normal functioning of an occupational therapy clinic. Let's look at what a typical day might be like in a truly computerized occupational therapy clinic.

Applied Dynamics of Computerization

Arriving for work on Monday morning you go to your workstation and turn on your computer. Your scheduler automatically starts and, in addition to showing you your patient schedule for the day, you see that you have a meeting with the burn unit coordinator at 1:00 p.m. You realize that your first patient is scheduled for an ADL screening, so you start your word processor and retrieve the template for an ADL screen from the hard drive and print the form. After completing the screening and the rest of the morning's patients, you have a few moments to enter the screening information into your database. You update the database with all of this morning's activity (thinking to yourself how much easier it is to have most of the information concerning your treatment plans pop up just by entering the patient identifier into the database). Two of the patients you have seen this morning are worker's compensation cases, and their case managers want the daily notes on a weekly basis. You query the database and select the records for the first patient relating to the previous week's notes. Then, using the fax software on your computer, you send the notes to the case manager and mark the database that the records were sent.

Now, it is time to go to the meeting with the burn unit coordinator. You have been working on a project for coordination of services relating to burn patient care. Now that all the final plans have been made, it is time to inform everyone about the changes to the burn protocol. Using your desktop publishing program, you create a neat little memo that is sure to catch everyone's attention. You uplink the memo onto the LAN (local area network, a system that enables computers in an office to share files and send messages to one another) sending it to all of your colleagues in the OT department. While on the computer, you check both your in-house and Internet email. (Wasn't it really nice of Dr. Smith to send you a note thanking you for taking such good care of that patient he referred last month.) You also get the memo that the OT supervisor has called a staff meeting for 4:00 p.m. this afternoon. Before leaving the station, you pop onto the web and print that new research article on hemiplegia that you heard about in the online therapists chat session last Thursday night.

In the afternoon, you have a new patient to see. The occupational therapy department has received the patient identifier for the new patient, so you log onto the Community Health Information Network (CHIN) and have the network download the patient's record. On reviewing the record, you note that patient has had several strokes in the past and has been seen by a local outpatient OT for ADL training and a local PT for gait training 2 years ago. Her local pharmacy notes show that she is still on medications relating to the stroke. Her primary care physician saw her 2 weeks ago after a fall at home and noted that she had a nondisplaced fracture of the radius. He placed her into a cast and referred her to the OT department for AROM exercises to the upper extremity to make sure she regains the motion in her hand and elbow while she is in the cast. Once again, after opening the desktop publisher, you print the appropriate evaluation forms in preparation for seeing the patient. After evaluating the patient, you decide that Codman's Shoulder exercises would also be appropriate for this patient to start at home. From your computer, you print a personalized home exercise sheet using a template you created in the word processor that pictures the Codman's exercises, lists the repetitions for the patient to complete and includes a tracking sheet that the patient can bring back on the next visit for your review.

During the afternoon OT staff meeting, the supervisor handed out last month's productivity graphs (she creates them with her spreadsheet) and went over the material utilization reports. She also asked that anyone having an interest in the new Cardiac Rehab Program please send her an email so that she can forward it to the Cardiac Rehab Coordinator.

Finally, making it to the end of another productive day, you spend a few minutes updating the database with today's patient information (simply changing the pertinent information and indicating which treatments were performed) and connect to the LAN to retrieve tomorrow's patient schedule. You print the daily encounter record (complete with the correct codes and times in treatment automatically supplied by the database) and post them to the OT office for entry into the financial database. Checking the scheduler one last time, it reminds you that your cousin's birthday is tomorrow, so you've got to pick up a nice card and gift on your way home today. It occurs to you that getting the day-to-day "paperwork" has become much less stressful since your hospital decided to go to the computerized systems. Remembering how hard it was to get clear orders, looking through those bulky charts, and having no information from other services, you wonder how you got through a day.

With time and effort, many of these applications can be made to fit your specific needs and requirements. Many of these applications can be acquired in groups called "suites" that provide easy transfer of information among the various applications in the group.

Other Considerations

All over-the-counter software can be made to function within the concept of the "computerized zones" mentioned earlier; however, they do not meet the requirements needed to produce a true computer-based medical record in that they are not designed to automatically gather, and identify all of the information concerning one patient.

Because of some of the difficulties encountered in attempting to modify existing applications to meet the requirements of a typical occupational therapy clinic, vendors have started designing software that will more specifically meet the needs of our profession. There are many different software packages/systems available on the market today, some of which are more comprehensive than others. They do not typically handle both patient information and financial information however. A summary of some of the systems illustrates this point. (See Table 14.2).

*Note: There is not enough room to list all the various applications and vendors that may produce software that could be or is specifically useful to occupational therapists. The intent of the table is to illustrate the availability of products on the market. (The listing of a product does not signify an endorsement by the author or The American Occupational Therapy Association, Inc.)

Table 14.2 Summary of Available Systems

Vendor	Product	Type of Application	Summary of
Cedaron PO Box 2100 Davis, CA 95617 (800)-424-1007 916-795-6000 Fax: 916-795-6003	Dexter® WorkStation	Patient Assessment, Evaluation and Documentation for the Upper and Lower Extremity	27 computerized examinations for the upper and lower extremity incl. Motor and strength tests, Physical Exams, Sensory Tests and Impairment Calculation
Greenleaf Medical System 3145 Porter Drive Bldg. A202 Palo Alto, CA 800-925-0925 http://www.greenleaf.com	EVAL®	Assessment/Evaluation Management	23 Computerized examinations and impairment calculation for the hand and upper extremity
	ORCA® for Hand Therapy	Computerized Outcomes Data Management Patient Documentation Management	21 examinations and questionnaires for assessment of patient pathology, impairment and functional limitations for hand therapists
	PT ORCA®	Computerized Outcomes Data Management and Patient Documentation Management	17 examinations for assessment of patient pathology for physical therapy
	WholePerson Premiere®	Patient Management for the Spine and Lower Extremity	15 orthopedic evaluations, 10 neurological evaluations
Precedent Systems 800-488-5668	Marathon	Practice Management	Business Applications Scheduling Staff Productivity
	Ghostwriter	Computerized Charting System	Demographics Clinical Info Measurement Data
FOTO, Inc. PO Box 11444 Knoxville, TN 37939 800-482-3686 423-450-9699 423-450-9484 (Fax)	FOTO™A, B, C (Focus on Therapeutic Outcomes)	Outcomes Database for OT or PT	Standardized questionnaire forms for Outcomes Data
	CADI™ (Computer Assisted Data Input/Integration Software	Automated Computerized Outcomes Reporting	Standardized questionnaire forms for Outcomes Data Computerized Charting
American Society of Hand Therapists	UENet®	Outcomes Database	Federated Database for Outcomes Reporting for Hand Therapy

Platform/OS	Printed Reports	Interface/Comments
PC/Windows	Demographics, Measurement Data, Initial Notes, Progress Notes, Discharge Summary, Permanent Partial Impairment Rating	Keyboard Specialized Evaluation Equipment. Ability to interact with the UENet database *Modular system that allows for different configurations
Macintosh	Demographics, Measurement Data, Permanent Partial Impairment Rating	Keyboard, Specialized Evaluation Equipment
Macintosh PC/Windows	Demographics, Initial Notes, Measurement Data, Progress Notes, Discharge Summary, Questionnaire Summary	Keyboard MessagePad Personal Digital Assistant (Pen Based) Ability to interact with the UENet database. Ability to interact with EVAL
PC/Windows	Demographics, Initial Notes, Measurement Data, Progress Notes, Discharge Summary	Keyboard, MessagePad 2000 Personal Digital Assistant (Pen-Based)
Macintosh	Demographics Initial Notes, Measurement Data, Progress Notes, Discharge Summary	Keyboard, Specialized Evaluation Equipment
PC/Windows	Business Summaries	Keyboard
PC/Windows	Automated Reporting, Demographics, Progress Notes, Measurement Data, Discharge Summary	Keyboard, Ability to interact with Marathon to produce automated billing from clinical data
Mail/Fax Data Integrate with CADI'	Utilization Review for Practice Management, Staffing, Discharge Data Sheet, Comparison to National Aggregates	May be integrated with CADI™ Software
PC/Windows	Intelligent software for information entry. Provides immediate information listed for FOTO™	Requires PC owned/purchased by user
	Utilization Review, Comparison to National Aggregates	Participation is by subscription. Must utilize computerized documentation system authorized as a UENet protocol

Conclusion

During the past several years, the medical community has increased the pace at which it is moving toward computerized documentation, and inevitably toward the goal of the electronic health record. The feasibility and probability of reaching the goal have increased dramatically during the past decade. It is noteworthy that other information intense industries, such as banking and insurance, typically spend 5-7.5 percent of their annual budgets on information technology while healthcare typically spends less than 2 percent (Council on Competitiveness, 1996). The percentage is quickly changing as healthcare begins the process of moving clinical documentation into the technological era.

While the tasks involved in moving healthcare into the realm of the electronic health record are not easy, they are inevitable. The process is starting, and we must be prepared and knowledgeable concerning the issues and other players within this environment if we are to properly represent our needs. Our ability to promote occupational therapy as a viable medical service to the larger healthcare environment and provide quality service depends on our ability to continue to meet the new challenge computerization offers.

References

Integration of Health Information Systems: The Highway to Health—Part I. In Highway to Health: Transforming US Healthcare in the Information Age. Council on Competitiveness, 1996a. *Drug Benefit Trends, 8*(2): 11-13, 17-18, 24-26, 28.

Integration of Health Information Systems: The Highway to Health—Part II. In Highway to Health: Transforming US Healthcare in the Information Age. Council on Competitiveness, 1996b. *Drug Benefit Trends, 8*(11): 22-26, 29, 36.

What is an electronic patient record? Medical Records Institute. (1995). Http://www.medrecinst.com/levels.html.

15. Legal Issues in Documentation: Fraud, Abuse, and Confidentiality

Kathryn D. McCann, JD, and
Thomas Steich, JD

As we document the case of each patient or client, the immediate purposes of our notes, such as good communication with other health care providers, are obvious. The authors discuss how crucial accurate and thorough documentation is for reasons that may not be so obvious. They also discuss fraud and abuse laws that are relevant to clinical documentation and related business practices.

Kathryn D. McCann is Regulatory Counsel for the Department of Government Relations of the American Occupational Therapy Association.

Thomas Steich is General Counsel for the American Occupational Therapy Association.

This chapter provides an overview of the major fraud and abuse laws applicable to the federal health programs, as well as a discussion of federal and state laws related to the creation, maintenance, and release of medical records. As a result of increased emphasis on health care fraud and abuse, occupational therapy practitioners and the facilities in which they work must be increasingly diligent in their business practices related to documentation and billing of services. It is crucial that occupational therapy practitioners equip themselves with at least a basic understanding of these laws. In the absence of some rudimentary understanding of these issues, health care practitioners can be implicated unwittingly in prohibited activities. Those who act in deliberate ignorance or reckless disregard of the truth are not immune from sanction or prosecution. Fraudulent intent may be inferred from patterns of conduct or circumstantial evidence (Regional Office Manual [HCFA-Pub.23-2]).

The fraud and abuse laws are complex and continually evolving, and their interpretation by the courts can vary. In any situation where an occupational therapy practitioner is entering into a financial or legal relationship with another health care provider/entity, or is otherwise confronted with a specific legal issue, it is imperative that the occupational therapy practitioner retain legal counsel. This chapter is not intended to be exhaustive. For example, we do not review specific case law, nor do we discuss corporate compliance programs, which are extremely important tools adopted by companies to police possible health care fraud within their own corporate structure.

Much of the content of this chapter focuses on the Medicare program. The primary reason for this is the fact that the Medicare program has a substantial body of established laws and regulations that is frequently adopted, in whole or in part, by other insurers and policy makers. It is imperative that occupational therapy practitioners familiarize themselves with laws and regulations governing medical records, billing, and related business practices. Even if you are working in an environment that does not require you to be involved in the day-to-day aspects of billing for your services, you should have some knowledge of how your services are being billed and reimbursed. If claims for your services are being denied, you should be privy to why they are being denied and, in most cases, these denials should be appealed. The importance of appealing denied claims cannot be overstated and goes beyond the necessity of obtaining proper reimbursement for your professional services. [If a health care provider does not dispute a carrier or intermediary's determination that a service was medically unnecessary, they are vulnerable to allegations that they have knowingly submitted claims for services that they knew, or should have known, were not reasonable and necessary.] If providers do not appeal these decisions, they are vulnerable to allegations of fraud and/or abuse with regard to present and future claims for services. In the current climate, billing errors and disputes have the potential of becoming allegations of fraud or abuse.

General Record Keeping Considerations

The creation of accurate and thorough clinical documentation is important for a myriad of reasons. Some of these reasons are obvious, such as the need to communicate with other health care providers and the importance of carefully documenting care in the event a malpractice claim must be defended. Proper and complete documentation is becoming increasingly important in obtaining proper reimbursement for services, given increased scrutiny of claims in medical review processes. Sound documentation is also crucial in appealing denied claims. Stricter fraud and abuse laws, as well as the dramatic increase in the enforcement of these laws, further necessitate documentation of health care services in a manner that supports that the type, frequency, and duration of the services were reasonable and necessary. In addition, documentation must support the level of skill needed to safely and effectively provide the service. In other words, an occupational therapist's documentation must clearly explain why the professional skill and judgment of an occupational therapy practitioner was necessary.

Good record keeping can help to avoid or win medical malpractice lawsuits. Most lawsuits are filed many years after the medical was provided. Juries find it difficult to believe that care was rendered if it is not documented. Careless documentation that contains silly errors or that lacks clarity is extremely problematic if you have to defend against charges of fraud in an administrative, civil, or criminal proceeding. Even unintentional mistakes can get health care practitioners into trouble. You can provide the best care to your patients, but if your documentation does not reflect and support that care, you have nothing with which to defend yourself in the event of legal action.

When preparing documentation, at a minimum, observe the following practices:

- Be clear and provide accurate and thorough information.

- In addition to documenting the plan of care, evaluation/re-evaluations, treatments, patient progress (or reasons for lack of progress), be sure to document why the treatment was medically necessary at the level of care at which it was furnished (in other words, explain why the professional skill and judgment of an occupational therapy practitioner was necessary).

- Institute some type of internal audit system to double-check entries in the clinical records and bills.

- Appeal denied claims, when appropriate.

- Complete documentation at the time of treatment or as soon as possible thereafter. The more time that elapses between treatment and recording, the greater the possibility of error.

- Make sure other supporting documentation is in the clinical record, such as the physician's orders.

- Date and initial all entries, including corrections made to the clinical record.

- Use factual, objective phrases. Avoid subjective phrases. For example, "Patient makes verbal claims that he is an alien" conveys objective information, whereas "Patient is crazy" is subjective. Use quotations to document unusual or bizarre behavior.

- Record broken appointments and patient "no shows" with reasons given by the patient, and describe any attempts to reschedule appointments.

Avoid the following practices:

- Avoid changing a record after the fact without clarifying when and by whom the change was made, as well as the nature of the change.

- Avoid cosigning another person's notes, unless you supervised that person in the provision of occupational therapy services.

- Avoid criticizing another health care provider in a written record.

- Avoid making judgmental statements about a patient or patient's family.

- Do not assume the patient will not see the medical records.

The Medical Record as a Legal Document

There are numerous laws with slight variations and professional standards that govern documentation. Both state and federal laws require health care providers to maintain records on the patients or clients they treat. Requirements related to documentation are contained in various bodies of law, such as the federal Medicare conditions of participation, state practice acts, or confidentiality statutes. Each practitioner must be responsible for identifying and meeting the specific requirements in his or her state.

Effective documentation is essential for third party payment. It itemizes type, frequency, and duration of services. The practitioner must be able to provide information on the specific therapeutic interventions provided to the patient. Without proper medical records to support the claims submitted to the payer, reimbursement will be denied. In cases where it appears, due to improper documentation, that claims were submitted for medically unnecessary services or services that were not provided, a payer will deny reimbursement. Payers will also pursue recovery of past payments. If a payer suspects fraud or abuse in billing for services and medical records are found to be inaccurate, fictitious, or "doctored" to generate improper payments, providers may be subject to administrative, civil, or criminal penalties. The federal government has significantly increased its enforcement authority in the area of health care fraud and abuse against federal programs such as Medicare, Medicaid, and the Civilian Health and Medical Program of the Uniformed Services (CHAMPUS).

Private insurers also have the authority to pursue various administrative actions, such as the recoupment of money for improperly paid claims. Medicare coverage criteria specify that there must be an expectation that the patient's condition will improve significantly in a reasonable, and generally predictable, period of time. Documentation must describe a skilled service. As previously noted, it is incumbent upon the occupational therapist to explain why the skills of an occupational therapy practitioner were required to perform the service.

If occupational therapy practitioners follow the guidelines established by the payer and adhere to documentation standards set forth by the AOTA, the likelihood that the reasonableness and necessity of the services will be questioned is greatly diminished. If the payer to whom you are submitting claims does not have written policies regarding documentation, you should follow Medicare's rules since those rules provide very specific guidelines for documenting medical necessity, evaluations, plans of care, treatments, and patient progress.

Since the establishment of the Medicare and Medicaid programs in 1965, Congress has frequently enacted new legislation and amended existing statutes to facilitate the prevention, discovery, and prosecution of fraud and abuse in these programs. Numerous statutes provide a range of civil and criminal penalties for fraudulent and abusive activities against Medicare, Medicaid, and other public health programs. The laws most frequently used by the government to proceed against persons and organizations suspected of program-related offenses include the Medicare-Medicaid Anti-Fraud and Abuse Amendments (including the Anti-Kickback Statute), the False Claims Act, the physician self-referral ("Stark") laws, and a range of administrative actions, such as the imposition of civil monetary penalties and assessments, and exclusion from participation in the Medicare and Medicaid programs.

Medicare and Medicaid Fraud and Abuse

Over the past several years insurers and government agencies have increased their scrutiny of health care providers. This heightened scrutiny has been focused on the reasonableness and necessity of the services health providers furnish to patients, how these services are documented and billed, and the myriad of financial and legal relationships amoung health care providers.

Congress continues to expand and revise the fraud and abuse laws and to allocate additional resources to the prevention, investigation, and prosecution of fraud and abuse in the Medicare, Medicaid, and CHAMPUS programs. The federal government has many options for proceeding against parties suspected of wrongdoing against federal health care programs. There are three broad categories of actions the government may take against someone suspected of fraud or abuse, including administrative proceedings, civil actions, and criminal actions. The penalties that may be imposed through each of these processes vary and could result in exclusion from participation in federal health care programs, restitution, imposition of civil monetary penalties, and imprisonment.

States also have increased their prevention and enforcement activities through enactment of legislation designed to reduce, detect, and prosecute fraud and abuse in the health care system. Many of the state laws mirror federal legislation. For example, many states have enacted physician self-referral laws similar to those applicable under the Medicare and Medicaid programs.

THE DISTINCTION BETWEEN FRAUD AND ABUSE – The words "fraud" and "abuse" are not synonymous. For an act to be deemed fraudulent, a false statement or misrepresentation of a material fact must have been made "knowingly," "willfully," and "intentionally." An example of fraud is the submission of a claim for services that the provider knows were never furnished to the patient. Another example of fraud is the willful misrepresentation of the nature of the services provided, such as billing for a more complicated procedure or service than that actually furnished. This practice is often referred to as "upcoding." Other examples of fraud include, but are not limited to, receiving a kickback for the referral of a Medicare patient, repeated viola-

Legal Issues in Documentation: Fraud, Abuse, and Confidentiality

tions of the limiting charge rules, and repeated violations of the participation agreement a provider has with Medicare. In general, fraudulent activity involves making false statements or misrepresentations of material facts in order to obtain program benefits for which no entitlement would otherwise exist.

The term abuse generally describes practices that are inconsistent with sound medical and business practices that result in unnecessary costs to the Medicare or Medicaid programs. Unlike fraud, the "knowingly and willfully" standard with respect to an individual's intent does not apply in cases of abuse. However, if a provider repeatedly engages in an abusive practice, it may rise to the level of fraud if it can be shown that the party knowingly and willfully continued to engage in the abusive practice. Examples of abusive practices include, but are not limited to, furnishing and receiving payment for services that do not meet recognized standards of care, overutilization of services, excessive charges for services, billing Medicare patients at a higher rate than non-Medicare patients, and repeatedly billing in excess of the limiting charge.

THE MEDICARE-MEDICAID ANTI-FRAUD AND ABUSE AMENDMENTS OF 1977 — In 1977 Congress enacted the Medicare-Medicaid Anti-Fraud and Abuse Amendments (Public Law No. 95-142). These amendments to Section 1128B of the Social Security Act contained a variety of measures to assist the government in both the prevention and detection of fraudulent and abusive practices in the Medicare and Medicaid Programs. This statute upgraded most fraudulent acts from misdemeanors to felonies and increased the maximum penalties that can be imposed on persons convicted under the law. The Medicare-Medicaid Anti-Fraud and Abuse Amendments established penalties for the following acts:

1. knowingly and willfully making false statements or representations of material facts in connection with the application or receipt of Medicare benefits or payments

2. knowingly concealing an event related to an initial or continued right to benefits or payments with an intent to fraudulently obtain benefits

3. knowingly and willfully converting benefits or payments to a use other than for the benefit of the person entitled to receive the payment or benefit (42 U.S.C. §1320a-7b).

A later amendment to the Medicare-Medicaid Anti-Fraud and Abuse Amendments prohibits payments made in return for or intended to induce the referral of Medicare or Medicaid business. This later amendment is commonly cited as the Anti-Kickback Statute.

THE ANTI-KICKBACK STATUTE AND THE SAFE HARBOR REGULATIONS — Section 1128B(b) of the Social Security Act is commonly referred to as the Anti-Kickback Statute. Effective in 1980, the Anti-Kickback Statute amended the 1977 laws by prohibiting the knowing and willful solicitation or receipt of anything of value (remuneration) for referring a person for a service or item for which payment may be made under Medicare or Medicaid. In other words, individuals or entities that knowingly and willfully offer, pay, solicit, or receive remuneration (e.g., kickback, bribe, rebate), in order to induce business reimbursed under Medicare or Medicaid, are guilty of a felony and, upon conviction, are subject to fines and/or imprisonment. The Anti-Kickback Statute is an intent-based statute that prohibits conduct that is knowing and willful.

Because of the broad scope of the Anti-Kickback Statute, there was concern among health care providers that many common, many nonfraudulent business practices could conceivably be considered violations of the law. As a result of this concern, Congress enacted the Medicare and Medicaid Patient and Program Protection Act of 1987 (Public Law No. 100-93). This Act directed the Department of Health and Human Services to promulgate regulations that describe business arrangements that would be immune from criminal prosecution or civil sanctions under the Anti-Kickback provisions. Those payment practices and business arrangements that will not be prosecuted or be a basis for exclusion from the Medicare program are known as "safe harbors".

The safe harbor regulations were first published in 1991. Those regulations cover the following payment and business practices:

- investment interests
- space rental
- equipment rental
- personal services and management contracts
- sale of a practice
- referral services
- warranties
- discounts
- employees
- group purchasing organizations
- waiver of beneficiary deductible and coinsurance payments.

The Health Insurance Portability and Accountability Act of 1996 (HIPAA) (Public Law No. 104-191) added an additional exception to the Anti-Kickback Statute. This new exception permits remuneration, pursuant to a written agreement, between a Medicare health maintenance organization (HMO) or competitive medical plan (CMP) and an individual or entity. The new exception established by the HIPAA also applies to certain risk-sharing arrangements if the written agreement places the individual or entity at substantial financial risk for the cost or utilization of the services the individual or entity is obligated to provide.

Compliance with the safe harbor regulations is voluntary. However, parties to a business arrangement who wish to seek immunity from administrative sanctions and criminal prosecution should ensure that the business arrangement or payment practice in question satisfies the specific criteria set forth in the applicable safe harbor rule. If a business transaction fits within one of the safe harbors, the parties will not be subject to administrative sanctions or prosecution. A transaction that does not fit within one of these safe harbors may be riskier, but it is not necessarily illegal if the requisite intent ("knowing and willful") does not exist.

As noted above, each safe harbor regulation sets forth specific rules. A business arrangement or payment practice has to be analyzed within the context of those rules in order to determine whether the parties will be immunized from criminal prosecution or civil sanctions. By way of an uncomplicated example, let us assume an occupational therapist in independent practice wants to rent office space from a physician. This same physician plans to refer Medicare beneficiaries to the occupational therapist. A question may be raised regarding the rental payments made by the occupational therapist to the physician. If this arrangement were scrutinized, the inquiry that likely would be made is whether the rental payments made by the occupational therapist to the physician constitute remuneration in return for the physician referring Medicare patients to the occupational therapist. Any remuneration in return for referring an individual to a person for the furnishing of services for which payment may be made under Medicare, in whole or in part, is suspect. Depending on how this business relationship is constructed, the arrangement could potentially be in violation of the Anti-Kick-back Statute. The rules for the space rental safe harbor prescribe that: a) there must be a signed, written lease agreement for a term of at least 1 year that specifies the premises covered; and b) the total amount of payments must be set out in advance and must be based on fair market value. The definition of fair market value does not allow the rental charge to be based on the proximity or convenience of the property to persons in a position to generate Medicare-related business. This principle of an "arms-length transaction" appears in many of the safe harbor regulations. For purposes of this example, the occupational therapist's rental payments should be based on the "going rate" for similar property in the area and should not reflect the value or volume of potential referrals from the physician. The occupational therapist and physician should sign a lease agreement (for a term of at least 1 year) that describes the premises covered by the lease and that sets forth the rental payments the occupational therapist will make to the physician.

Keep in mind that this example is an oversimplification of the analysis that must be performed in making the determination as to whether a business practice qualifies for immunity under the space rental safe harbor. Further, this example does not address how the arrangement may be scrutinized under the physician self-referral laws or other federal and state fraud and abuse laws. Analysis of business arrangements under these laws is extremely fact specific. Legal counsel should be obtained before entering into such an arrangement.

PHYSICIAN SELF-REFERRAL LAWS – The Omnibus Budget Reconciliation Act (OBRA) of 1990 (Public Law No. 101-508) amended the Social Security Act by prohibiting physicians from making referrals to entities for the furnishing of clinical laboratory services for which Medicare would pay, if the physician (or a member of the physician's immediate family) has a financial relationship with the entity providing lab services. A financial relationship is generally defined as an ownership or investment interest or a compensation arrangement. The physician self-referral prohibition established by OBRA 1990 is commonly referred to as "Stark I." In addition to clinical laboratory services, the Omnibus Budget Reconciliation Act of 1993 extended this prohibition to several other designated health services, including:

- occupational therapy
- physical therapy
- radiology or other diagnostic services
- radiation therapy
- durable medical equipment
- parenteral and enteral nutrients, equipment, and supplies
- prosthetics and orthotics
- home health services
- outpatient prescription drugs
- inpatient and outpatient hospital services.

The OBRA 1993 amendments are commonly known as "Stark II". The Stark laws are contained in Section 1877 of the Social Security Act (42 U.S.C. §1395nn).

The Stark laws do not prohibit financial relationships between physicians and entities furnishing designated health services. What is prohibited is the referral of patients for services for which Medicare will pay, if such a financial relationship exists. The submission of a claim under a prohibited referral is also prohibited.

The Stark law contains several exceptions to the blanket prohibition against physician self-referrals. Each exception contains specific criteria that must be satisfied to assure that the referrals are not proscribed under the law. Some of the general exceptions apply to both ownership and compensation arrangements, and other exceptions relate exclusively to certain ownership or investment interests or compensation arrangements.

Determining what type of financial relationship exists between a physician and an entity that provides designated health services, and whether any of the exceptions apply, is a complex analytical task. Practitioners who have questions on the structure of a relationship and its implications under the Stark laws should seek legal counsel.

Unlike the intent-based Anti-Kickback Statute where an act must be knowing and willful, the Stark law is a strict liability statute, which means that the government does not have to demonstrate a party's intent to violate the law. The Stark law can be violated in two ways. First, a physician who makes a referral to an entity for the furnishing of a designated health service for which Medicare would pay would be in violation of the law if the physician (or a member of the physician's immediate family) has a financial relationship with the entity, unless one of the exceptions applies. Second, the Stark law is violated if an entity that furnishes designated health services submits a Medicare claim pursuant to a prohibited referral. Let us assume, for example, that a physician with an ownership interest in an outpatient clinic that furnishes therapy services refers a Medicare beneficiary to that clinic for occupational therapy services. Let us further assume that none of the exceptions under the Stark law applies in this particular instance, which means that the physician has violated the law by making a prohibited referral. If the clinic submits a claim for the occupational therapy services to the Medicare program, then the clinic has also violated the Stark law, because it has submitted a claim to the Medicare program pursuant to a prohibited referral.

One of the general exceptions under the Stark law, applicable to both ownership interests and compensation arrangements, is the in-office ancillary services exception. Many physicians and group practices rely on this exception to protect what otherwise would be considered prohibited referrals. This exception applies to all of the designated health services except DME (excluding infusion pumps) and parenteral and enteral nutrients and supplies. In order to qualify for this exception, the designated health services:

1. Must be furnished personally by the referring physician or another physician in the same group practice, or by individuals who are directly supervised by the referring physician or another physician in the same group practice

2. Must be furnished (a) in a building in which the referring physician (or another physician in the same group) furnishes services unrelated to the furnishing of designated health services or (b) where the referring physician is a member of a group practice, the designated health service may be furnished in another building used by the group practice for the centralized provision of the group's designated health services. (Note that the criteria for the in-office ancillary exception vary somewhat for clinical lab services provided by a group practice).

In addition, the designated health services must be billed by the physician performing or supervising the services, by a group practice of which the physician is a member, or by an entity that is wholly-owned by the physician or group practice. In the example used above, the referral would not be prohibited if we assume that:

1. The occupational therapy services were performed by occupational therapy practitioners who were directly supervised by the referring physician or another physician in the group practice.

2. The clinic where the occupational therapy practitioners furnished the services is in a building used by the group practice for the centralized provision of therapy services.

3. The services were billed to the Medicare program using the billing number assigned to the group practice to which the referring physician belongs.

At the time of publication of this chapter, the Department of Health and Human Services had not yet issued final regulations implementing the Stark II law.

THE CIVIL FALSE CLAIMS ACT – The False Claims Act (Title 31 of the United States Code) contains prohibitions against knowingly filing false or fraudulent claims against the government. Under the False Claims Act either the government or a private person, on behalf of the government, may bring a civil action against an individual who has violated the Act by knowingly submitting a false claim to the government. Actions brought by private persons are known as "qui tam" or "whistleblower" actions. Under the False Claims Act, qui tam plaintiffs share in any proceeds that are recovered as a result of the suit.

THE CRIMINAL FALSE CLAIMS ACT – Prior to the passage of the Health Insurance Portability and Accountability Act (HIPAA) of 1996 (Public Law No. 104-191), the false claims provisions contained in the Criminal False Claims Act (Title 18 of the United States Code) were not specifically applicable to health care. Nonetheless, Title 18 had been used prior to enactment of the HIPAA to prosecute fraud and abuse in the Medicare and Medicaid programs. The HIPAA amended Title 18 to specifically include various federal health care offenses including, but not limited to, false statements relating to health care matters and the obstruction of criminal investigations of health care offenses. The offenses contained in Title 18 are punishable by significant fines and terms of imprisonment.

CIVIL MONETARY PENALTIES AND ASSESSMENTS – Pursuant to §1128A of the Social Security Act, the Secretary of Health and Human Services is authorized to impose civil money penalties and assessments against a person or organization for a variety of practices involving the submission of false claims or other improper requests for payment. Civil money penalties and assessments may be imposed if a person knew, or should have known, that the claim was false or fraudulent. Civil money penalties may be imposed in lieu of, or in addition to, criminal proceedings. Individuals and organizations subject to civil money penalties may also be suspended from participation in the Medicare and Medicaid programs.

PROGRAM EXCLUSION – The Secretary of Health and Human Services also has broad authority for excluding providers from the Medicare and Medicaid programs. There are two types of exclusion authority: mandatory and permissive. Persons or entities subject to mandatory exclusion include those convicted of a program-related crime, a criminal offense related to patient neglect and abuse, a felony related to health care fraud or a controlled substance felony. The minimum period of mandatory exclusion is 5 years. The Secretary's permissive exclusion authority may be invoked on several grounds. Examples include misdemeanor convictions for health care fraud, misdemeanor convictions for controlled substance offenses, and convictions for nonhealthcare criminal offenses relating to fraud, theft, embezzlement, breach of fiduciary duty or other financial misconduct of a program funded in whole, or in part, by a government agency. There are two types of permissive exclusions. Derivative exclusions are based on actions previously taken by a licensing board, court, or other agency. Nonderivative exclusions are based on determinations of misconduct that are initiated by the Department of Health and

Human Service's Office of the Inspector General. The exclusion period pursuant to a permissive exclusion can vary but is generally 3 years.

THE HEALTH INSURANCE PORTABILITY AND ACCOUNTABILITY ACT OF 1996 – The Health Insurance Portability and Accountability Act of 1996 (HIPAA) (Public Law No. 104-191) significantly expanded measures to combat fraud and abuse. One of the most important features of HIPAA was the extension of the Medicare-Medicaid anti-fraud and abuse amendments to all federal health care programs. This means that any plan or program that provides health benefits and is funded, in whole or in part, by the United States government (with the exception of the Federal Employment Health Benefit Program) is governed by the same laws that govern the Medicare and Medicaid programs. The HIPAA provided that, effective January 1, 1997, a civil monetary penalty (CMP) may be imposed if an individual knowingly submits, or causes the submission of, a false or fraudulent claim to any federal healthcare program. The person submitting the claim must have actual knowledge that the claim is false or must act in deliberate ignorance or reckless disregard of the truth of the information on the claim. The HIPAA increased the assessment that will be imposed on an individual who submits a false claim to three times the amount claimed for the service and increased the fine to $10,000 for each service or item on the false claim.

The HIPAA instructed the Secretary of Health and Human Services to establish a national health care fraud and abuse control program, to be coordinated with the U.S. Department of Justice. This program provides mechanisms for coordination among federal, state, and local law enforcement agencies for the prevention, investigation and prosecution of health care fraud and abuse. The HIPAA also provided for a Medicare Integrity Program whereby the Secretary will have the authority to contract with private entities to carry out functions that have traditionally been handled by Medicare carriers and fiscal intermediaries.

The HIPAA also contained a directive that the Secretary of Health and Human Services provide guidance to health care providers in the form of additional safe harbor regulations, fraud alerts, and advisory opinions. The 4 year requirement that the Secretary issue advisory opinions is a significant, and controversial, new development. Under this provision of the law, parties to a business arrangement or activity that may subject them to sanctions under certain fraud and abuse laws may request a binding opinion from the Office of the Inspector General (OIG) of the Department of Health and Human Services. The advisory opinions are limited in scope, however, to the arrangement described in the request, are only binding on the parties requesting the opinion, and cannot be relied upon by others. In addition, some matters are not subject to advisory opinions, such as determinations on the fair market value for goods, services, or property.

Other important features of the HIPAA related to fraud and abuse include changes to the Secretary's exclusion authority, establishment of an additional exception to the Anti-Kickback Statute for certain risk sharing arrangements, incorporation of certain healthcare fraud activities into the criminal statutes, and stricter penalties for physicians who inappropriately certify that a Medicare beneficiary is eligible for the home health benefit.

THE BALANCED BUDGET ACT OF 1997 – In addition to the sweeping changes in Medicare reimbursement contained in the Balanced Budget Act of 1997 (BBA), (Public Law No. 105-33), the legislation contained a number of changes to the fraud and abuse laws. The BBA added a "three strikes and you're out" provision to the law. Anyone convicted of three health care related offenses will be permanently excluded from the federal health care programs (Balanced Budget Act of 1997, Subtitle D, Chapter 1, Section 4301 amending §1128(c)(3) of the Social Security Act). The law also contains a nondiscrimination provision related to post-hospital referrals to home health services. This provision requires hospitals to furnish Medicare beneficiaries with a list of home health agencies that serve the area in which the patient resides (Balanced Budget Act of 1997, Subtitle D, Chapter 2, Section 4321, amending §1861(ee)(2)of the Social Security Act). Other BBA changes to the fraud and abuse laws include the imposition of civil money penalties for certain offenses (Balanced Budget Act of 1997, Subtitle D, Chapter 1, Section 4304, amending §1128A(a) of the Social Security Act), a requirement that some types of providers (e.g., home health agencies) obtain a surety bond (Balanced Budget Act of 1997, Subtitle D, Chapter 2, Section 4312, amending §1834(a) of the Social Security Act), and expansion of the advisory opinion process to include certain physician self-referral provisions (Balanced Budget Act of 1997, Subtitle D, Chapter 2, Section 4314, amending §1877(g) of the Social Security Act).

Patient Confidentiality Laws

A majority of states have enacted medical records confidentiality statutes to protect confidential information involving personal medical records, hospital records, and research records from disclosure. Most states also have enacted physician-patient and psychotherapist-patient privilege statutes to protect confidential information from disclosure. In interpreting these statutes, courts balance the patient's right to confidentiality with the need for protecting the public's health and safety.

The government's need for access to patient information can sometimes conflict with the patient's right of privacy. In balancing the government's interests in accessing information (such as in fraud investigations) against the patient's privacy interests, courts sometimes allow disclosure of patient medical records. Although some courts have attempted to limit the extent of the information disclosed, few have provided specific standards to protect patient records from unwarranted disclosure of confidential information. Some states have narrow exceptions to the physician-patient privilege statutes that permit the disclosure of information, usually to the Department of Public Health or other state entity. These exceptions generally involve an investigation of a complaint against a physician or other health care practitioner. In some cases a patient's right to confidentiality is deemed to be waived if a patient places his or her medical condition at issue in a lawsuit. State patient confidentiality laws are usually divided into those governing research records and those governing personal medical records.

CONFIDENTIAL RESEARCH RECORDS – A confidential research record is any record, report, statement, note, or other information that is assembled or obtained for research or study and names or otherwise identifies any person. Its custody and use are generally restricted. The confidential record may only be used for the research and study for which it was assembled or obtained.

The records can only be disclosed to persons engaged in the research or project. The only exception allowing for disclosure to others is an aggregate summary that does not disclose the identity of any person who is the subject of the confidential record. Confidential research record laws usually apply to public health departments and drug abuse agencies and their agents.

PERSONAL MEDICAL RECORDS — DISCLOSURE AND RETENTION – Laws regulating the disclosure of personal medical records generally apply to any provider of medical care, whether the provider is an individual or an organization. What constitutes a medical record depends on the legal definitions found in state law. At a minimum, the definition covers every record of medical care that a health care provider or facility maintains that clearly identifies an individual patient (e.g., name, sex, Social Security number) and contains information on the individual's past and present health status, reports of examinations and evaluations, care plans, treatments, progress notes, and discharge summaries.

Currently, states do most of the regulating in the area of health information privacy. However, the Health Insurance Portability and Accountability Act of 1996 (HIPAA) contained a mandate that the Secretary of the Department of Health and Human Services submit a report to Congress detailing recommendations on privacy standards of individually identifiable health information. State laws generally: provide for mandatory disclosures under limited circumstances; prohibit disclosures unless authorized by the individual on whom the record is kept; and establish timelines and procedures for the destruction of medical records. Health care providers owe a duty to their patients to not disclose information obtained during the course of treatment. In general, a patient's clinical records cannot be disclosed without the patient's consent. Some exceptions to this general rule include release of information for purposes of peer review activities, release of information pursuant to legal proceedings or a lawful request by the government, or pursuant to a medical research protocol. In the absence of a statute to the contrary, or absent a serious danger to the patient or others, a patient's written authorization must be obtained prior to releasing medical records.

Many state laws provide that records of an adult patient may not be destroyed for 5 years after the record is made. The records of a minor patient may not be destroyed for 5 years after the record is made or until the patient attains the age of 21, whichever is later, unless the parent or guardian is notified.

The Medicare regulations that set forth the conditions of participation for providers specify standards for the maintenance, release, and retention of clinical records. In general, the Medicare regulations prescribe that clinical records be maintained in accordance with accepted professional standards. The clinical record should contain sufficient information to identify the patient, to justify the diagnosis and treatment, and to record the results of the care. The clinical records of patients should be completely and accurately documented, readily accessible, and systematically organized to facilitate retrieval. In addition, providers must ensure that the clinical records are safeguarded against loss, destruction, or unauthorized use. Written procedures should govern the use and removal of records and include conditions for the release of information from the clinical record. A patient's written consent is required for release of information which is not authorized by law (See, for example, Medicare Conditions for Coverage for Independently Practicing Therapists, 42 C.F.R. §486.161 and Medicare Conditions of Participation for Comprehensive Outpatient Rehabilitation Facilities, 42 C.F.R. §485.60).

With respect to the retention of records, Medicare regulations generally prescribe that clinical records be retained for a period of time not less than:

1. That determined by state law, or
2. In the absence of state law:
   a. 5 years after the date of discharge or,
   b. In the case of a minor, 3 years after the patient reaches the age of majority under state law, or 5 years after the date of discharge, whichever is longer (see, for example, Medicare Conditions of Participation for Rehabilitation Agencies, 42 C.F.R. §485.721).

Conclusion

In the rapidly changing health care environment it is crucial that occupational therapy practitioners have an awareness and understanding of the state and federal laws and regulations related to documentation, billing, and related business practices. With heightened scrutiny of health care providers and increased enforcement of the fraud and abuse laws, health care professionals must not only provide the highest possible standard of care, but they must also protect themselves by exercising extreme care and diligence in documenting and billing the care they provide. The best defense to a charge of fraudulent or abusive conduct or to a malpractice claim is accurate, carefully prepared documentation.

References

United States Code, Title 42

United States Code, Title 31

United States Code, Title 18

Code of Federal Regulations, Title 42

16. Ethical Issues in Documentation

S. Maggie Reitz, PhD, OTR/L, and Penny Kyler, FAOTA

This chapter provides a discussion of the important relationship of documentation to ethical issues. The American Occupational Therapy Association has made a serious effort through its Code of Ethics and other documents to give ethical issues the prominence they deserve.

S. Maggie Reitz is an associate professor in the occupational therapy department, Towson University, Towson, Maryland.

Penny Kyler is Ethics Program Manager of the American Occupational Therapy Association.

The preceding chapter discussed the legal aspects of documentation. That discussion was based on current laws and statutes that have developed over time from ethical principles, most commonly from principles of justice. Dilemmas of justice usually focus on competition among different activities, each of which wants a share of limited resources. The American Occupational Therapy Association's (AOTA's) *Occupational Therapy Code of Ethics* is based upon the principles of justice, veracity, beneficence, as well as others, and it serves to guide both the practice of occupational therapy and the documentation of that practice. This chapter briefly discusses the historical interest of occupational therapy in quality documentation and familiarizes the reader with various ethical principles promoted by AOTA and AOTA's Standards and Ethics Commission (SEC). Most importantly, the chapter outlines a process for resolving ethical dilemmas and concludes with a discussion of actual documentation issues in a case study format.

The importance of gaining both knowledge and skill in documentation has long been appreciated by the profession of occupational therapy. As early as 1948, *The American Journal of Occupational Therapy* (*AJOT*) published an article on documentation (Booth, 1948). Through the years, articles on the legal and ethical aspects of documentation (Gleave, 1960) as well on specific documentation skills (Carr, 1969; Overs, 1964) and reimbursement (Foto, 1988; Thomesen, 1996) have appeared in the *AJOT*. More recently, other AOTA publications have provided readers with articles on specific aspects of documentation. These articles can be relevant and applicable to current practitioners, both as clinicians and managers of occupational therapy services.

The AOTA's *Code of Ethics* requires members of the association to examine the quality of both their practice and the documentation that reflects components of that practice. In recent years, financial constraints and the resulting increased scrutiny by managed care companies and fiscal intermediaries have further stimulated interest in documentation issues.

Increasing numbers of items published on documentation have appeared in AOTA publications. A computer search of OT Bibsys, (the bibliographic database of AOTA/AOTF) discovered over 240 entries for documentation. Articles appeared on documentation and reimbursement, Medicare, mental health, managed care, home health, and many other facets of occupational therapy (OT) practice. Documentation is an increasingly visible and integral task in the occupational performance of OT practitioners.

Prior to reading the case studies, the reader should become familiar with the AOTA's *Code of Ethics* (1994) (see Appendix A) and *Reference Guide to the Code of Ethics* (AOTA, 1996), the SEC's *Enforcement Procedure for Occupational Therapy Code of Ethics* (AOTA, 1996) (see Appendix B), AOTA's *Core Values and Attitudes of Occupational Therapy* (Kanny, 1993) (see Appendix C), and NBCOT's *Procedures for Disciplinary Action* (Appendix D). The reader should also become familiar with a systematic process for resolving ethical issues. A detailed discussion of ethical theories, principles, and general terms can be found in the May 1988 *AJOT* special issue on ethics, as well as the "Everyday Ethics" video workshop and companion guide (AOTA, 1995).

There are different ways to analyze ethical dilemmas. One process will be described and demonstrated in this chapter. Even when individuals use the same process, they may arrive at different conclusions based on their value systems. Therefore, therapists must be conscious of potential conflicts in values, viewpoints, and needs among health care providers (Hansen, 1988). It is important for each therapist to consciously examine the dilemmas that arise and consider a variety of possible courses of action prior to making a decision. Action should not be taken on impulse. When highly regarded values are threatened, people tend to react in an immediate and exaggerated manner (Everly, 1990); this action frequently results in responses that may seem irrational to others and may be hard to defend. A more professional response to an ethical dilemma will be formulated if the decision:

- has been carefully analyzed and executed

- is consistent with the therapist's personal value system

- is compatible with the laws and regulations to which the therapist is bound

- is executed only after all available options are considered.

Table 16.1 Steps in an ethical reasoning process

1. Gather all additional pertinent information
First, identify the "players" or participants in the dilemma. Next, gather information regarding the specific dilemma and review the AOTA's Code of Ethics, the Enforcement Procedure of AOTA's SEC, as well as the code of ethics and the documentation guidelines of the institution/workplace. Documentation and practice guidelines of fiscal intermediaries should also be reviewed.

2. Identify conflicting values and neutral territory
Time needs to be taken to identify possible conflicting values between the participants, as well as values that may be compatible if not identical. Locating this neutral territory of shared values may facilitate the resolution of the dilemma.

3. Identify all possible alternative actions
All alternatives should be listed—even those that at the beginning may seem risky or inappropriate. The commitment to the final choice of action might be strengthened by a clear understanding of the reasons for and consequences of the alternative actions. The therapist may also find this preparation helpful if it becomes necessary to defend the final choice to others.

4. Determine both positive and negative consequences of each action
A realistic appraisal of the costs and benefits of each possible action should be listed so they can be reviewed at length.

5. Weigh the actions and their consequences to determine the best possible course of action
Sufficient time should be taken to carefully weigh the total positive and negative consequences of each action and all possible combinations of actions to select an action that is both "right" and defensible.

Sources: Adapted from Aroskar, 1980; Hansen, Kamp, & Reitz, 1988

The case studies in this chapter use a five-step process (Aroskar, 1980; Hansen, Kamp, & Reitz, 1988), outlined in Table 16.1. This process uses one of several possible matrices available to assist in ethical decison making. During the process of resolving ethical dilemmas it is important to be open and receptive to contrasting points of view. Competent therapists should be aware of their value systems and the potential areas of conflict within their particular workplaces. Therapists are also responsible for being familiar with all federal and state laws and regulations that govern their practice.

When a dilemma arises, the occupational therapist should first identify the "players" involved. Next, all necessary information about legal and professional standards should be gathered. The therapist must become familiar with the laws and regulations that pertain to the particular issue and practice area. Occupational therapy personnel should also be knowledgeable of facility policies on documentation and reimbursement. Copies of the following should be obtained for guidance: AOTA's *Code of Ethics*, the AOTA's *Reference Guide to the Code of Ethics*, and the *Enforcement Procedure* of AOTA's SEC. Individuals should also be familiar with the occupational therapy practice act that governs practice in the state where they are providing services and the National Board for Certification in Occupational Therapy's (NBCOT) *Procedures for Disciplinary Action* (see Appendix D) After all additional pertinent and accessible information has been gathered, the occupational therapist should determine whether any conflicting values among participants can be identified.

Application of Ethical Reasoning Process

If an employer determines that treatment is no longer cost-effective, regardless of the patient's progress as measured and documented by the therapist, the therapist must choose among conflicting values. The therapist may be caught between the value of upholding a duty to the patient, the principle of nonmaleficence (that is, doing no harm), and the value of upholding a duty to an employer. This dilemma revolves around the utilitarian theory of ethics, most commonly described as the greatest good for the greatest number.

It is not always possible to identify conflicting values initially. The true nature of a dilemma will become more apparent when the conflicts are identified. Most often, ethical dilemmas are complex, and a variety of values are involved. It may be helpful to identify those areas where conflicting parties share similar values and goals. Locating this neutral territory or middle ground is an important first step. Once it has been identified, a collaborative problem-solving effort that allows mutual respect for differing values is possible.

The next step in the ethical reasoning process consists of listing all possible actions or responses to the dilemma. Skills in problem solving are an asset here. The quality of the final resolution of the dilemma is dependent upon the variety and comprehensiveness of alternative actions that can be developed.

Next, the consequences—both benefits and risks—of each possible action should be determined. Finally, all options and their consequences should be weighed and balanced. The action that best coincides with the therapist's value system should be selected as the optimal course of action. By following this or a similar ethical reasoning process, a thoughtful solution can be articulated and defended. This process will be applied in the following two case analyses. The analyses are not exhaustive but rather are illustrative examples used for educational purposes.

Dilemmas that have a documentation component are one of the most frequently occurring calls to the Ethics Program Manager at AOTA. These case studies were discussed informally with other experts in the field, and their feedback was used in the development of the lists of possible alternative actions.

Case Study One

The director of occupational therapy announced at a staff meeting that occupational therapy personnel will be cosigning notes for the art and dance therapists in the future. When asked why, she said this practice would ensure that these services would be reimbursed as occupational therapy by third party payers and that the facility needed to ensure that adequate funds were provided by reimbursement mechanisms in order to provide quality services. One therapist was concerned about the legal and ethical implications of this new policy. What should this therapist do?

First, the therapist should gather additional pertinent facts and information from all parties involved, as well as the appropriate documents. The therapist can initiate this process by reviewing AOTA's *Code of Ethics* and *Reference Guide*. In addition, the therapist should review the documentation guidelines of the third party payers involved. It may also be helpful to investigate the ethical code and standards of practice of the art and dance therapists. When discussing ethics there are opposing views, *not* a "right" view and a "wrong" view. However, when fraud is present (i.e., billing a non–occupational therapy service as occupational therapy), the issue becomes a legal one. Fraudulent billing is something most state regulatory boards, the AOTA, and the NBCOT either implicitly or explicitly cover under unprofessional conduct. The U.S. Office of the Inspector General of Health and Human Services has vigorously investigated Medicare fraud by improper documentation of billing for services not rendered by occupational therapy. However, the manner in which both the dilemma and the original problem are resolved (i.e., reimbursement for non–occupational therapy services) depends on ethical reasoning. Possible alternative actions may vary depending on personal and institutional values and viewpoints.

The next step in the ethical reasoning process is to construct a table similar to Table 16.2, which displays steps 3 and 4 in the ethical reasoning process for the case study. The primary tools needed for the final analysis of the ethical dilemma are displayed in this table. Sufficient time should be spent studying the options outlined in the table, weighing the value of each alternative action, and determining which action or combination of actions would be most consistent with the therapist's personal value system and the AOTA's Code of Ethics. Gathering the appropriate information and educating people about the ramifications of their behavior or proposed behavior (Action #3) are often sufficient to resolve ethical dilemmas. The other alternative actions listed in table 16.2 should be considered only as last resorts.

Table 16.2 Case study one: Analysis of alternative actions

Action	**Consequences**
1. Follow the director's proposal without asking any questions or seeking additional information.	**Positive:** Less risk in the short term. **Negative:** Risk of engaging in illegal and unethical conduct; in opposition to AOTA's *Code of Ethics*—Principles 4A, 4B, 4D, & 5C; against personal values.
2. Report the director immediately to reimbursement agencies.	**Positive:** Fraudulent billing will be stopped/not initiated. **Negative:** In opposition to AOTA's *Code of Ethics*—Principles 4B and 6C; disruptive to relationship with supervisor.
3. Request to meet with the director after reviewing the following additional information: Third party Payment Guidelines AOTA's Code of Ethics AOTCB's Procedures for Disciplinary Action Art/Dance Therapy Code of Ethics/Standards of Practice	**Positive:** Supported by AOTA's *Code of Ethics*—Principles 4B, 4D, 5C, & 6; increases personal knowledge of ethics, codes of ethics and regulations, and enhances ability to educate supervisor. **Negative:** May be risky if director is not in agreement; meeting may become confrontational.
4. If the director is prepared to rescind the policy, provide support as needed and develop possible alternative strategies. For example: • Investigate if OTRs periodically evaluate patients' progress. Can this service be legally billed? (This may be an additional source of reimbursed services.) • Investigate whether co-led groups (i.e., OTR and art/dance therapists) can be billed for. • Conduct quality assurance studies to determine the effectiveness of art/dance therapy in this setting by collecting data as to whether patients who receive art and dance therapy and OT meet treatment goals and are discharged quicker than those just receiving OT.	**Positive:** Supported by AOTA's *Code of Ethics*—Principles 4B, 4D, 5D, and supportive of director. **Negative:** May be risk in terms of job security.

Table 16.2 (continued)

• Contact the professional associations for art/dance therapy to determine if the hospital can assist in their efforts to become a reimbursable service. • If any art or dance therapists express an interest in graduate school, introduce them to OT schools with degrees for non-OTs.	**Positive:** Supported by AOTA's *Code of Ethics*—Principles 4B and 4D supportive of director. **Negative:** May be risk in terms of job security.
5. If the director does not take action, discuss issue with hospital administrator.	**Positive:** Supported by AOTA's *Code of Ethics*—Principles 3B, 5, & 6; increases understanding of codes. **Negative:** Risk to job security; disloyalty to director.
6. Inform the director that you are prepared to make a report to the appropriate regulatory board (i.e., state regulatory board, AOTA's SEC commission, or NBCOT). Follow through with report if necessary.	**Positive:** Supported by AOTA's *Code of Ethics*—Principles 4D and 6. **Negative:** Risk to job security; disloyalty to director.
7. If the hospital does not take action, meet again with the administrator and inform him or her that you are prepared to report the hospital to the reimbursement agency's fraud section. If action is still not taken, follow through with report.	**Positive:** Supported by AOTA's *Code of Ethics*—Principle 4B. **Negative:** Risk to job security; disloyalty to director and hospital.
8. If the director does not take action, quit without taking any action.	**Positive:** Remove personal risk of legal repercussions. **Negative:** Disloyalty to director and patients; in opposition to AOTA's *Code of Ethics*—Principle 6.

A general rule in resolving ethical dilemmas is that attempts to resolve the dilemma should begin at the level closest to the participants. Attempts should be made to resolve this particular dilemma with the director before escalating the situation by reporting the director to the appropriate regulatory board (e.g., state regulatory board, AOTA's SEC, or NBCOT). The AOTA has jurisdiction only over its members. If the director is not a member of the AOTA, it would be inappropriate to make a report to the AOTA's SEC; however, since she is a registered occupational therapist, it would be appropriate to contact the NBCOT. The benefits of resolving dilemmas prior to reporting to an external authority include:

- increasing the probability that the dilemma may be resolved quickly

- providing an approach compatible with Principles 4A and 4B of the AOTA's *Code of Ethics*, which state that therapists are responsible for abiding by applicable regulations and laws and policies as well as informing employers and employees of those laws and regulations that affect occupational therapy services (AOTA, 1994, p. 795)

- educating the staff and administration concerning the effects of ethical dilemmas on practice

- enhancing the therapist's credibility (i.e., the fact that the therapist "went through channels") if the disagreement is escalated.

In one possible resolution of this case, the therapist, after carefully studying the options, attempts to educate the director regarding the issues of fraud (see Table 16.2—Action #3). In selecting this action, the therapist has weighed the value of upholding duties to: the employer (i.e., director and institution), the profession's code of ethics, and the law. At first it may seem that these values are in conflict; however, all of these values support Action #3. Principle 4B of the AOTA's *Code of Ethics* clearly gives the therapist guidance in selecting this option. It is important that the therapist establish a collaborative rather than a confrontational tone when meeting with the director and/or hospital administration. The common goal of providing quality treatment while maintaining fiscal responsibility should be stressed. Furthermore, it is important during the resolution of any ethical dilemma to find middle ground or a common goal, which can enhance collaboration and the potential for a successful resolution.

The majority of cases can be satisfactorily resolved using this approach. If, however, this strategy proves unsuccessful, the therapist needs to carefully weigh the other possible courses of action presented in Table 16.2. These alternative actions (Actions 6 through 8) should be used only as a last resort after repeated unsuccessful attempts to educate the director and the hospital administration. Greater potential consequences include the possibility of: (a) limiting treatments and services that may jeopardize the institution's accreditation and reimbursement sources because of illegal practices and (b) losing a job or engaging in fraudulent billing and losing one's credentials to practice occupational therapy.

If the hospital adopts the proposed policy—resulting in the director being engaged in fraud—the therapist is bound by the AOTA's *Code of Ethics* to report the director's behavior to an appropriate regulatory body (AOTA's SEC, NBCOT, or state regulatory board). The AOTA and NBCOT have no jurisdiction over the hospital administrator or the hospital as a whole. The AOTA's Code of Ethics supports the therapist in reporting the hospital administration to the appropriate authorities (the fraud section of the fiscal intermediaries). Prior to reporting either party, the therapist should inform both the director and the hospital administrator of this plan and provide them with the opportunity to reconsider their decisions.

This is one of many possible resolutions of this hypothetical dilemma. Occupational therapists, who are skilled in problem solving, communication, and task analysis, can be extremely

Table 16.3 Case study two: Analysis of alternative actions

Action	Consequences
1. Follow administrator's directions without asking any questions or seeking additional information.	**Positive:** Less risk for job security. **Negative:** Risk of engaging in illegal or unethical conduct in opposition to AOTA's *Code of Ethics*—Principle 1, Principles 1C, 1D, 3E, 4A against personal values.
2. State that you have concerns about the legality and ethics of this solution. Suggest you meet again after you have reviewed the possible ramifications.	**Positive:** Supported by AOTA's *Code of Ethics*—Principles 4, 4B, and 5C. **Negative:** May be risk to job security if administrator is not concerned about legal or ethical issues.
3. Quit after determining that fraud could be involved (i.e., if service provided by a non-OT is billed as OT)	**Negative:** In opposition to AOTA's *Code of Ethics*—Principles 5C and 4A; administrator's solution may be instituted upon your departure, putting staff and patients at risk.
4a. Investigate alternate strategies to present to administrator. For example: • Investigate cost of an on-call OTR/temporary OTR. • Suggest that the use of aides be restricted to maintenance therapy, which cannot be billed as OT; when the patients are re-evaluated by an OTR, that session can be charged as OT. • Investigate a policy of priority scheduling. • Investigate possibility of decreasing frequency of therapy sessions to ensure that all priority patients are treated, with technicians to provide carry-over activities on the days that patients do not receive therapy.	**Positive:** Displays leadership skills and skills in resolving ethical dilemmas through problem solving. **Negative:** Takes time away from other administrative and clinical duties.

Table 16.3 (continued)

Action	Consequences
4b. Meet with the administrator and present alternative actions (see 4a, above) and additional concerns, such as: What is the cost in terms of both time and money, to train these aides? What duties will they be competent to perform? How will their competency be determined? How will their activities be documented and charged for? Since additional training will be required, will this be viewed as a promotion? Will the salary of the technicians increase from that of their current job? Are there opportunities for further career upward mobility? Will this be a cost-effective solution if implemented in a legal fashion?	**Positive:** Supported by AOTA's *Code of Ethics*—Principles 1C, 1D, 3C, 3E, and 4A. **Negative:** May be risk to job security if administrator is not concerned about legal or ethical issues; meeting may become confrontational.
5. If administrator wants to institute his solution, including fraudulent billing, resign.	**Positive:** Supported by AOTA's *Code of Ethics*—Principles 4B, 5A, & 6. **Negative:** Risk of losing job reference; lack of fidelity to staff and patients.
6. If administrator wants to institute his solution, including fraudulent billing, meet again and inform administrator that you are prepared to report him to the fraud sections of the appropriate third party payers. Follow through with reports if issue is not resolved.	**Positive:** Supported by AOTA's *Code of Ethics* Principles 4B, 4D, 5C, and 6C. **Negative:** Risk of losing job.

adept at resolving both dilemmas and management crises in an ethical and cost-effective manner. The proposed alternative strategies that could be substituted for the process of having the registered occupational therapists cosign the notes (Action #4) demonstrate an example of this problem-solving approach.

Case Study Two   The manager of occupational therapy in an outpatient setting in which two of six therapists are on maternity leave was informed by one of the remaining therapists that he was moving out of state in 2 weeks. The OT service had a full caseload and a waiting list. The manager approached the administrator of the outpatient service to request temporary staff. The administrator suggested that the manager train three nursing aides from the inpatient service to provide skilled occupational therapy service until the two therapists on maternity leave returned to work. The administrator stated, "Once the therapists return, you can select the aide with the best performance record as a permanent occupational therapy technician. This way the hardest worker will receive a promotion and you won't be short staffed. Quite a satisfactory arrangement, don't you agree?" How should the manager respond?

Now that the reader is familiar with the format and process of ethical reasoning that is being used, the rest of the case will be presented in a more concise form. Table 16.3 lists the alternative actions and consequences for the second case.

It is important for the chief to refrain from making premature judgments (for example, "All the administrator ever thinks about is money!") or allowing inital impressions to cloud the analysis of the dilemma (e.g., "I guess they have checked into the legalities and I'd better go along or I'll be out the door"). The manager should take the time to logically consider the dilemma. As a manager, the occuptional therapist's actions will ultimately affect more than just herself. Again, the first step would be to gather additional pertinent information listed in Table 16.3— Action #2.

By following an ethical reasoning process, the manager found that Principle 5C of the AOTA's *Code of Ethics* (AOTA, 1994) prohibits fraudulent communication and that billing services provided by individuals who are neither certified nor licensed as an occupational therapy practitioner can be considered fraudulent under Medicare guidelines. It also became clear that both the manager and aides would be committing fraud if the services provided by aides were billed as occupational therapy services.

After reviewing the values and goals of occupational therapy and the administrator's goals, several creative solutions became apparent, which are listed in Table 16.3—Action #4a. Several questions—aside from the question of billing—also came into focus as the manager examined the issue (see Table 16.3—Action #4b). In the majority of cases, having clear, predetermined, and well-articulated questions and alternative solutions when meeting with superiors can lead to successful and productive outcomes. Only as a last resort should more vigorous actions be required.

Competent documentation can be a powerful tool both in communicating a patient's response to therapy and also in educating other health care providers and fiscal intermediaries to the value of occupational therapy. Incompetent, unethical, or fraudulent documentation puts the therapist at risk of facing legal repercussions and diminishes the credibility and potential of the profession as a whole. Documentation must not be viewed as a nuisance, waste of time, luxury, or purely intellectual/academic exercise. It is an integral part of ethical, competent clinical practice.

References

American Occupational Therapy Association. (1991). *Reference guide: Occupational therapy code of ethics*. Bethesda, MD: Author.

American Occupational Therapy Association. (1994). Occupational therapy code of ethics. *American Journal of Occupational Therapy, 42*, 1037-1038.

American Occupational Therapy Association. (1995). *Everyday Ethics*. Video workshop and companion guide. Bethesda, MD: Author.

American Occupational Therapy Association. (1995). Position Paper: Use of Occupational Therapy Aides in Occupational Therapy Practice. Bethesda, MD: Author.

American Occupational Therapy Association/American Occupational Therapy Foundation (1996). OTBibsys: A bibliographic database. Bethesda, MD: Author.

American Occupational Therapy Association Standards and Ethics Commission. (1996). *Enforcement procedure for occupational therapy code of ethics*. Bethesda, MD: Author.

Aroskar, M. (1980). Anatomy of an ethical dilemma: The practice. (Part II). *American Journal of Nursing, 80*, 661-663. Bethesda, MD: Author.

Booth, M. (1948). An occupational therapist's guide for progress notes: Which facts and why. *American Journal of Occupational Therapy, 2*, 15-19.

Carr, S. (1969). Documentation of services. *American Journal of Occupational Therapy, 23*, 335-338.

Everly, C. (1990, January 29). *Personality*. Lecture presented in a graduate course, HLTH 650: Health Problems in Guidance, at the University of Maryland at College Park.

Foto, M. (1988). Nationally speaking–Managing changes in reimbursement patterns, Part 2. *American Journal of Occupational Therapy, 42*, 629-631.

Gleave, G. M. (1960). Legal aspects of medical records. *American Journal of Occupational Therapy, 14*, 180-182.

Hansen, R. (1988). Nationally speaking—Ethics is the issue. *American Journal of Occupational Therapy, 42*, 279-281.

Hansen, R., Kamp, L., & Reitz, S. (1988). Two practitioners' analyses of occupational therapy practice dilemmas. *American Journal of Occupational Therapy, 42*, 312-319.

Kanny, E. (1993). *Core Values and Attitudes of Occupational Therapy*. Bethesda, MD: American Occupational Therapy Association.

Kyler-Hutchison, P. (1988). Ethical reasoning and informed consent in occupational therapy. *American Journal of Occupational Therapy, 42*, 283-287.

Overs, R. (1964). Writing work evaluation reports: Core or challenge. *American Journal of Occupational Therapy, 18*, 63-65.

Thomesen, M. (1996). The Resource Utilization Group Systems of Nursing Home Reimbursement Policies: Influences on Occupational Therapy Practice. *American Journal of Occupational Therapy, 50*, 790-797.

Occupational Therapy Code of Ethics

The American Occupational Therapy Association's Code of Ethics is a public statement of the values and principles used in promoting and maintaining high standards of behavior in occupational therapy. The American Occupational Therapy Association and its members are committed to furthering people's ability to function within their total environment. To this end, occupational therapy personnel provide services for individuals in any stage of health and illness, to institutions, to other professionals and colleagues, to students, and to the general public.

The Occupational Therapy Code of Ethics, is a set of principles that applies to occupational therapy personnel at all levels. The roles of practitioner (registered occupational therapist and certified occupational therapy assistant), educator, fieldwork educator, supervisor, administrator, consultant, fieldwork coordinator, faculty program director, researcher/scholar, entrepreneur, student, support staff, and occupational therapy aide are assumed.

Any action that is in violation of the spirit and purpose of this Code shall be considered unethical. To ensure compliance with the Code, enforcement procedures are established and maintained by the Commission on Standards and Ethics. Acceptance of membership in the American Occupational Therapy Association commits members to adherence to the Code of Ethics and its enforcement procedures.

PRINCIPLE 1. – Occupational therapy personnel shall demonstrate a concern for the well- being of the recipients of their services. (beneficence)

    A. Occupational therapy personnel shall provide services in an equitable manner for all individuals.

    B. Occupational therapy personnel shall maintain relationships that do not exploit the recipient of services sexually, physically, emotionally, financially, socially or in any other manner. Occupational therapy personnel shall avoid those relationships or activities that interfere with professional judgment and objectivity.

    C. Occupational therapy personnel shall take all reasonable precautions to avoid harm to the recipient of services or to his or her property.

    D. Occupational therapy personnel shall strive to ensure that fees are fair, reasonable, and commensurate with the service performed and are set with due regard for the service recipient's ability to pay.

PRINCIPLE 2. – Occupational therapy personnel shall respect the rights of the recipients of their services. (e.g., autonomy, privacy, confidentiality)

    A. Occupational therapy personnel shall collaborate with service recipients or their surrogate(s) in determining goals and priorities throughout the intervention process.

B. Occupational therapy personnel shall fully inform the service recipients of the nature, risks, and potential outcomes of any interventions.

C. Occupational therapy personnel shall obtain informed consent from subjects involved in research activities indicating they have been fully advised of the potential risks and outcomes.

D. Occupational therapy personnel shall respect the individual's right to refuse professional services or involvement in research or educational activities.

E. Occupational therapy personnel shall protect the confidential nature of information gained from educational, practice, research, and investigational activities.

PRINCIPLE 3. – Occupational therapy personnel shall achieve and continually maintain high standards of competence. (duties)

A. Occupational therapy practitioners shall hold the appropriate national and state credentials for providing services.

B. Occupational therapy personnel shall use procedures that conform to the Standards of Practice of the American Occupational Therapy Association.

C. Occupational therapy personnel shall take responsibility for maintaining competence by participating in professional development and educational activities.

D. Occupational therapy personnel shall perform their duties on the basis of accurate and current information.

E. Occupational therapy practitioners shall protect service recipients by ensuring that duties assumed by or assigned to other occupational therapy personnel are commensurate with their qualifications and experience.

F. Occupational therapy practitioners shall provide appropriate supervision to individuals for whom the practitioners have supervisory responsibility.

G. Occupational therapists shall refer recipients to other service providers or consult with other service providers when additional knowledge and expertise are required.

PRINCIPLE 4. – Occupational therapy personnel shall comply with laws and Association policies guiding the profession of occupational therapy. (justice)

A. Occupational therapy personnel shall understand and abide by applicable Association policies; local, state, and federal laws; and institutional rules.

B. Occupational therapy personnel shall inform employers, employees, and colleagues about those laws and Association policies that apply to the profession of occupational therapy.

C. Occupational therapy practitioners shall require those they supervise in occupational therapy related activities to adhere to the Code of Ethics.

D. Occupational therapy personnel shall accurately record and report all information related to professional activities.

PRINCIPLE 5. – Occupational therapy personnel shall provide accurate information about occupational therapy services. (veracity)

A. Occupational therapy personnel shall accurately represent their qualifications, education, experience, training, and competence.

B. Occupational therapy personnel shall disclose any affiliations that may pose a conflict of interest.

C. Occupational therapy personnel shall refrain from using or participating in the use of any form of communication that contains false, fraudulent, deceptive, or unfair statements or claims.

PRINCIPLE 6. – Occupational therapy personnel shall treat colleagues and other professionals with fairness, discretion, and integrity. (fidelity, veracity)

A. Occupational therapy personnel shall safeguard confidential information about colleagues and staff.

B. Occupational therapy personnel shall accurately represent the qualifications, views, contributions, and findings of colleagues.

C. Occupational therapy personnel shall report any breaches of the Code of Ethics to the appropriate authority.

Author:
Commission on Standards and Ethics (SEC)
Ruth Hansen, PhD, OTR, FAOTA, Chairperson

Approved by the Representative Assembly: 4/77
Revised: 1979, 1988, 1994
Adopted by the Representative Assembly: 7/94

NOTE: This document replaces the 1988 *Occupational Therapy Code of Ethics* that was rescinded by the 1994 Representative Assembly.

Enforcement Procedure for Occupational Therapy Code of Ethics

I. PREAMBLE

A. – The American Occupational Therapy Association and its members are committed to furthering individual's ability to function fully within their total environment. To this end, the occupational therapy practitioner renders services to clients in all phases of health and illness, to institutions, to other professionals and colleagues, to students, and to the general public.

The American Occupational Therapy Association's Code of Ethics is a public statement of the values and principles to use as a guide in promoting and maintaining high standards of behavior in occupational therapy. AOTA and its members are committed to furthering people's ability to function within their total environment. To this end, occupational therapy personnel provide services for individuals in any stage of health and illness, to institutions, to other professionals and colleagues, to students, and to the general public.

The Occupational Therapy Code of Ethics is a set of principles that applies to occupational therapy personnel at all levels. The roles of practitioner (registered occupational therapist and certified occupational therapy assistant), educator, fieldwork educator, supervisor, administrator, consultant, fieldwork coordinator, faculty program director, researcher/scholar, entrepreneur, student, support staff, and occupational therapy aide are assumed.

Any action that is in violation of the spirit and purpose of this code shall be considered unethical. To ensure compliance with the code, enforcement procedures are established and maintained by the Commission on Standards and Ethics (SEC). Acceptance of membership in the AOTA commits members to adherence to the Code of Ethics and its enforcement procedures. As preamble to the official procedures, the SEC urges particular attention to the following issues:

B. PROFESSIONAL RESPONSIBILITY – All occupational therapy personnel have an obligation to maintain the standards of ethics of their profession and to promote and support these same standards among their colleagues. Each member must be alert to practices which undermine these standards and be obligated to take whatever remedial action is required. At the same time, members must carefully weigh their judgments of unethical practice to ensure that they are based on objective evaluation and not on personal bias or prejudice.

C. JURISDICTION – The American Occupational Therapy Association shall have jurisdiction over all members of the Association in the monitoring and enforcement of the Occupational Therapy Code of Ethics. The Code applicable to any complaint shall be that version or edition in force at the time the alleged act or omission was committed. If the date of the alleged act or omission cannot be determined, then the act or omission shall be judged by the code in force on the date of the complaint.

D. Disciplinary Action

Disciplinary action for members of the Association shall be limited to reprimand, censure, suspension, or revocation from the Association. These are defined as follows:

- Reprimand - a formal expression of disapproval of conduct communicated privately by letter from the Chairperson of the SEC.
- Censure - a formal expression of disapproval that is public.
- Suspension - removal of membership for a specified period of time.
- Revocation - permanent denial of membership.

Final disciplinary actions of censure, suspension, and revocation are reported in official publications of the Association.

E. Dismissal of Complaints

SEC may dismiss a complaint for any of the following:

1. No Violation. The SEC finds the individual against whom the complaint is filed has not violated the Occupational Therapy Code of Ethics. (e.g., accusing someone of being rude.)
2. Corrected Violation. The SEC determines that any violation it might find has been or is being corrected.
3. Insufficient Evidence. The SEC determines there is insufficient fact, evidence, or detail to support a finding of an ethics violation.
4. Absolute Time Limit/Not Timely Filed. The SEC determines that the alleged violation of the Occupational Therapy Code of Ethics occurred more than 10 years prior to the filing of the complaint.
5. Lack of Jurisdiction. The SEC determines that it has no jurisdiction over the defendant or complaint. (e.g., a complaint against a non-member.)
6. Subject to Jurisdiction of Another Authority. The SEC determines that the complaint is based on matters which are already covered by another authority, jurisdiction, or are regulated by law (e.g., accusing a superior of sexual harassment at work; accusing someone of anti-competitive practices.)
7. Advice of Counsel. On the advice of counsel, or other advice, that no further action should be taken on the complaint.

F. Advisory Opinions

1. The SEC may issue advisory opinions on ethical issues to inform and educate the membership. These opinions shall be publicized to the membership.

2. Educative Letter

The SEC determines that the allegations in the complaint are not unethical, however they do not fall completely into the prevailing standards of practice or good professionalism, the SEC may send a letter to educate the complainant and respondent regarding standards of practice and/or good professionalism.

G. CONFIDENTIALITY

Strict confidentiality shall be maintained by all who are involved in the reporting, monitoring, reviewing, and enforcing of alleged infractions of the Occupational Therapy Code of Ethics. The maintenance of confidentiality, however, shall not interfere with the provision of proper notice to all parties involved in the disciplinary proceedings as determined by the Commission on Standards and Ethics. Likewise, final decisions of the Judicial Council and the Appeals Panel will be publicized as described in these procedures.

II. DISCIPLINARY PROCEDURES
A. COMPLAINT

Complaints stating an alleged violation of the Association's Occupational Therapy Code of Ethics may originate from any individual or group within or outside the Association. All complaints must be in writing, signed by the complainant(s), and submitted to the Chairperson of the Standards and Ethics Commission at the address of the Association's National Office. All complaints shall be timely and shall identify the person against whom the complaint is directed (hereafter the respondent), the ethical principles which the complainants believe have been violated and, an explanation of the alleged violations. If available, supporting documentation should be attached.

B. SUA SPONTE COMPLAINTS

1. The SEC may file a sua sponte complaint and thereby initiate a disciplinary inquiry against a member of the AOTA whose actions violate the Code of Ethics if the SEC receives or discovers through public records any of the following actions by other authorities including but not limited to: (a) a felony conviction, (b) findings of malpractice, (c) revocation, suspension, or surrender of a license to practice, (d) censure or monetary fine of an individual licensed to practice (e) finding of academic misconduct, or (f) actions by a duly authorized tribunal or administrative hearing procedure.

2. The SEC may initiate a sua sponte complaint from other information discovered.

C. CONTINUATION OF COMPLAINT PROCESS

If a member fails to renew membership or fails to cooperate with the ethics investigation, the SEC shall continue to process the complaint noting in its report the circumstances of the respondent's resignation from membership or his/her failure to cooperate. Failure to renew membership or to cooperate with the investigation shall not deprive the SEC of jurisdiction.

D. Rules of Evidence

Formal rules of evidence which are employed in legal proceedings do not apply to these "Procedures for Disciplinary Action." The Judicial Council and the Appeals Panel can consider any evidence which they deem appropriate and pertinent. The Judicial Council may take additional material evidence at any time while the matter is pending before it. In general, appeals brought before the Appeals Panel shall be limited to the Judicial Council proceedings. In the interest of fairness, the Appeals Panel may take additional material evidence not submitted to the Judicial Council.

III. INVESTIGATION

A. Acknowledgment and Review of Complaint

Within 90 days of receipt of a complaint the SEC shall make a preliminary assessment of the complaint and decide whether or not an investigation is warranted.

If, in its preliminary review of the complaint, the SEC determines that an investigation is not warranted, the individual filing the complaint will be so notified. The respondent will be notified that a complaint was received. No records will be maintained.

If an investigation is required, the SEC Chairperson shall, within 15 days, do the following:

(1) Notify the Ethics Program Manager (EPM) at the AOTA National Office who will serve to investigate the complaint.

(2) Notify the respondent (by certified, return receipt mail) that a complaint has been received and an investigation is being conducted. A copy of the complaint shall be enclosed with this notification.

(3) Notify the complainant that an investigation is being conducted.

B. Conflict of Interest

The investigator shall (1) never have had a substantial professional relationship with either the complainant or the respondent; and (2) not have a conflict of interest with either the complainant or the respondent. In the event that the EPM does not meet these criteria, the SEC Chairperson shall appoint an alternate investigator.

C. Response to Complaint

1. The respondent shall be given 30 days from receipt of the notification to respond verbally and/or in writing to the Investigator and must be given full opportunity to refute all charges.

Apart from the complainant and the charged party (respondent), no other persons will participate in the investigation without prior approval of the respondent.

2. The complainant shall be made aware of any new evidence submitted to the investigator, being given a copy of it and shall have fourteen days in which to submit a rebuttal. Thereafter, the record shall be closed.

3. Failure to Act or Participate in Cases - Failure of the respondent to cooperate with the investigation (1) shall not prevent continuation of the Enforcement Procedures of the Code of Ethics and (2) shall in itself constitute a violation of the Occupational Therapy Code of Ethics.

D. INVESTIGATOR TIMELINE

The investigation process will be completed within 90 days of the appointment of the investigator. The investigator shall report to the SEC unless the SEC determines special circumstances which warrant additional time for the investigation. The Investigator's report shall state findings regarding the validity of the complaint.

E. RETENTION AND REFERRAL OF COMPLAINT

The SEC may at any time refer a matter to the National Board for Certification in Occupational Therapy (NBCOT), state regulatory boards, or other recognized authorities (authority) for appropriate action. Upon such referral to the appropriate authority, the SEC shall (a) retain jurisdiction; (b) stay any action until SEC receives notification of a decision by that authority. A stay in conducting an investigation shall not constitute a waiver of SEC jurisdiction.

F. NOTIFICATION OF STAYED ACTION

The SEC shall send written notification of a stayed case. Such notification will be sent by certified mail to the complainant and the respondent.

IV. STANDARDS AND ETHICS COMMISSION REVIEW AND DECISION

A. The Commission on Standards and Ethics shall review the Investigator's report and shall render a decision within 90 days of receipt of the report whether a formal charge by the Association is warranted. The SEC may, in the conduct of its review, take whatever further investigatory actions it deems necessary.

B. Acceptance of SEC Decision

If the respondent accepts the charge and disciplinary action as the result of the preliminary investigation, the SEC Chairperson notifies all parties involved and carries out the disciplinary action. The disciplinary action shall be publicized.

If the respondent refutes the allegation, the President of the Association shall be so notified in writing by the SEC Chairperson.

C. Filing of Formal Charges

If the SEC decides that a formal charge is warranted, the respondent to the complaint is notified of the SEC's decision to file a formal charge and the recommended disciplinary action. The respondent can choose at this time to admit to the violation, accept the disciplinary action, and relinquish the right to a hearing by the Judicial Council. The respondent has two (2) weeks from receipt of the SEC's decision to notify the Chairperson of his or her decision.

V. THE JUDICIAL COUNCIL

A. PANEL SELECTION

The Judicial Council, comprised of three members in good standing of the Association, shall be appointed by the President of the Association within 30 days of the notification to hear the formal charges against the respondent and decide on the merits of the case. Members appointed shall (1) never have had a substantial professional relationship with either the complainant or the respondent; and (2) not have a conflict of interest with either the complainant or the respondent.

B. HEARING

Thirty days in advance of the hearing, the Judicial Council shall notify in writing all parties of the date, time, and place for the hearing. Within 20 days of notification of the hearings, the respondent charged by the Association may submit to the Council a response to the Association's charges.

C. SUPPORT PERSONNEL

Legal counsel shall represent the Association at the hearing.

The respondent may be represented by legal counsel. Full opportunity to refute all charges shall be afforded. All parties shall have the opportunity to confront and cross-examine witnesses. Testimony may be presented by others than those who are parties to the charge. A record of the hearing shall be made.

D. DECISION

1. Within 15 days after the hearing, the Judicial Council shall notify the President of the Association of its decision, which shall include whatever disciplinary action might be required.

2. Within 10 days of notice from the Judicial Council, the President shall notify all parties, and the original complainant, of the Council's decision. Within 30 days after the notification of the Council's decision any individual or individuals judged deserving of disciplinary action may appeal the judgment to the Executive Board of the Association. (See below) If no

appeal is filed, the President shall notify appropriate bodies within the Association and make any other notifications deemed necessary.

VI. APPEAL PROCESS

Appeals shall be written, signed by the appealing party, and sent by certified mail to the Executive Director at the Association's National Office. The basis for the appeal shall be fully explained in this document.

A. APPEAL PANEL

The Vice-President, Secretary, and Treasurer of the Association shall constitute the Appeals Panel. In the event of vacancies in these positions or the existence of a potential conflict of interest, the Vice-President shall appoint replacements drawn from among the other Board members. The President and Chairperson of SEC shall not serve on the Appeals Panel.

B. GROUNDS FOR APPEAL

The appeal must relate to issues and procedures that are part of the record of the hearing before the Judicial Council. The appeal may also address the substance of the disciplinary action.

1. The Executive Director shall forward any letter of appeal to the Appeals Panel within 15 days of receipt.

2. Within 45 days after the appeal is received by the appeals panel, the Panel shall determine whether a hearing is required. If the Panel decides that a hearing is necessary, timely notice for such hearing shall be given to the appealing party. Participants at the hearing shall be limited to the appealing party and legal counsel (if so desired), legal counsel for the Association, and any others approved in advance by the Appeals Panel.

C. DECISION

Within 45 days after receipt of the appeal, if there is no hearing, or within 15 days after the appeals hearing, the Appeals Panel shall notify the President of the Association of its decision. The President shall immediately notify the appealing party, the original complainant, and appropriate bodies of the Association. The President shall make any other notifications deemed necessary.

For Association purposes, the decision of the Appeals Panel shall be final.

VII. NOTIFICATION

All notification referred to in this procedure shall be in writing and shall be by certified, return-receipt mail.

VIII. RECORDS AND REPORTS

At the completion of this procedure all records and reports shall be returned to the Ethics Program Manager. The original records and reports which form the initial basis for the complaint, actual evidence, and disposition of the complaint shall be filed in the confidential file of the Executive Director of the Association. All other copies shall be destroyed.

IX. PUBLICATION

Final decisions of the Judicial Council will be publicized only after all appeals have been exhausted.

Approved by the Representative Assembly, April 1996

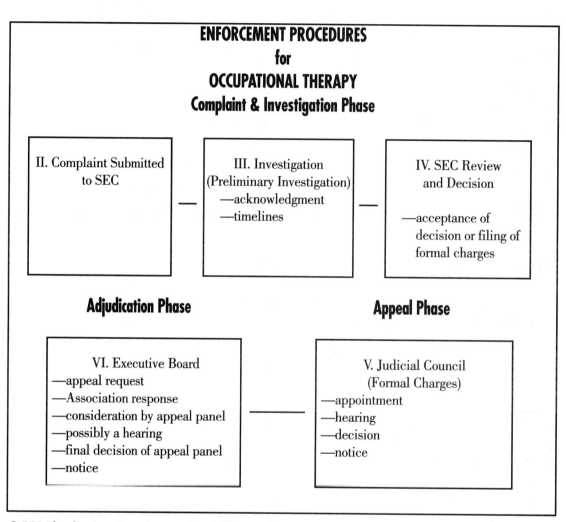

ENFORCEMENT PROCEDURES
for
OCCUPATIONAL THERAPY
Complaint & Investigation Phase

II. Complaint Submitted to SEC	III. Investigation (Preliminary Investigation) —acknowledgment —timelines	IV. SEC Review and Decision —acceptance of decision or filing of formal charges

Adjudication Phase   **Appeal Phase**

VI. Executive Board —appeal request —Association response —consideration by appeal panel —possibly a hearing —final decision of appeal panel —notice	V. Judicial Council (Formal Charges) —appointment —hearing —decision —notice

Core Values and Attitudes of Occupational Therapy Practice

Elizabeth Kanny, MA, OTR
for Standards and Ethics Commission
Ruth A. Hansen, PhD, OTR, FAOTA, Chairperson (1988-1994)

INTRODUCTION

In 1985, the American Occupational Therapy Association funded the Professional and Technical Role Analysis Study (PATRA). This study had two purposes: to delineate the entry-level practice of OTRs and COTAs through a role analysis and to conduct a task inventory of what practitioners actually do. Knowledge, skills, and attitude statements were to be developed to provide a basis for the role analysis. The PATRA study completed the knowledge and skills statements. The Executive Board subsequently charged the Standards and Ethics Commission (SEC) to develop a statement that would describe the attitudes and values that undergird the profession of occupational therapy. The SEC wrote this document for use by AOTA members.

The list of terms used in this statement was originally constructed by the American Association of Colleges of Nursing (AACN) (1986). The PATRA committee analyzed the knowledge statements that the committee had written and selected those terms from the AACN list that best identified the values and attitudes of our profession. This list of terms was then forwarded to SEC by the PATRA Committee to use as the basis for the Core Values and Attitudes paper.

The development of this document is predicated on the assumption that the values of occupational therapy are evident in the official documents of the American Occupational Therapy Association. The official documents that were examined are: (1) "Dictionary Definition of Occupational Therapy" (April 1986), (2) *The Philosophical Base of Occupational Therapy* (AOTA, Resolution C #531-79), (3) *Essentials and Guidelines for an Accredited Educational Program for the Occupational Therapist* (AOTA, 1991a), (4) *Essentials and Guidelines for an Accredited Educational Program for the Occupational Therapy Assistant* (AOTA, 1991b), and (5) *Occupational Therapy Code of Ethics* (AOTA, 1988). It is further assumed that these documents are representative of the values and beliefs reflected in other occupational therapy literature.

A *value* is defined as a belief or an ideal to which an individual is committed. Values are an important part of the base or foundation of a profession. Ideally, these values are embraced by all members of the profession and are reflected in the members' interactions with those persons receiving services, colleagues, and the society at large. Values have a central role in a profession, and are developed and reinforced throughout an individual's life as a student and as a professional.

Actions and *attitudes* reflect the values of the individual. An attitude is the disposition to respond positively or negatively toward an object, person, concept, or situation. Thus, there is an assumption that all professional actions and interactions are rooted in certain core values and beliefs.

Seven Core Concepts

In this document, the *core values and attitudes* of occupational therapy are organized around seven basic concepts-altruism, equality, freedom, justice, dignity, truth, and prudence. How these core values and attitudes are expressed and implemented by occupational therapy practitioners may vary depending upon the environments and situations in which professional activity occurs.

Altruism is the unselfish concern for the welfare of others. This concept is reflected in actions and attitudes of commitment, caring, dedication, responsiveness, and understanding.

Equality requires that all individuals be perceived as having the same fundamental human rights and opportunities. This value is demonstrated by an attitude of fairness and impartiality. We believe that we should respect all individuals, keeping in mind that they may have values, beliefs, or life styles that are different from our own. Equality is practiced in the broad professional arena, but is particularly important in day-to-day interactions with those individuals receiving occupational therapy services.

Freedom allows the individual to exercise choice and to demonstrate independence, initiative, and self-direction. There is a need for all individuals to find a balance between autonomy and societal membership that is reflected in the choice of various patterns of interdependence with the human and nonhuman environment. We believe that individuals are internally and externally motivated toward action in a continuous process of adaptation throughout the life span. Purposeful activity plays a major role in developing and exercising self-direction, initiative, interdependence, and relatedness to the world. Activities verify the individual's ability to adapt, and they establish a satisfying balance between autonomy and societal membership. As professionals, we affirm the freedom of choice for each individual to pursue goals that have personal and social meaning.

Justice places value on the upholding of such moral and legal principles as fairness, equity, truthfulness, and objectivity. This means we aspire to provide occupational therapy services for all individuals who are in need of these services and that we will maintain a goal-directed and objective relationship with all those served. Practitioners must be knowledgeable about and have respect for the legal rights of individuals receiving occupational therapy services. In addition, the occupational therapy practitioner must understand and abide by the local, state, and federal laws governing professional practijs.

Dignity emphasizes the importance of valuing the inherent worth and uniqueness of each person. This value is demonstrated by an attitude of empathy and respect for self and others.

We believe that each individual is a unique combination of biologic endowment, sociocultural heritage, and life experiences. We view human beings holistically, respecting the unique interaction of the mind, body, and physical and social environment. We believe that dignity is nurtured and grows from the sense of competence and self-worth that is integrally linked to the person's ability to perform valued and relevant activities. In occupational therapy we emphasize the importance of dignity by helping the individual build on his or her unique attributes and resources.

Truth requires that we be faithful to facts and reality. Truthfulness or veracity is demonstrated by being accountable, honest, forthright, accurate, and authentic in our attitudes and actions. There is an obligation to be truthful with ourselves, those who receive services, colleagues, and society. One way that this is exhibited is through maintaining and upgrading professional competence. This happens, in part, through an unfaltering commitment to inquiry and learning, to self-understanding and to the development of an interpersonal competence.

Prudence is the ability to govern and discipline oneself through the use of reason. To be prudent is to value judiciousness, discretion, vigilance, moderation, care, and circumspection in the management of one's affairs, to temper extremes, make judgments and respond on the basis of intelligent reflection and rational thought.

Summary

Beliefs and values are those intrinsic concepts that underlie the core of the profession and the professional interactions of each practitioner. These values describe the profession's philosophy and provide the basis for defining purpose. The emphasis or priority that is given to each value may change as one's professional career evolves and as the unique characteristics of a situation unfold. This evolution of values is developmental in nature. Although we have basic values that cannot be violated, the degree to which certain values will take priority at a given time is influenced by the specifics of a situation and the environment in which it occurs. In one instance dignity may be a higher priority than truth; in another prudence may be chosen over freedom. As we process information and make decisions, the weight of the values that we hold may change. The practitioner faces dilemmas because of conflicting values and is required to engage in thoughtful deliberation to determine where the priority lies in a given situation.

The challenge for us all is to know our values, be able to make reasoned choices in situations of conflict, and be able to clearly articulate and defend our choices. At the same time, it is important that all members of the profession be committed to a set of common values. This mutual commitment to a set of beliefs and principles that govern our practice can provide a basis for clarifying expectations between the recipient and the provider of services. Shared values empowers the profession and, in addition, builds trust among ourselves and with others.

REFERENCES:

American Association of Colleges of Nursing. (1986). *Essentials of College and University Education for Professional Nursing*. Final report, Washington, DC.

American Occupational Therapy Association. (April 1986). Dictionary definition of occupational therapy. Adopted and approved by the Representative Assembly April 1986 to fulfill Resolution #596-83. (Available from: AOTA, 4720 Montgomery Lane, PO Box 31220, Bethesda, MD 20824-1220.)

American Occupational Therapy Association. (1988). Occupational Therapy Code of Ethics. *American Journal of Occupational Therapy, 42*, 795–796.

American Occupational Therapy Association. (1991a). Essentials and Guidelines for an Accredited Educational Program for the Occupational Therapist. *American Journal of Occupational Therapy, 45*, 1077–1084.

American Occupational Therapy Association. (1991b). Essentials and Guidelines for an Accredited Educational Program for the Occupational Therapy Assistant. *American Journal of Occupational Therapy, 45*, 1085–1092.

Resolution C #531-79– The philosophical base of occupational therapy. (1979). *American Journal of Occupational Therapy, 33* (11), 785.

Approved by the Representative Assembly June, 1993

FROM: *The American Journal of Occupational Therapy*, December 1993, Vol. 47, No. 12, 1085–1086.

PROCEDURES FOR DISCIPLINARY ACTION

Section A. Preamble

In exercising its responsibility for promoting and maintaining standards of professional conduct in the practice of occupational therapy, the National Board for Certification in Occupational Therapy ("NBCOT" formerly known as "AOTCB") has adopted these procedures for the investigation and adjudication of complaints concerning persons who have been certified by the NBCOT as Occupational Therapists, Registered, Certified Occupational Therapy Assistants, or who have applied for such certification. These procedures are intended to enable the NBCOT, through its Disciplinary Action Committee ("DAC"), to act fairly in the performance of its responsibilities to the public as a certifying agency, and to ensure that the rights of individuals against whom complaints have been made are protected.

The purpose of the disciplinary action program - The central purpose of the NBCOT's disciplinary action program is the protection of the public from those practitioners whose professional performance or fitness to practice reflects incompetence, breaches of ethics, or impairment. The disciplinary action program is not intended to be solely punitive; it is also intended to be rehabilitative, providing insofar as possible incentive to practitioners to engage in the safe, proficient and/or competent practice of occupational therapy.

Rules of Evidence - Formal rules of evidence which are employed in legal proceedings do not apply to disciplinary action proceedings. The NBCOT's Disciplinary Action Committee and the Appeals Panel may consider any evidence which they deem appropriate and pertinent.

Advisory Opinion - On its own initiative, or at the request of others, the NBCOT Disciplinary Action Committee may issue advisory opinions on the interpretation and application of the disciplinary program. This is a mechanism for obtaining an opinion before the fact or in relation to a hypothetical situation. All advisory opinions shall be in writing, approved by the NBCOT Directors and signed by the President of the NBCOT.

Jurisdiction - The DAC shall have jurisdiction over all who are certified or who have applied to take the NBCOT Certification Examination for Occupational Therapist, Registered ("OTR") or Certified Occupational Therapy Assistant ("COTA").

Section B. Grounds for Discipline — The grounds for disciplinary action for failure to engage in the safe, proficient and/or competent practice of occupational therapy are:

1. Incompetence — Engaging in conduct which evidences a lack of knowledge of, or lack of ability or failure to apply, the prevailing principles and/or skills of the profession for which the individual has been certified.

2. Unethical Behavior — Violating prevailing ethical standards of the profession relating to

the safe, proficient and/or competent practice of occupational therapy, including:

   a. Making false statements or providing false information in connection with an application for certification.

   b. Misrepresenting one's credentials (education, training, experience, competence).

   c. Engaging in false, misleading or deceptive advertising.

   d. Obtaining or attempting to obtain compensation by fraud or deceit.

   e. Violating any federal or state statute or law which relates to the practice for which the individual has a certificate.

   f. Engaging in assault and battery of patients or others with whom the practitioner has a professional relationship.

   g. Engaging in sexual misconduct or abuse involving patients or others with whom the practitioner has a professional relationship.

   h. Being convicted of a crime, the circumstances of which substantially relate to the practice of occupational therapy or indicate an inability to engage in the practice of occupational therapy safely, proficiently and/or competently.

   i. Otherwise violating the prevailing standards of the profession relating to the safe, proficient and/or competent practice of occupational therapy.

3. Impairment — The inability to engage in the practice of occupational therapy safely, proficiently and/or competently as a result of substance abuse, or physical or psychological disability. This includes, but is not limited to:

   a. Engaging in professional practice while one's ability to practice is impaired by alcohol or other drugs.

   b. Engaging in practice while one's ability to practice is impaired by reason of physical or mental disability or disease.

   c. Being adjudicated mentally incompetent by a court.

SECTION C. SANCTIONS

The Disciplinary Action Committee may impose any one or more of the following sanctions:

1. Ineligibility for certification, which means that an individual is barred from becoming certified by the NBCOT, either indefinitely or for a certain duration.

2. Reprimand, which means a formal expression of disapproval which shall be retained in the certificant's file but shall not be publicly announced.

3. Censure, which means a formal expression of disapproval which is publicly announced.

4. Probation, which means continued certification is subject to fulfillment of specified condi-

tions, e.g., monitoring, education, supervision, and/or counseling.

5. Suspension, which means the loss of certification for a certain duration, after which the individual may be required to apply for reinstatement.

6. Revocation, which means permanent loss of certification.

All sanctions other than reprimand and ineligibility for certification shall be announced publicly, in accordance with Section D. 3. All sanctions other than reprimand shall be disclosed in response to inquiries in accordance with Section D. 3.

Section D. Disciplinary Procedures

1. Initiation of the Disciplinary Process

The disciplinary action process shall be initiated upon receipt by the DAC of information that appears to be relevant to an individual's fitness to practice or otherwise constitute grounds for disciplinary action under these procedures. Ordinarily, this will occur when a complaint is received by the DAC from an individual or group; however, the DAC may also commence a disciplinary action process without such a complaint upon receipt of information that indicates that there may be grounds for disciplinary action. For purposes of these procedures, this shall also be considered a complaint.

2. Investigation

The Chair of the Disciplinary Action Committee shall make a preliminary assessment of each complaint and, in consultation with the Disciplinary Action Committee Staff ("Staff") decide whether a formal investigation is warranted. The Chair of the DAC may dismiss complaints which are frivolous or outside the DAC's jurisdiction, but any such dismissal shall be reported to the full DAC at the next scheduled meeting.

If the Chair of the DAC determines that a formal investigation is warranted, the Staff shall immediately notify the subject of the complaint of the investigation. This notification shall be in writing and shall include a description of the complaint and the identity of the complainant. The notice shall be sent by certified mail. The subject of the complaint shall have 30 days from the date notification is sent to respond in writing to the complaint. The Staff may extend this period up to an additional 30 days upon request, provided sufficient justification for the extension is given.

Any complaint received by the DAC more than 60 days prior to the DAC's next scheduled meeting shall be placed on the agenda for that meeting. Complaints received less than 60 days prior to the DAC's next scheduled meeting shall be placed on the agenda for the following DAC meeting.

The Staff shall be responsible for conducting the formal investigation. In discharging this responsibility, he/she may utilize the services of other NBCOT personnel, legal counsel, independent investigators and/or others as the Staff deems appropriate.

The Staff shall provide a written report on its investigation to the DAC prior to the meeting at which the complaint will be on the DAC's agenda. If the investigation is complete, the report shall include the basis for Staff's findings, as well as any written responses, or other materials submitted by the subject of the complaint.

In cases where a state regulatory board has taken disciplinary action against an individual, the Staff will contact the state regulatory board for information and will include this information in the report to the DAC.

Failure by the subject of a complaint to respond to the disciplinary action proceedings shall be sufficient grounds for the imposition of sanctions by the DAC.

If the subject of a complaint seeks to forfeit his/her certification, the complaint may be dismissed within the discretion of the DAC. If the complaint is dismissed, public notice of the circumstances of the dismissal, including the existence of the complaint, may be given in accordance with Section D. 3 of these procedures.

3. DISCIPLINARY ACTION COMMITTEE REVIEW AND DECISION

The DAC shall review the report of the Staff and, based upon the available information, either (a) dismiss the complaint; (b) direct the Staff to obtain additional information; (c) stay the proceedings pending completion of related litigation or state disciplinary action; or (d) make a preliminary determination of disciplinary action. If the DAC makes a preliminary determination of disciplinary action, it shall also schedule a hearing.

The Staff shall give the subject of the complaint written notice of the DAC's action. If the DAC has made a preliminary determination of disciplinary action, the notice shall state the grounds for the preliminary determination, the proposed sanction and the time, date and place of the scheduled hearing.

The subject of the complaint may be represented at the hearing by his/her legal counsel, or any other individual of his/her choosing. The subject of the complaint shall be solely responsible for all of his/her own expenses related to the hearing. The subject of the complaint may waive his/her right to a hearing by accepting the DAC's preliminary determination of disciplinary action and proposed sanction.

Following the hearing, the DAC shall notify in writing the complainant and the subject of the complaint of its decision. The DAC's decision shall take effect immediately unless otherwise provided by the DAC.

If an individual's certification is suspended or revoked, or he/she is placed on probation or censured, all occupational therapy state regulatory boards and occupational therapy state associations shall be notified and an announcement included in one or more publications of general circulation to persons engaged or otherwise interested in the profession of occupational therapy. The NBCOT may also disclose such disciplinary actions, as well as ineligibility for certification, to others as it deems appropriate, including, persons inquiring about the status of an individual's certification, employers, insurers and the general public.

4. APPEALS PROCESS

Within thirty (30) days after the notification of the DAC's decision, any individual(s) sanctioned by the DAC may appeal the decision to the NBCOT Directors. A notice of appeal, which must be in writing and signed by the appealing party, shall be sent by the appealing party to the NBCOT Directors in care of the Executive Director. The grounds for the appeal shall be fully explained in this notice.

The President shall form an Appeals Panel within 30 days after receipt of the notice of appeal. The Appeals Panel shall be comprised of three NBCOT Directors and shall include at least one OTR or one COTA and one public member. Members of the DAC who participated in any aspect of the DAC proceedings related to the complaint shall not serve on the Appeals Panel.

An appeal must relate to evidence, issues and procedures that are part of the record of the DAC hearing and decision. The appeal may also address the substance of the disciplinary action. However, the Panel may in its discretion consider additional evidence.

Within 15 days after the notice of appeal is received by the Appeals Panel, the Panel shall either decide the appeal or schedule a hearing. If a hearing is scheduled the appealing party shall be given at least 30 days notice of the hearing. The appealing party may be represented at the hearing by legal counsel or any other individual of his/her choosing. The appealing party shall be solely responsible for all of his/her own expenses related to the hearing. Within 15 days after the appeals hearing, the Panel shall notify the President of its decision.

The President shall promptly notify the appealing party of the Appeals Panel's decision. The decision of the Appeals Panel shall be final.

5. NOTIFICATION

All notifications referred to in these procedures shall be in writing and shall be by certified, return receipt mail unless otherwise indicated.

6. RECORDS AND REPORTS

At the completion of this procedure, all records and reports shall be returned to the Staff. The complete files in the disciplinary proceedings shall be carefully reviewed and everything discarded except information on the initial basis for the challenge, the actual evidence in resolving the proceeding, and the disposition of the case.

7. Expedited Action

The DAC or, in the case of an appeal, the Appeals Panel, may expedite a matter by shortening any notice or response period provided for under these procedures if the DAC or Appeals Panel determines in its sole discretion that shortening the period is appropriate in order to protect against the possibility of harm to recipients of occupational therapy services.

8. Amendment to Procedures

These procedures may be amended at any time by the NBCOT Directors.

Amended: June 1989
Amended: October 1989
Amended: August 1991
Amended: July 1993
Amended: March 1995

The National Board for Certification in Occupational Therapy, Inc. ("NBCOT" formerly known as "AOTCB") is a national organization that certifies qualified persons as occupational therapists, registered (OTRs) and as certified occupational therapy assistants (COTAs). The NBCOT's goal is to promote the health, safety and welfare of the public by establishing, maintaining and administering standards, policies and programs for certification and registration of occupational therapy personnel.

The NBCOT has jurisdiction over all individuals who are certified by NBCOT as occupational therapists (OTRs) and occupational therapy assistants (COTAs), as well as over those individuals who have applied to take the certification examinations. In its efforts to protect the public from those OTRs and COTAs and examination candidates who are incompetent, unethical or impaired, the NBCOT has developed procedures* for the investigation and adjudication of complaints.

The central principle which defines the scope of disciplinary action procedures is "safe, proficient and/or competent practice of occupational therapy". Thus, an individual who is accused of billing patients for occupational therapy services at a rate which is not "based on cost analysis" and is not "commensurate with services rendered" might be subject to consideration by the AOTA's Standards and Ethics Commission as a violation of the AOTA's Code of Ethics. However, such conduct would not necessarily fall within the NBCOT's scope since individual billing rates and setting of fees alone usually do not relate to safe, proficient and/or competent practice of occupational therapy. On the other hand, submitting bills for services unrendered may fall within NBCOT's scope, since this does relate to safe, proficient practice of OT, inasmuch as the patient's health or rehabilitation may be jeopardized due to unrendered services. Additionally, the patient's access to service from a third party payor may be affected because services were billed which were not provided.

Other examples of practices more or less likely to involve the principle of "safe, proficient and/or competent practice" are provided in Attachment A. Actions that may be illegal or morally offensive are not by reason of that fact alone within the scope of the Disciplinary Action Committee; they must clearly relate to and involve the safe, proficient and/or competent practice of occupational therapy.

It is the intent of the Disciplinary Action Committee to act fairly in the performance of its responsibilities to the public and to ensure that the rights of individuals against whom complaints have been made are protected.

Disciplinary Action and State Regulation – NBCOT's disciplinary actions are independent of sanctions for disciplinary action by state regulatory agencies. However, NBCOT routinely advises regulatory bodies when it receives a complaint against an individual in a regulated state and of its decision concerning the complaint. Normally, when a complaint is under active consideration by a state regulatory body, the Disciplinary Action Committee chooses to stay action until the state has taken action on the case.

* See NBCOT 'Procedures for Disciplinary Action'; also, the brochure entitled 'Disciplinary Action: A Process to Protect The Public'.

Ethical Issues in Documentation

Attachment A

Likely to involve "Safe, Proficient and Competent Practice of Occupational Therapy"	Less likely to involve "Safe, Proficient and Competent Practice of Occupational Therapy"
• Current drug addiction	• Felony conviction for use of controlled substances several years ago
• Not renewing state license for several years; not complying with state's continuing education requirements	• Failure to renew state license promptly
• Walking off job while a patient is waiting for a splint to be completed	• Quitting a job without notice to employer
• Engaging in sexual activity with a patient	• Sexual activity between consenting adults in a non-professional relationship
• Providing less frequent and shorter duration occupational therapy than agreed to in a student's Individual Education Plan (IEP)	• Signing a student's Individual Education Plan (IEP) when another therapist completed the evaluation
• Advertising treatment which makes false claims about the value of the treatment	• Advertising treatment which contains a testimonial or endorsement by another person
• Conviction of DWI while driving a group of patients	• Conviction of a single incidence of DWI, unrelated to job requirements
• Providing incorrect home program instructions to a patient	• Providing correct home program instruction using wrong terminology
• Practicing outside the scope of practice as defined by state law	• Non-payment of student loans

17. Alternative Documentation

Sandy Hanebrink, OTS

One of the most important components of an occupational therapy practitioner's daily functions is documentation. It is a source of information about expected outcomes; and it provides a record of treatment, a continous feedback on the client's response to treatment, and therefore is a source of information for evaluating the effectiveness of care. Additionally, it provides data for reimbursement, quality assurance, research, education, treatment innovations, and program promotion. The implications are significant if a practitioner can not or has difficulty documenting services.

Sandy Hanebrink wrote this chapter while completing a Level II fieldwork affiliation with the American Occupational Therapy Association.

ortunately for practitioners with disabilities or other limitations there are alternatives to the use of traditional documentation methods. This chapter will provide a general overview of ideas, examples, suggestions, and resources on alternative documentation methods that can help an occupational therapy practitioner to maximize his or her performance. The inclusion of these methods and/or techniques does not constitute an endorsement by the author or the American Occupational Therapy Association, Inc.

Alternative Documentation Methods

Addressing the individual needs of the facility or person is paramount in choosing an alternative documentation method. This places human performance at the core of the decision-making process. Several factors should be considered in selecting an alternative method or technique:

- the characteristics of the practitioner's disability (if applicable) and his or her resultant needs
- the needs of the staff
- the documentation requirements and system of the facility
- the cost of the adaptation/modifications.

Some methods can range from no-cost to very expensive to implement. For the most part, however, with the exception of the high-technology areas, alternative documentation methods are relatively inexpensive (see Table 17.1).

COGNITIVE LIMITATIONS – For those practitioners with limitations or difficulties with organizational skills, distractibility, processing written material, and other documentation interpretation problems, there are a variety of alternative documentation methods and/or techniques available. Process modification can be as simple as providing a quiet, unintrusive environment for documentation or additional time to complete the documentation; or using a dictation or a computerized system. Including photographs and video as part of documentation can be useful. Using another individual (such as a reader), may be necessary for clinicians with processing problems such as dyslexia.

Table 17.1

Frequent Breaks	$0
Hand Exercises	$0
Relocation of Work Activities	$0
Wrist Rests	$20
Arm/Elbow Supports	$200
Alternative Keyboards	$180 - $2,000

Source: President's Committee on Employment of People with Disabilities.

Having a quiet environment for documentation does not necessarily mean setting aside a special room for documentation only. It could mean establishing a list of offices or vacant rooms available for chart review and documentation purposes. Additional time needed by a clinician to effectively complete documentation may be accommodated by careful patient scheduling. Dictation services are already available at a number of facilities and can enhance documentation efficiency. Photography and video are also becoming more widely used in a variety of clinics as an integral form of documentation.

Some facilities incorporate multimedia techniques with computerized systems. With any of these scenarios or suggestions, it is important to remember that human performance is the focus. Increasing function, maximizing skills, and accomplishing the goals of each individual clinician and the facility are the intended outcomes. Choosing the technique that meets the needs of clinicians has to be done on a case-by-case basis. It is important to note that if an alternative documentation technique is helpful for one clinician, it probably will benefit other clinicians as well.

MOBILITY LIMITATIONS – Alternative documentation for clinicians with mobility limitations is a prime example of what works for one may work for all. Mobility limitations may include dexterity problems secondary to carpal tunnel syndrome, arthritis, spasticity, paralysis, amputations, tendon injuries, fractures, or simple poor penmanship. Other limitations include difficulties with standing, walking, moving, or balance dysfunction associated with temporary or permanent conditions. Effective documentation for these individuals may be directly related to the environment or setting where the work is being done. For example, the work station itself may require modification such as lowering or raising shelves, files, or desk tops. Furniture may need to be arranged to provide safe and functional access. Seating and positioning can be adjusted to provide better access to equipment, to reduce barriers secondary to the disability, to decrease fatigue, and to improve overall function. The area of ergonomic seating has emerged as a specialization and has grown rapidly in recent years. According to the Hewlett-Packard Company, ergonomic sitting posture includes:

1. chair adjusted to keep body supported in an upright position

2. back rest adjusted to fit the lumbar region of spine

3. chair height allowing adequate leg clearance

4. keyboard/work surface maintained at elbow level

5. top of screen at or below eye level

6. feet able to rest firmly on the ground or supported by a footrest (Cook & Hyssey, 1995).

Other alternative documentation methods include the use of assistive technology. There are a variety of tools and aids available, such as split keyboards, adaptive keyboards, keyguards, adaptive computer mouse, on-screen keyboards, voice activated computer systems, dictation services, typing aids, personalized computer systems, and facility-based computer systems. Using photography and video as well as the assistance of other individuals to carry out physical tasks are options for practitioners with mobility limitations.

VISUAL LIMITATIONS – Specific accommodations for clinicians who are visually impaired or blind include enlarged print in charts, enlarged print software programs, audio copies of charts, braillers, readers, writers, dictation services, and computerized voice recognition systems.

COMPUTER METHOD AND TECHNIQUES – Documentation is increasingly becoming computerized. From individualized techniques to total facility network systems, computers are replacing the traditional handwritten documentation format.

Commercial programs are available for rate enhancement modifications. Word predict, on screen key boards, voice activation programs, templates, and foreign language interpretation or translation programs are examples of the technology that is available. Desktop and portable scanners, printers, or laptop and notebook computers can be used for effective documentation in facilities that may or may not have large centralized computer systems. Clinicians may use scanners to copy facility forms or documents into a laptop system. By creating and using personal templates and macros, the clinician can efficiently input necessary information onto the scanned documents, and the document then can be printed and added to the permanent medical record.

Macros allow the clinician to group computer commands together as a unit and execute them with one or two keystrokes. This technique helps maintain uniform documents and filing in the charts. This technique may be beneficial to the home health or traveling practitioner who visits many locations with a variety of documentation forms. The clinician uses the appropriate form and uses macros with commonly used goals and other documentation items to efficiently and consistently document the client's progress. This in turn gives the clinician more time to provide quality care.

A similar technique can be used with facility network systems. Many facilities use a combination of dictation services that are transcribed and input onto their network systems. Clinicians proofread and approve the documentation, which then becomes a part of the permanent record and is available to be accessed by authorized personnel. This process can take from 2 to 5 days. Using the same macro procedures as described above, the documentation can be uploaded into the facility network system in much less time.

Conclusion

Alternative documentation methods are effective ways to improve efficiency, accuracy, timeliness, and consistency of documentation. They will result in organized, legible, clear, concise, accurate, complete, and current treatment records. All the purposes for documentation—providing a serial and legal record of the treatment process, serving as an information source for care, facilitating communication among health care professionals, and furnishing data for education, research, and reimbursement—will be met.

Any accommodations, modifications, methods, or techniques used must be in compliance with local, state, and federal statutes and facility standards. Alternative documentation is essential to the provision of reasonable accommodation, and choosing the technique or method that meets the needs of practitioners with disabilities has to be done on a case-by-case basis. Yet, all occupational therapy practitioners, with and without disabilities, may benefit from the use of alternative document methods and techniques. These methods and techniques are an advantage to employees, employers, and the overall general operation of the department and facility.

References

Church, G., & Glennen, S. (1992). *The handbook of assistive technology*. San Diego, CA: Singular Publishing Group.

Cook, A. M., & Hyssey, S. M.. (1995). *Assistive technologies: Principles and practice*. St. Louis, MO: Mosby-Year Book.

Nagler, M. (Ed.). (1993). *Perspectives on disability* (2nd ed.) Palo Alto, CA: Health Markets Research.

New York State Department of Civil Service. (1996). *Working with people with disabilities*.

President's Committee on Employment of People with Disabilities. (1993). *ADA and the healthcare professional*. Washington, DC: Author.

Thompson-Hoffman, S., & Storck, I. F. (Eds). (1991). *Disability in the United States: A portrait from National Data*. New York: Springer Publishing.

The following resources were compiled by the author to assist the reader with alternative documentation. She wishes to acknowledge the work of A.M. Cook and S.M. Hyssey, whose data on resources are published in *Assistive Technology: Principles and Practice* (1995), St. Louis, MO: Mosby, Inc.

BRAILLE INPUT-OUTPUT DEVICES:

APH Pocket Braille
American Printing House for the Blind
The APH Pocket Braille is a portable computer with braille input and synthesized speech output. The system can be connected to Apple II series, Commodore, IBM, Tandy, and Texas Instruments computers through a serial port. It also can send information directly to braille embosser printers.

Braille Mate
Telesensory Braille Mate is a portable braille computer with an 8-dot braille keyboard, an 8-dot braille cell, and a built-in speech synthesizer. It can use grade 1 or grade 2 braille input. Grade 2 braille is printed into standard text. Braille Mate can serve as an input system for IBM PC or compatible computers.

Braille 'n Speak
Blazie Engineering
This is a portable computer system that can be used as a braille word processor. It has talking features, a calculator, clock, calendar, computer terminal, and telephone directory. The Braille 'n Speak can be connected to most computers through a serial port.

Braillex IB40 and IB80
Adhoc Reading Systems, Inc.
The Braillex is a 40- or 80-cell braille output printer system for IBM computers.

Braillo 200, Braillo 400S, and Braillo 90 Printers
American Thermofoam Corp.
These printers provide braille print for a variety of computer systems. The 200 is designed for high-speed printing with IBM computers. The 400S is a high-speed printer that also collates and can be used with IBM, Apple II series, and Tandy computers. The 90 is a small personal printer designed for use with the Apple II series of computers and IBM.

Keybraille
Humanware
Keybraille is used with MS-DOS series computers. It provides a 5-cell Braille display that indicates line, column, and screen attributes of the operating software.

Marathom Brailler
Enabling Technologies

This braille embosser printer can be used with Apple II series, IBM, Macintosh, Commodore, Tandy, and Texas Instruments computers.

Nomad
Syntha/Voice Computers

Nomad is a portable IBM-XT-compatible laptop computer with synthesized speech output and the option of a braille or Qwerty keyboard. It is equipped with a cursor tracking screen reading program, and 2400-baud modem.

Notex
Adhoc Reading Systems

This is a small, portable Braille notebook computer. The system has 24-cell braille output, braille input, and word processor and calculator software.

Xerox/Kurzweil Personal Reader
Xerox Imaging Systems

This device "reads" printed materials and converts them into synthetic speech. It can be used for computer data entry via an RS 232 interface and can provide Braille output.

COMPUTER ACCESS DEVICES:

AID+ME
Computability

The AID+ME provides alternate access methods for IBM, Commodore, Apple II, and Macintosh computers. Any input device can be used, including Powerpad, Touch window, expanded keyboards, communication aids with serial output, and joystick.

Disk Guide
Extensions for Independence Prentke Romich TASH

A disk guide attaches to the front of a disk drive to help align computer disks with the drive opening. It is available in 3.5-inch or 5.25-inch sizes for a variety of computers.

Dragon Dictate
Dragon Systems

Dragon Dictate is a voice-operated accessing system for IBM-compatible computers. It can transparently operate any software application. The voice recognition software is designed to "learn" a user's speech patterns in a relatively short period of time. It also relies on word-prediction strategies. The recognition "dictionary" has up to 21,000 words at one time.

Free Wheel
Pointer Systems

Free Wheel is a small head-mounted optical pointer that controls cursor movement on Macintosh and PC computers. The software places a keyboard image on the computer screen which is used to operate standard software. The PC version allows access via joystick, mouse, or single-switch options.

Info Window Display
IBM

The Info Window Display is an IBM color monitor for PC and PS2 computers with built-in touch window capabilities.

Kurzweil Voice System and Kurzweil Voice Report
Kurzweil Applied Intelligence

The Kurzweil systems are voice-recognition input systems for IBM PC, AT, and XT computers. The Voice System recognizes up to 1,000 words, and can operate a variety of software including spreadsheets, word processing, and databases. The Voice Report is designed as a word processing system. It recognizes up to 5,000 words and can store macros that are triggered by a single word or phrase.

Magic Wand Keyboard
In Touch Systems

This device is a miniature alternative keyboard for IBM computers. The user touches a hand-held "wand" on the keyboard to operate it. The keyboard plugs directly into the keyboard socket of any IBM or compatible computer.

Touch Window
Edmark

The Touch Window is a transparent screen that mounts over the monitor display of Apple II series, IBM, and Tandy computers. Software written for Touch Window allows the user to touch the screen to control the cursor.

Voice Key
TASH

Voice Key is a speech recognition system designed for IBM series computers. It has a 512-word or phrase capacity.

Voice Navigator
Articulate Systems

The Voice Navigator provides spoken voice control for Macintosh computers. It operates transparently and provides any keyboard function including mouse emulation. New voice commands can be added for special software applications.

20/20+
Optalec

This high-resolution computer monitor for IBM series computers provides enlarged text output.

Diconix 150 Plus
Adhoc Reading Systems

The Diconix is a small inkjet portable printer that weighs less than 4 pounds. It can be attached to IBM computes and some communication aids.

Vista
Telesensory

Vista enlarges computer screen text and graphics 3 to 16 times. It is designed for use with IBM series computers. Three-button mouse is used to control the screen image and a screen cursor.

SOFTWARE:

Access 190
Adaptive Communication Systems

Access 190 is a RAM-resident software program written for IBM series computers. It offers one-key computer functions, variable keystroke timing delays, word and letter prediction, and voice output when an external synthesized-speech system is connected. It can be accessed by the standard keyboard, single-switch scanning, or joystick controls.

Arctic Focus
Arctic Technologies

This software program enlarges the text and graphics on IBM series computers. A graphics adapter card is required.

Braille-Talk
GW Micro

This program for Apple II series and IBM computers translates any text file into Grade I or II Braille for printer output.

Brikeys Utility
Enabling Technologies Company

This RAM-resident utility gives a user a "pop up" braille keyboard that overrides the regular keyboard. It operates on IBM series or Tandy computers.

Easy Access
Apple Computer Inc.

This program is included in the system disk of Macintosh computers. It allows one-finger typists a "Sticky Key" option that bypasses having to press multiple keys at once and a keyboard mouse emulation function.

EZ Keys/EZ Wiz
Words+

This software program provides keyboard assistance for IBM series computers. This RAM-resident program offers word prediction and abbreviation expansion for slow typists.

PC Assisted Keyboard
DADA

The PC Assisted Keyboard is a software program that has functions for one-finger typists. It has key redefinition, sticky key, and macro customization features. It operates on IBM series computers.

Screen Doors
Madenta Communications Prentke Romich

Screen Doors is a keyboard emulation program for Macintosh computers. It provides an on-screen keyboard that can be accessed using a mouse, joystick, or Headmaster pointing system. Word-prediction features are included in the software.

Screenkeys
Berkley Systems

ScreenKeys is an alternate computer input program for Macintosh computers. A graphic image of the keyboard is pictured on the computer monitor. Any pointing access device can be used to access the screen keyboard.

Verbal Operating System
Computer Conversations

This IBM-series program provides synthesized speech output of all keyboard and computer screen actions. The system tracks the program cursor throughout all application programs. It includes a word processor.

Verbal View
Computer Conversions

Verbal View is a computer screen magnification program. It can enlarge the print to fill six, three, or two lines and has options for changing character and background colors. It was written for IBM series computers equipped with color graphics boards.

REFERRAL SOFTWARE:

Assistive Device Locator System (ADLS)
Academic Software

ADLS is a menu-driven program that lists thousands of assistive technology products in over 660 categories. It is available on floppy disks for Apple II series and IBM series computers. The program is updated annually for a minimum fee.

Hyper-ABLEDATA

Trace Research and Development

Hyper-ABLEDATA is an assistive technology database with over 15,000 products listed in hardware and software categories. The software is available in CD-ROM or in disk form for use on a hard drive system. Because Hyper-ABLEDATA uses HyperCard stacks, it currently operates only on Macintosh computers.

CUSTOM SOFTWARE

Research Corporation Medical

C & S Research has generic documentation Management Solutions and billing software systems as well as writing custom software specific for individual practice.

Marla Productions

Marla Productions has generic documentation and billing software systems.

SCANNERS

Color Flatbed

Mustek

MFS600IIEP-—Features: color capability, 26-Bit; greyscale; IBM compatible; OCR Technology included; TWAIN Compliant; 1 year parts and labor warranty.

Desktop

Storm Software

460618 (internal & external)—color capability; greyscale, 256 levels; up to 1200 DPI resolution; maximum scanning size 5"x7"; IBM compatible; TWAIN compliant; 1 year parts and labor warranty.

7357334400 (PRIMAX)-—Features: 24-bit True Color; 256 Greyscale and Black and White; 600 DPI (200 optical resolution) up to 1200 DPI enhanced resolution; maximum scanning size 5"x7"; IBM compatible; Macintosh compatible; PowerPC; TWAIN compliant.

Hand-Held

Logitec

9601060100(Scanman Color 2000)-—Features: 24-bit color; 8-bit (256)Gray Scale; 400x800dpi; maximum scanning width 4.1"; IBM compatible; OCR technology included; TWAIN compliant; 2 year warranty.

Sheet Feed

Mustek

MFS-12000C (Page color)-— Features: color compatible; 256 greyscale; 300x600dpi resolution; maximum scanning size 8.5"x14"; IBM compatible; OCR Technology included; TWAIN compliant; 1 year parts and labor warranty.

Organizations

Accessability Resource Center
1056 E. 19th Avenue
B-410
Denver, CO 80218-1088
(303) 861-6250

Alaska Center for Adaptive Technology
PO Box 6069
Sitka, AK 99835
(907) 747-6960

American Foundation for Technology
Assistance
Rt 14, PO Box 230
Morgantown, NC 28655
(704) 433-9697

American Foundation for the Blind
15 W 16th Street
New York, NY 10011
(212) 620-2000

Center for Computer Assistance to the
Disabled
617 Seventh Avenue
Fort Worth, TX 76104
(817) 870-9082

Center for Technology and Human
Disabilities
2301 Argonne Drive
Baltimore, MD 21218
(301) 554-3046

Clearinghouse on Computer Accommodation
(COCA)
KGDO, 18th and F Streets, NW
Room 2022
Washington, DC 20405
(202) 523-1906

Closing the Gap, Inc.
PO Box 68
Henderson, MN 56044
(612) 248-3294

Committee on Personal Computers and the
Handicapped (COPH-2)
PO Box 7701
Chicago, IL 60680-7701
(708) 866-8195

Compute Able Network
PO Box 1706
Portland, OR 97207
(503) 645-0009

Computer Access Center
2425 16th Street, Room 23
Santa Monica, CA 90405
(213) 450-8827

Direct Link for the Disabled
PO Box 1036
Solvang, CA 93463
(805) 688-1603

Easter Seal Systems' Computer Assisted
Technology (CATS)
c/o Technology Related Loan Fund Officer
5120 South Hyde Park Blvd.
Chicago, IL 60615
(312) 667-8400

Electronic Industries Foundation
Rehabilitation Engineering Center
1901 Pennsylvania Avenue, NW
Suite 700
Washington, DC 20006
(202) 955-5826

Health Research Center
1 Dupont Circle
Suite 800
Washington, DC 20036-1193
(202) 727-3866

IBM National Support Center for Persons
with Disabilities (IBM-NSCPD)
PO Box 2150
Atlanta, GA 30055
(800) 426-2133

International Society for Augmentative and
Alternative Communication (ISAAC)
PO Box 1762
Sta. R.
Toronto, Ontario M4G 4A3
Canada
(416) 737-9308

Job Accommodation Network (JAN)
West Virginia University
918 Chestnut Ridge Road
Suite 1
PO Box 6080
Morgantown, WV 26506-9901
(800) 526-7234

National Easter Seal Society
5120 S. Hyde Park Boulevard
Chicago, IL 60615-1146
(312) 667-8400

National Federation for the Blind
1800 Johnson Street
Baltimore, MD 21230
(301) 659-9314

National Institute for Rehabilitation
Engineering (NIRE)
PO Box 841
Butler, NJ 07405
(201) 838-2500

National Organization on Disability (NOD)
910 16th Street, NW
Suite 600
Washington, DC 20006
(202) 293-5968

National Spinal Cord Injury Association
600 W. Cummings Park
Suite 2000
Woburn, MA 01801
(617) 935-2722

National Technology Center
c/o American Foundation for the Blind
15 West 16th Street
New York, NY 10011
(212) 620-2000

U.S. Equal Employment Opportunity
Commission (EEOC)
ADA Service Office
1801 L Street, NW
Washington, DC 20507
(800) 669-3362 (V) for free publications
(800)800-3302 (TT)
(800)669-4000 (V) for technical assistance

Volunteers for Medical Engineering
c/o UMBC TEC
5202 Westland Boulevard
Baltimore, MD 21227
(301) 455-6395

Databases

Abledata
181 E. Cedar Street
Newington, CT 06111
(203) 667-5405

Accent on Information
PO Box 700
Bloomington, Il 61702
(309) 378-2961

Access/Abilities
PO Box 458
Mill Valley, CA 94942
(415) 388-3250

Compuserve
5000 Arlington Centre Boulevard
PO Box 20212
Columbus, OH 43220
(614) 457-8600

Publications

Assistive Technology: A Funding Workbook
RESNA Press
1101 Connecticut Avenue, NW
Suite 700
Washington, DC 20036
(202) 857-1199

Augmentative Communication News
One Surf Way
Suite 215
Monterey, CA 93940
(408) 649-3050

Closing the Gap
PO Box 58
Henderson, MN 56044
(612) 248-3294

Computer-Disability News
National Easter Seal Society
5120 S. Hyde Park Boulevard
Chicago, IL 60615
(312) 667-8400

Directory of Computer and High Technology
GrantsResearch Grant Guides
Department 3A
PO Box 1214
Loxahatchee, FL 33470
(407) 795-6129

Direct Link
Independent Living Center
617 Seventh Avenue
Fort Worth, TX 76104
(817) 870-9082

Financial Aid for the Disabled and Their Families
References Service Press
1100 Industrial Road
Suite 9
San Carlos, CA 94070
(415) 594- 0743

Funding Book: The Many Faces of Funding
Phonic Ear, Inc.
250 Camino Alto
Mill Valley, CA 94941
(415) 383-4000

Mobility Ltd.
401 Linden Center Drive
Fort Collins, CO 80524
(303) 484-7969

Rehabilitation Technology Service Delivery
Directory
RESNA Press
Department 4813
Washington, DC 20061-4813
(202) 857-1199

Ability Research
PO Box 1721
Minnetonka, MN 55345
(612) 939-0121

American Printing House for the Blind
PO Box 6085
Louisville, KY 40206-0085
(502) 895-2405

AbleNet
1081 10th Avenue, S.E.
Minneapolis, MN 55414-1312
(612) 379-0956

American Therofoam Corporation
2311 Travers Avenue
City of Commerce, CA 90040
(213) 723-9021

AbleOffice
Center For Rehabilitation Technology, Inc.
Georgia Tech Univeristy
(440) 876-8580

Apple Computer, Inc.
One Infinite Loop, MS 38DS
Cupertino, CA 95014
800-600-7808

Academic Software
331 W. 2nd Street
Lexington, KY 40507
(606) 233-2332

Arctic Technologies
55 Park Street Suite 2
Troy, MI 48083
(313) 588-7370

ADAMLAB
33500 Van Born Rd
PO Box 807
Wayne, MI 48184
(313) 467-1415

Articulate Systems, Inc.
600 West Cummings Park
Suite 4500
Woburn, MA 01801
(617) 935-5656

Adaptive Communication System, Inc.
Box 12440
Pittsburgh, PA 15231
(412) 264-2288

AssisTech
PO Box 137
Stow, NY 14785
(716) 789-4197

Berkeley Systems
1700 Shattuck Avenue
Berkeley, CA 94709
(415) 540-5537

Blazie Engineering
3660 Mill Green Road
Street, MD 21154
(301) 879-4944

C & C Software
5713 Kentford Cir.
Wichita, KS 67220
800-521-6263

C & S Research Corporation
1001 West 9th Avenue   Suite A
King of Prussia, PA 19406
(610) 265-9118

Computability Corporation
400 Grand River
Suite 109
Novi, MI 48375
(800) 433-8872

Computer Conversations
6297 Worthington Road, SW
Alexandria, OH 43001
(614) 924-2885

Computerade Products
2346 Wales Drive
Cardiff, CA 92007
(619) 942-3343

DADA
249 Concord Avenue
Unit 2
Toronto, ON M6H 2P4
Canada
(416) 530-0038

Didatech Software, Ltd.
4250 Dawson Street Suite 200
Burnaby, BC V5C 4B1
Canada
800-665-0667

Digital Impact
6506 S. Lewis
Suite 250
Tulsa, OK 74136
800-775-4232

Don Johnston Incorporated
1000 N. Rand Road
Bldg. 115
Wauconda, Il 60084
800-999-4660

Dragon Systems, Inc.
320 Nevada Street
Newton, MA 02160
(617) 965-5200

Edmark Corporation
PO Box 3903
Bellevue, WA 98009-3903
(800) 426-0856

Enabling Technologies Co.
3102 S. E. Jay Street
Stuart, FL 34997
(407) 283-4817

Extensions for Independence
555 Veteran Boulevard
B-368
San Diego, CA 92154
(619) 423-7709

*Functional Assessment and Training
Consultants*
7701 N. Lamar
Suite 126
Austin, TX 78752
(512) 453-4593

GW Micro
310 Racquet Dr.
Fort Wayne, IN 46825
(219) 483-3625

Health Care Keyboard Company, Inc.
N60 W 1447 Kaul Avenue
Menomonee Falls, WI 53051
(414) 703-0170

Humanware, Inc.
6245 King Road
Suite P
Loomis, CA 95650
(916) 652-7253

*IBM National Support Center for Persons
with Disabilities*
PO Box 2150
Atlanta, GA 30055
(800) 426-2133
(800) 284-9482

In Touch Systems
11 Westview Rd.
Spring Valley, NY 10977
(914) 354-7431

Inkwell Systems
PO Box 1318
Talent, OR 97540
(541) 535-1210

Innovative Designs, Inc.
2464 El Camino Real
Suite 245
Santa Clara, CA 95051
(408) 985-9255

IntelliTools
55 Leveroni Court, Suite 9
Novato, CA 94949
(800) 899-6687

Keyboard Technology, Inc.
824 E. Rand Road #271
Arlington Heights, Il 60004
(847) 392-0514

Keytec, Inc.
1293 N. Plano Road
Richardson, TX 75081
(800) 624-4289

Kurzweil Imaging Systems, Inc.
185 Albany Street
Cambridge, MA 02139
(800) 343-0311

Marla Productions
524 Don Gaspar
Santa Fe, NM 87501
(505) 982-5321

Optelec USA, Inc.
6 Liberty Way
Westford, MA 01886
(800) 828-1056

Pointer Systems, Inc.
One Mill Street
Burlington, VT 05401
(800) 537-1562

Prentke Romich Company
1022 Heyl Road
Wooster, OH 44691
(800) 262-1984

Syntha-Voice Computers, Inc
800 Queenston Road
Suite 304
Stoney Creek, ON L8G IA7
Canada
800-263-4540

Talking Computer Products
100 Main
Wallace, KS 67761
(913) 891-3522

TeleSensory
455 North Bernardo
Mountain View, CA 94039-7455
(415) 960-0920

Trace Research and Development Center
Rm. S-151 Waisman Center
University of Wisconsin
Madison, WI 53705-2280
(608) 262-6966

Words+
40015 Sierra Highway
B-145
Palmdale, CA 93550-2117
(800) 869-8521

XEROX Imaging Systems, Inc.
185 Albany Street
Cambridge, MA 02139
(617) 864-4700

Appendices

MEDICARE MEDICAL REVIEW PART B
GUIDELINES FOR OCCUPATIONAL THERAPY

A3 3906. MR OF PART B INTERMEDIARY OUTPATIENT OCCUPATIONAL THERAPY (OT) BILLS

A. General.—The following is criteria for MR of OT services. Use the edits in Exhibit 1 to assist you in conducting focused MR within your budgeted levels. Conduct focused review using other selection criteria which you determine to be effective. If you choose to use any of the diagnostic edits listed in Exhibit I, do not change the visits and/or duration parameters without approval from CO. Conform to the MR requirements for all outpatient claims from rehabilitation agencies, SNFs, hospitals, and HHAs that provide OT in addition to home health services (bill types, hospital-12 and 13, SNF-22 and 23, HHA-34, rehabilitation agency, public health agency or clinic-74 and CORF-75). These criteria do not apply to OT services provided under a home health plan of care.

The criteria for MR case selection are based on ICD-9-CM diagnoses, elapsed time from start of care (at the billing provider) and number of visits. (See Exhibit 1.)

Denial of a bill solely on the basis that it exceeds the criteria in the edits is prohibited.

The edits are only for assisting you to select bills to review or for paying bills if they meet Level I criteria. Do not provide automatic coverage up to these criteria. They neither guarantee minimum nor set maximum coverage limits.

B. Use of OT Edits (Exhibit 1) Level I Review.—OT edits have been developed for a number of diagnoses. The diagnoses were selected on the basis that, when linked with a recent date of onset, there is a high probability that Medicare patients with these diagnoses will require skilled OT. The edits do not specify every diagnosis which may require OT, and the fact that a given diagnosis does not appear in the edits does not create a presumption that OT services are not necessary or are inappropriate. Do not approve or deny claims at Level I for medical necessity. Pay claims that suspend or pass the edits in Exhibit 1 without being subjected to Level II MR. However, refer all claims which meet your focused MR criteria to Level II MR.

For patients receiving OT services only (V57.2) during an encounter/visit, list the appropriate V code for the service first, and, if documented, list the diagnosis or problem for which the services are performed second. Program your system to read the diagnosis or problem listed second to determine if it meets the Level I OT edits.

EXAMPLE: Outpatient rehabilitation services, V57.2, for a patient with multiple sclerosis, 340. The V code will be listed first, followed by the code for multiple sclerosis (V57.2, 340). Edit for multiple sclerosis not the V code. Use this same procedure for V57.81 (Orthotic training) V57.89 (Other) and V57.9 (Unspecified rehabilitation procedure).

Evaluate bills at Level I based upon:

1. Facility and Patient Identification.—(Facility name, patient name, provider number, HICN, age.)

2. Diagnosis.—List the primary diagnosis for which OT services were furnished by ICD-9-CM code first. List other Dx(s) applicable to the patient or that influence care second.

3. Duration.—The total length of time OT services have been furnished (in days) from the date treatment was initiated for the diagnosis being treated at the billing provider (including the last day in the current billing period).

4. Number of Visits.—The total number of patient visits completed since OT services were initiated for the diagnosis being treated by the billing provider. The total visits to date (including the last visit in the billing period) must be given rather than for each separate bill (value code 51).

5. Date Treatment Started (Occurrence Code 44).—The date OT services were initiated by the billing provider for the primary medical Dx for which OT services are furnished.

6. Billing Period.—When OT services began and ended in the billing period (from/through dates).

C. Level II Review Process.—If a bill is selected for focused or intensified review, refer it to the Level II health professional MR staff. If possible, have occupational therapists review OT bills.

Once the bill is selected for focused MR, review it in conjunction with the medical information submitted by the provider.

1. Reimbursable OT Services.—Reimburse OT services only if they meet all requirements established by the Medicare guidelines and regulations. Each bill for OT services that is subjected to Level II MR must be supported with adequate medical documentation for you to make a determination. (For additional requirements see §§3101.9 and 3148.)

2. MR and Documentation.—When a claim is referred to Level II review, use the following pertinent data elements in addition to those used for Level I review:

   a. Medical History.—Obtain only the medical history which is pertinent to, or influences the OT treatment rendered, including a brief description of the functional status of the patient prior to the onset of the condition requiring OT, and any pertinent prior OT treatment.

   b. Date of Onset (Occurrence Code 11).—The date of onset or exacerbation of the primary medical diagnosis for which OT services are being rendered by the billing provider.

c. Physician Referral and Date.—

d. OT Initial Evaluation and Date.—

e. Plan of Treatment and Date Established.—

f. Date of Last Certification.—Obtain the date on which the plan of treatment was last certified by the physician.

g. Progress Notes.—Obtain updated patient status reports concerning the patient's current functional abilities/limitations.

The following explains specific Level II documentation principles:

3906.1 Medical History. – If a history of previous OT treatment is not available, the provider supplies a general summary regarding the patient's past relevent medical history recorded during the initial evaluation with the patient/family or through contact with the referring physician. Information regarding prior OT treatment for the current condition, progress made, and treatment by the referring physician is provided when available. The level of function prior to the current exacerbation or onset is described.

The patient's medical history as it relates to OT, includes the date of onset and/or exacerbation of the illness or injury. If the patient has had prior therapy for the same condition, use that history in conjunction with the patient's current assessment to establish whether additional treatment is reasonable.

The history of treatments from a previous provider is necessary for patients who have transferred to a new provider. For example, if surgery has been performed, obtain the type and date. The date of onset and type of surgical procedure should be specific for diagnoses such as fractures. For other diagnoses, such as arthritis, the date of onset may be general. Establish it from the date the patient first required medical treatment. For other types of chronic diagnoses, the history gives the date of the change or deterioration in the patient's condition and a description of the changes that necessitate skilled OT.

3906.2 Evaluation. – Approve an OT initial evaluation, (excluding routine screening) when it is reasonable and necessary for the therapist to determine if there is an expectation that either restorative or maintenance services are appropriate. Approve reevaluations when the patient exhibits a demonstrable change in physical functional ability, requiring reestablishment of appropriate treatment goals, or when reasonable and necessary, for ongoing assessment of the patient's rehabilitation needs. Approve initial evaluations or reevaluations that are reasonable and necessary based on the patient's condition, even though the expectations are not realized, or when the evaluation determines that skilled rehabilitation is not needed.

The OT evaluation establishes the physical and cognitive baseline data necessary for assessing expected rehabilitation potential, setting realistic goals, and measuring progress. The evaluation of the patient's functional deficits and level of assistance needed forms the basis for the OT goals. Objective tests and measurements are used (when possible) to establish base- line data.

The provider documents the patient's functional loss and the level of assistance requiring skilled OT intervention resulting from conditions such as:

- Activities of Daily Living (ADL) Dependence–The individual is dependent upon skilled intervention for performance of activities of daily living. These include, but are not limited to, signficant physical and/or cognitive functional loss, or loss of previous functional gains in the ability to:

  – Feed, eat, drink;

  – Bathe;

  – Dress;

  – Perform personal hygiene;

  – Groom; or

  – Perform toileting.

This could include management and care of orthoses and/or adaptive equipment, or customized therapeutic adaptations.

- Functional Limitation - The individual is dependent upon skilled OT intervention in functional training, observation, assessment, and environmental adaptation due, but not limited to:

  – Lack of awareness of sensory cues, or safety hazards;

  – Impaired attention span;

  – Impaired strength;

  – Incoordination;

  – Abnormal muscle tone;

  – Range of motion limitations;

  – Impaired body scheme;

  – Perceptual deficits;

  – Impaired balance/head control; and

  – Environmental barriers.

- Safety Dependence/Secondary Complications - A safety problem exists when a patient, without skilled OT intervention, cannot handle him/herself in a manner that is physically and/or cognitively safe. This may extend to daily living or to acquired secondary complications which could potentially intensify medical sequelae such as fracture nonunion, or skin breakdown. Safety dependence may be demonstrated by high probability of falling, lack of environmental safety awareness, swallowing difficulties, abnormal agressive/destructive behavior, severe pain, loss of skin sensation, progressive joint contracture, and joint protection/preservation requiring skilled OT intervention to protect the patient from further medical complication(s).

f the goal is to increase the patient's functional abilities and decrease the level of assistance needed, the initial evaluation must measure the patient's starting functional abilities and level of assistance required.

3906.3 PLAN OF TREATMENT. – The OT plan of treatment must include specific functional goals and a reasonable estimate of when they will be reached (e.g., 6 weeks). It is not adequate to estimate "1 to 2 months on an ongoing basis." The provider submits changes in the plan with the progress notes. The plan must include:

- Type of OT Procedures - Describes the specific nature of the therapy to be provided.

- Frequency of Visits - An estimate of the frequency of treatment to be rendered (e.g., 3x week).

The provider's medical documentation should justify the intensity of services rendered. This is crucial when they are given more frequently than 3 times a week.

- Estimated Duration - Identifies the length of time over which the services are to be rendered in days, weeks, or months.

- Diagnoses - Includes the OT diagnosis if different from the medical diagnosis. The OT diagnosis should be based on objective tests, whenever possible.

- Functional OT Goals (short or long-term) - Reflects the occupational therapist's and/or physician's description of what functional physical/cognitive abilities the patient is expected to achieve.

Assume that factors may change or influence the level of achievement. If this occurs, the occupational therapist or physician explains the factors which led to the change in functional goal(s).

- Rehabilitation Potential - The occupational therapist's and/or physician's expectation concerning the patient's ability to meet the established goals.

3906.4 PROGRESS REPORTS (TREATMENT SUMMARY FOR BILLING PERIOD). – The provider documents and reports:

- The patient's initial functional status;
- The patient's functional status and progress (or lack thereof) specific for this reporting period;

---

including clinical findings (amount of physical and/or cognitive assistance needed, range of motion, muscle strength, unaffected limb measurements, etc.); and

- The patient's expected rehabilitation potential.

Where a valid expectation of improvement exists, the services are covered even though the expectation may not be realized. However, in such instances, the OT services are covered only to the time that no further significant practical improvement can be expected. Progress reports or status summaries must document a continued expectation that the patient's condition will continue to improve significantly in a reasonable and generally predictable period of time.

"Significant," means a generally measurable and substantial increase in the patient's present level of functional independence and competence, compared to that when treatment was initiated. Do not interpret the term "significant" so stringently that you deny a claim simply because of a temporary setback in the patient's progress. For example, a patient may experience an intervening medical complication or a brief period when lack of progress occurs. The medical reviewer may approve the claim if there is still a reasonable expectation that significant improvement in the patient's overall safety or functional ability will occur. However, the provider should document the lack of progress and justify the need for continued skilled OT.

The provider must provide treatment information regarding the status of the patient during the billing period. The provider's progress notes and any needed reevaluation(s) must update the baseline information provided at the initial evaluation. If there is a change in the plan of treatment, it must be documented. Additionally, when a patient is continued from one billing period to another, the progress report(s) must reflect the comparisons between the patient's current functional status and that during the previous billing and/or initial evaluation.

Conduct a MR of claims with an understanding that skilled intervention may be needed, and improvement in a patient's condition may occur, even where a patient's full or partial recovery is not possible. For example, a terminally ill patient may begin to exhibit ADL, mobility and/or safety dependence requiring OT. The fact that full or partial recovery is not possible or rehabilitation potential is not present, does not affect MR coverage decisions. The deciding factor is whether the services are considered reasonable, effective, treatment for the patient's condition and they require the skills of an occupational therapist, or whether they can be safely and effectively carried out by nonskilled personnel. The reasons for OT must be clear, as well as its goals, prior to a favorable coverage determination. They often require Level III review.

It is essential that the provider documents the updated status in a clear, concise, and objective manner. Objective tests and measurements are stressed when they are practical. The occupational therapist selects the method to demonstrate current patient status. However, the method chosen, as well as the measures used, should be consistent during the treatment duration. If the method used is changed, the reasons for the change should be documented, including how the new method relates to the old. You must have an overview of the purpose of treatment goals in order to compare the patient's current functional status to that in previous reporting periods.

Documentation of the patient's current functional status and level of assistance required compared to previous reporting period(s) is of paramount importance. The deficits in functional ability should be clear. Occupational therapists must document functional improvements (or lack thereof) as a result of their treatments. Documentation of functional progress must be stated in objective, measurable terms. The following illustrate these principles and demonstrate that significant changes may occur in one or more of the assistance levels:

A. Change in Level of Assistance.—Occupational therapist's document assistance levels by describing the relationship between functional activities and the need for assistance. Within the assistance levels of minimum, moderate, and maximum there are intermediate gradations of improvement based on changes in behavior and response to assistance. Improvements at each level must be documented to compare the current cognitive and/or physicial level achieved to that previously achieved. While cognitive assistance often is the more severe and persistent disability, physical assistance often is the major obstacle to successful outcomes and subsequent discharge. Interpret the levels as follows:

1. Total Assistance.—Is the need for 100 percent assistance by one or more persons to perform all physical activities and/or cognitive assistance to elicit a functional response to an external stimulation.

An individual requires total assistance if the documentation indicates the patient is only able to initiate minimal voluntary motor actions and requires the skill of an occupational therapist to develop a therapeutic program or implement a maintenance program to prevent, or minimize, deterioration.

A cognitively impaired patient requires total assistance when documentation shows external stimuli are required to elicit automatic actions such as swallowing or responding to auditory stimuli. Skills of an occupational therapist are needed to identify and apply strategies for eliciting appropriate, consistent automatic responses to external stimuli.

2. Maximum Assistance.—Is the need for 75 percent assistance by one person to physicially perform any part of a functional activity and/or cognitive assistance to perform gross motor actions in response to direction.

Patients require such assistance if maximum OT physical support and proprioceptive stimulation is needed for performance of each step of a functional activity, every time it is performed.

A cognitively impaired patient, at this level, may need proprioceptive stimulation and/or one-to-one demonstration by the occupational therapist due to the patient's lack of cognitive awareness of other people or objects.

3. Moderate Assistance.—Is the need for 50 percent assistance by one person to per-

form physical activities or constant cognitive assistance to sustain/complete simple, repetitive activities safely.

A physically impaired patient requires moderate assistance if documentation indicates that moderate OT physical support and proprioceptive stimulation is needed each time to perform a functional activity.

The records submitted should state how a cognitively impaired patient requires intermittent one-to-one demonstration or intermittent cueing (physical or verbal) throughout the activity. Moderate assistance is needed when the occupational therapist/caregiver needs to be in the immediate environment to progress the patient through a sequence to complete an activity. This level of assistance is required to halt continued repetition of a task and to prevent unsafe, erratic or unpredictable actions that interfere with appropriate sequencing.

4. Minimum Assistance.—Is the need for 25 percent assistance by one person for physical activities and/or periodic, cognitive assistance to perform functional activities safely.

A physically impaired patient requires minimum assistance if documentation indicates that activities can only be performed after physical set-up by the occupational therapist or caregiver, and if physical help is needed to initiate, or sustain an activity. A review of alternate procedures, sequences and methods may be required.

A cognitively impaired patient requires minimal assistance if documentation indicates help is needed in performing known activities to correct repeated mistakes, to check for compliance with established safety procedures, or to solve problems posed by unexpected hazards.

5. Standby Assistance.—Is the need for supervision by one person for the patient to perform new procedures adapted by the therapist for safe and effective performance.

A patient requires such assistance when errors are demonstrated or the need for safety precautions are not always anticipated by the patient.

6. Independent Status.—Means that no physical or cognitive assistance is required to perform functional activities.

Patients at this level are able to implement the selected courses of action, demonstrate lack of errors and anticipate safety hazards in familiar and new situations.

B. Change in Response to Treatment Within Each Level of Assistance.— Significant improvement must be indicated by documenting a change in one or more of the following categories of patient responses:

1. Refusals.—The patient may respond by refusing to attempt an activity because of

fear or pain. The documentation should indicate the activity refused, the reasons, and how the OT plan addresses them.

These responses are often secondary to a change in medical status or medications. If the refusals continue over several days, the therapy program should be put on "hold" until the patient is willing to attempt functional activities.

For the cognitively impaired patient, refusal to perform an activity can escalate into aggressive, destructive or verbally abusive behavior if the therapist or caregiver presses the patient to perform. In these cases, a reduction in these behaviors is considered significant progress, but must be documented, including the skilled OT provided to reduce the abnormal behavior.

For the psychiatrically impaired patient, refusals to participate in an activity frequently are symptoms of the diagnosis. The patient should not be put on a "hold" status due to refusals. If the documentation indicates that the patient is receiving OT, is contacted regularly, and is actively encouraged to participate, medically review the claim to determine if reasonable and necessary skilled care has been rendered.

2. Inconsistency.—The patient may respond by inconsistently performing functional tasks from day-to-day or within a treatment session.

Approve the claim when the documentation indicates a significant progression in consistency of performance of functional tasks within the same level of assistance.

3. Generalization.—The patient may respond by applying previously learned concepts for performing an activity to another, similar activity. The records submitted should document a significant increase in scope of activities that the patient can perform, their type, and the skilled OT services rendered.

C. A New Skilled Functional Activity is Initiated.—Examples:

- Adding teaching of lower body dressing to a current program of upper body dressing;

- Increasing the ability to perform personal hygiene activities for health and social acceptance.

D. A New Skilled Compensatory Technique is Added.—(With or without adapted equipment.) Examples:

- Teaching a patient techniques such as one-handed shoe tying;

- Teaching the use of a button hook for buttoning shirt buttons.

E. Length of Time in Treatment.—The acceptable length of time in treatment for various disorders is determined by the patient's documented functional abilities and progress.

3906.5 LEVEL OF COMPLEXITY OF TREATMENT. — Base decisions on the level of complexity of the services rendered by the occupational therapist and not what the patient is asked to do. Examples:

A. Skilled OT.—The documentation must indicate that the severity of the physical/emotional/perceptual/cognitive disability requires complex and sophisticated knowledge to identify current and potential capabilities. In addition, consider instructions required by the patient and/or the patient's caregivers. Instructions may be required for activities that most healthy people take for granted. The special knowledge of an occupational therapist is required to decrease or eliminate limitations in functional activity performance. Occupational therapists must often address underlying factors which interfere with specific activities. These factors could be cognitive, sensory, or perceptual deficits.

The occupational therapist modifies the specific activity by using adapted equipment, making changes in the environment, altering procedures for accomplishing the task, and providing specialized assistance to meet the patient's current and potential abilities. Skilled services include, but are not limited to reasonable and necessary:

- Patient evaluations;

- Determinations of effective goals and services with the patient and patient's caregivers and other medical professsionals;

- Analyzing and modifying functional tasks;

- Determinating that the modified task obtains optimum performance through tests and measurements;

- Providing instructions of the task(s) to the patient/family/ caregivers; and

- Periodically reevaluating the patient's status with corresponding readjustment of the OT program.

A period of practice may be approved for the patient and/or patient's caregivers to learn the steps of the task, to verify the task's effectivnesss in improving function, and to check for safe and consistent performance.

3. Nonskilled OT.—When the documentation indicates a patient has attained the therapy goals or has reached the point where no further significant improvement can be expected, the skills of an occupational therapist are not required to maintain function at the level to which it has been restored. Examples of maintenance procedures:

- Daily feeding programs after the adapted procedures are in place;

- Routine exercise and strengthing programs;

- The practice of coordination and self-care skills on a daily basis; and

- Presenting information on energy conservation or pacing, butnot having the patient perform the activity.

You may approve a claim because the patient requires the judgment and skills of the occupational therapist to design a safe and effective maintenance program and make periodic checks of its effectiveness. The services of an occupational therapist in carrying out the established maintenance program are not reasonable and necessary for the treatment of illness or injury and may not be approved.

3906.6 REPORTING ON NEW EPISODE OR CONDITION. – Occasionally, a patient who is receiving or who has received OT services, experiences a new illness. The provider must document the significance of any change to the patient's functional capabilities. This may be through pre and post episodic nursing notes or physician reports. If the patient is receiving treatment, it might be lengthened. If the patient had completed treatment a significant change in the patient's functional status must be documented to warrant a new treatment plan.

3906.7 OTHER MR CONSIDERATIONS. –

A. Pain.—Consider documentation describing the presence or absence of pain and its effect on the patient's functional abilities in MR decisions. A description of its intensity, type, changing pattern, and location at specific joint ranges of motion materially aids correct decisions. Documentation should describe the limitations placed upon the patient's ADL, mobility and/or safety, as well as the subjective progress made in the reduction of pain through treatment.

B. Therapeutic Programs.—The objective documentation should support the skilled nature of the program, and/or the need for the design and establishment of a maintenance OT program. The goals should be to increase functional abilities in ADL, mobility or patient safety. Documentation should indicate the goals and type of program provided.

Approve claims when the therapeutic program, because of documented medical complications, the condition of the patient, or complexity of the OT employed, must be rendered by, or under, the supervision of an occupational therapist. For example, while functional ADL may be performed safely and effectively by nonskilled personnel, fracture nonunion, severe joint pain, or other medical or safety complications may warrant skilled occupational therapist intervention to render the service and/or to establish a safe maintenance program. In these cases, the complications and the skilled services they require, must be documented by physician orders and/or occupational therapist notes. For correct MR decisions, the patient's losses and/or dependencies in ADL, mobility and safety must be documented. The possibility of adverse effects from the improper performance of an otherwise unskilled service does not make it a skilled service unless documentation supports why skilled OT is needed for the patient's medical condition and/or safety.

Approve the establishment and design of a maintenance exercise program to fit the patient's level of ADL, function, and any instructions to supportive personnel and/or family members need to safely and effectively carry it out. Reevaluation may be approved when reasonable and necessary to readjust the maintenance program to meet the changing needs of the patient. There must be justification for readjusting a maintenance program, e.g., loss of previous functional gains.

C. Cardiac Rehabilitation Exercise.—Occupational therapy is not covered when furnished in connection with cardiac rehabilitation exercise program services (see Coverage Issues Manual 35-25) unless there is also a diagnosed noncardiac condition requiring it, e.g., a patient who is recuperating from an acute phase of heart disease may have had a stroke which requires OT. (While the cardiac rehabilitation exercise program may be considered by some a form of OT, it is a specialized program conducted and/or supervised by specially trained personnel whose services are performed under the direct supervision of a physician.)

D. Transfer Training.—The documentation should describe the patient's functional limitations in transfer ability that warrant skilled OT intervention. Documentation includes the special transfer training needed to perform functional daily living skills and any training needed by supportive personnel and/or family members to safely and effectively carry it out. Approve transfer training when the documentation supports a skilled need for evaluation, design and effective monitoring and instruction of the special transfer technique for safety and completion of the activities of daily living or mobility.

Documentation that supports only repetitious carrying out of the transfer method once established, and monitored for safety and completion does not show covered care.

E. Fabrication of and Training in Use of Orthoses, Prostheses and Adaptive Equipment.—Approve reasonable and necessary fabrication of orthoses, prostheses, adaptive equipment, and reasonable and necessary skilled training needed in their safe and effective use, if documentation indicates the need for the device and training in its use.

F. OT Forms.—Documentation may be submitted on a specific form you require or may be copies of the provider's record. However, your form must capture the needed MR information. If you choose to require a particular form, show the OMB clearance number. The information submitted must be complete. If it is not, return the bill for the additional information. The information you require to review the bill is that which is required by an occupational therapist to properly treat a patient.

G. Certification and Recertification.—OT services must be certified and recertified by a physician and must be furnished while the patient is under the care of a physician. OT services must be furnished under a written plan of treatment established by the physician or a qualified occupational therapist. If the plan is established by an occupational therapist, it must be reviewed periodically by the physician.

The plan of treatment must be established (reduced to writing by either professional or the provider when it makes a written record of oral orders) before treatment is begun. When outpatient OT services are continued under the same plan of treatment for a period of time, the physician must certify at least at 30-day intervals that there is a continuing need for them. Obtain the recertification when reviewing the plan of treatment since the same interval of at least 30 days is required for review of the plans. A recertification must be signed by the physician, who reviewed the plan of treatment. Any changes to the treatment plan established by the occupational therapist must be in writing and signed by the therapist or by the attending physician. The physician may change a plan of treatment established by the occupational therapist. However, the occupational therapist may not alter a plan of treatment established by a physician.

3906.8 OCCUPATIONAL THERAPY AVAILABILITY. – Two or more disciplines may provide therapy services to the same patient. There may also be occasions where these services are duplicative. In many instances, the description of the services appears duplicative, but the documentation proves that they are not. Some examples where there is not a duplication include:

A. Transfers.—PT instructs the patient in transfers to achieve the level of safety with the techniques. OT utilizes transfers as they relate to the performance of daily living skills (e.g., transfer from wheelchair to bathtub).

B. Pulmonary.—PT instructs the patient in an adapted breathing technique. OT carries the breathing retraining into activities of daily living.

C. Hip Fractures/Arthroplasties.—PT instructs the patient in hip precautions and gait training. OT reinforces the training with precautions for activities of daily living, e.g., lower extremity dressing, toileting, and bathing.

D. CVA.—PT utilizes upper extremity neurodevelopmental (NDT) techniques to assist the patient in positioning the upper extremities on a walker and in gait training. OT utilizes NDT techniques to increase the functional use of the upper extremity for dressing, bathing, grooming, etc.

3906.9 FOCUSED MR ANALYSIS. – The HCFA edits may assist you in identifying OT claims for focused MR. Perform regular evaluations of provider claims which pass or fail the edits. Change your focused review claims selection based on the results of the evaluation. For example, a provider billing at an aberrantly consistent rate just below the edit parameters is subject to intensified review.

Develop procedures for focused MR based on each of the following trends or characteristics:

- Edits with high charges per aggregate bill charges;
- Providers billing a higher than average utilization of specific diagnostic codes that fall just below the edit parameters; and

- Specific principal DX codes, such as those with longer visits and duration; those representing the most frequent denials in pre-pay MR; special codes, e.g., 585, Chronic Renal Failure; 733.1, Senile Osteoporosis; and 290.0-290.9, Senile and Presenile Organic Psychotic Conditions; and/or certain edit groups such as 17, 19, and 29 in one quarter and others in the next quarter.

3906.11 FORMS HCFA-700/701, OUTPATIENT REHABILITATION SERVICES FORMS.—

A. General.—The outpatient rehabilitation services forms, Forms HCFA- 700/701, are combined medical review (MR), certification/recertification, plan of treatment (POT) forms for outpatient Part B, physical therapy (PT), occupational therapy (OT) and speech language pathology (ST). The forms' design promotes national consistency in reporting and reducing unnecessary requests for additional medical records. HCFA will not mandate use of the hard copy Forms HCFA 700/701. However, some providers have made significant investments in the use of these forms. Therefore, intermediaries must accept hard copy versions of the Forms HCFA-700/701 if the provider chooses to use them. Providers complete the Form HCFA-700 only for initial bills. For interim-to-discharge bills, the provider completes the Form HCFA-701.

Use the forms as a source of supporting medical information. Request Forms HCFA-700/701 when you need supporting medical information to help determine whether services are reasonable and necessary, noncovered services.

Base payment and denial decisions on information contained in these forms. However, request additional information when you need additional medical information to support a decision. A denial determination may not be made solely on the reviewer's general inferences about beneficiaries with similar diagnoses or on data related to utilization. Instead, reviewers must make determinations based upon clear objective clinical evidence concerning the beneficiary's unique medical condition and individual need for care.

Do not routinely require providers to submit the Forms HCFA-700/701. Request only the Form HCFA-700 for initial bills. Obtain the Form HCFA-701 for subsequent bills. Obtain photocopies of prior months Forms HCFA-700/701 only when you need them for coverage determinations.

> NOTE: If your system can retrieve previously submitted Forms HCFA-700/701 information/data, inform providers not to send copies.

Providers must complete all applicable items on the forms. However, if an item is blank but you can make a coverage determination, process the claim. Providers may complete items with "N/A," not applicable, when the item does not apply (e.g., no hospitalization occurred). If you need the information for a coverage decision in an item marked as "N/A" (or left blank), request the information from the provider.

Obtain completed Forms HCFA-700/701 from acute hospitals, skilled nursing facilities (SNFs), home health agencies (HHAs), comprehensive outpatient rehabilitation facilities (CORFs), rehabilitation agencies, public health agencies, and clinics (bill types 12, 13, 22, 23, 34, 74, and 75). Obtain a separate form for each therapy discipline (revenue code) billed. For example, if a patient received treatment by two services (i.e., PT and OT), the provider must submit two forms. You may also use these forms for outpatient hospital cardiac rehabilitation (CR), respiratory therapy (RT), or psychiatric services (PS). CORFs may also use the forms for skilled nursing (SN) and medical social services.

B. Electronic Media Claims (EMC).—Providers submitting batch attachments must use the current version of the UB-92 flat file record type (RT) 77 by October 1, 1996. This information may be sent with claim data or independent of claim data. See Addenda A, B,and D and §3908.1 for further instructions. Require providers to notify you before submitting records independent of the claim and test as appropriate. Require the provider to maintain the information to support the EMC format in the beneficiary's medical record, whether hard copy, or electronic. Request additional information to support a decision only as necessary.

3906.12 Instructions for Completion of Form HCFA-700, Plan of Treatment for Outpatient Rehabilitation. —

The provider is to submit the following information on the Form HCFA-700:

1. Patient's Name.—This item indicates the patient's last name, first name, and middle initial as shown on the health insurance card.

2. Provider Number.—This item indicates the six digit number issued by Medicare to the provider. The number contains two digits, a hyphen, and four digits (e.g., 00-7000).

3. HICN.—This item indicates the numeric plus alpha indicator(s) as shown on the patient's health insurance card, certification award, utilization notice, temporary eligibility notice, or as reported by the SSO.

4. Provider Name.—This item indicates the name of the Medicare billing provider.

5. Medical Record Number.—This item indicates the patient's medical/clinical record number issued by the billing provider.

6. Onset Date.—This item indicates either the onset date of the primary medical diagnosis (if it is a new diagnosis) or the date of the most recent exacerbation of a previous diagnosis. If the exact day is not known, "01" is used for the day (e.g., 120192). This date must match Occurrence Code 11 on the UB-92.

7. SOC (Start of Care) Date.—This item indicates the six digit month, day, and year on which rehabilitation services began at the billing provider, i.e., MMDDYY (061392). The SOC date is the first Medicare billable visit (normally the date of initial evaluation). This date

remains the same on subsequent claims until the patient is discharged or the claim is denied. A provider may suspend services and later resume them under the same SOC date in accordance with its internal procedures. The SOC date may also reflect a re-initiation after discharge or denial if for an exacerbation. For PT, the SOC date must correspond to Occurrence Code 35 on the UB-92, for OT code 44, for SLP code 45, and for CR code 46.

8. Type.—The provider checks this item for the type of therapy furnished, i.e., PT, OT, SLP, for outpatient hospital CR, RT, or PS. CORFs may also check skilled nursing (SN) and/or medical social services (SW).

9. Primary Diagnosis .—This item indicates the medical diagnosis (DX) that has resulted in the therapy disorder and which is most closely related to the current plan of care for therapy. The diagnosis may or may not be related to the patient's most recent hospital stay but must relate to the services furnished by the provider. If more than one diagnosis is treated concurrently, the provider enters the diagnosis that represents the most intensive services (over 50 percent of rehabilitation effort for the revenue code billed). The primary DX may change on subsequent forms if the patient develops an acute condition or an exacerbation of a secondary diagnosis requiring intensive services different than established on the initial plan of treatment (POT). In all such instances, the date treatment started at the billing provider remains the same until the patient is discharged.

10. Treatment Diagnosis.—This item indicates the DX for which rehabilitative services were furnished (e.g., for SLP the treatment DX is a communication disorder). For example, while cerebrovascular accident (CVA) may be the primary medical DX, aphasia might be the SLP treatment DX. If the treatment DX is the same as the medical DX, the word "same" is used in this item.

11. Visits From Start of Care.—This item indicates the cumulative total visits that were completed since the start of services at the billing provider for the treated DX through the last visit on the bill. This total corresponds to the UB-92 Value Code 50 for PT, 51 for OT, 52 for SLP, or 53 for CR.

12. Plan of Treatment/Functional Goals.—

    A. Functional goals.—This item indicates the initial short and long-term goals in measurable, objective, and functional terms. Included are the functional levels (or safety levels) the patient is expected to achieve upon discharge as a result of therapy services. Also, indicated are the levels the patient is to achieve outside of the therapeutic environment. Time-oriented goals are entered when applicable. For example, communicate basic physical needs and emotional status within weeks (as a functional goal for SLP).

    B. Plan.—This item indicates the initial overall plan of care, type, and specific nature of rehabilitation procedures that are to be furnished (i.e., treatment the therapist is using — procedures or modalities used).

13. Signature.—The signature (or name) and professional designation of the professional who established the plan of treatment is entered in this item. A qualified therapist or speech/language pathologist may establish the POT for PT, OT, or SLP.

14. Frequency/Duration.—This item indicates the frequency of treatment the provider expects to furnish per day, week, or month. Also, projected is the length of time the provider expects to furnish services. This is to be expressed in days, weeks, or months (e.g., 3/Wk x 4 Wks).

15. Physician's Signature.—The physician signs and dates this item if the Form HCFA-700 is to be used as the physician's certification. If you use an alternative signed certification form, the "On File" box should be checked (Item 18). Identify the period of certification in Item 17 on the HFCA-700. When certification is not required, the provider uses "N/A."

Rubber signature stamps are not acceptable as the physician signature. The provider must keep the form containing the physician's original signature on file at the provider site.

16. Date.—This item indicates the date the physician signed the form in 6 digits (i.e., month, day, and year).

17. Certification.—This item indicates the six digit month, day, and year (i.e., MMDDYY 061592-071592) which identifies the period covered by the POT. The "From" date for the initial certification must match the SOC date. The "Through" date can be up to, but never exceed, 30 days (60 days for CORFs). The "Through" date is repeated on a subsequent recertification as the next sequential "From" date. Services delivered on the "Through" date are covered in the next recertification period.

18. On File.—This box is checked if the provider uses the form for certification. The provider is to enter the name of the physician who certified the POT that is on file at the billing provider. If certification is not required for the type of service checked in Item 8, the name of the physician who referred or ordered the service should be entered, but the "On File" box is not to be checked.

19. Prior Hospitalization.—This item indicates the six digit month, day, and year (inclusive dates) of the most recent hospitalization that is pertinent to the patient's condition or primary DX billed (date from 1st day of admission through discharge day). The provider enters "N/A" if this is not applicable. If the period is not known, they enter "N/A."

20. Initial Assessment.—This item indicates a brief historical narrative of the injury or illness and the reason(s) for referral as they relate to the primary or treatment DX. The providers use the following guidelines when constructing their narrative:

- Describe pertinent functional deficits and clinical findings and problems found on the initial assessment.

- Use objective, measurable terminology such as tests and measurements;

- Assess the patient's activities of daily living (ADL), range of motion (ROM), strength, functional abilities, psychological status, level of assistance required, and pertinent speech-language functional deficit findings. Include tests administered with scores;

- Relate pertinent safety precautions and medical complications that may affect a patient's progress or attainment of goals and which require skilled intervention;

- List the patient's rehabilitation potential, cognitive status that affects functional ability, and psychological, respiratory, cardiac tests and measurements, as appropriate; and

- Document audiologic results, vision status, and use or status of amplification for patients receiving speech reading services.

21. Functional Level.—This item indicates the patient's functional physical, cardiac, respiratory, or psychological status reached at the end of the claim period. The provider is to compare results to that shown on the initial assessment (Item 20). Record functional levels and progress in objective terminology. Include test results and measurements as appropriate. Record information about any change in functional level related to the goal(s) of treatment. When only a few visits have been made (e.g., evaluation) and when there is no change in function, the training/treatment furnished and the patient's response to the visit(s) are recorded.

The provider checks the box titled "Continue Services" if services were continued. The provider checks the box titled "DC Services" if services were discontinued (e.g., if the patient was discharged).

22. Service Dates.—This item indicates the "From/Through" dates that represent this billing period. If the provider uses this form for certification (with the exception of CORFs), this billing period should be monthly. The "From/Through" dates in field 22 on the UB-92 must match the dates in this item. Providers may not use "00" in the date, e.g., 010892 for January 8, 1992.

3906.13 Instructions for Completion of Form HCFA-701, Updated Plan Progress for Outpatient Rehabilitation. – The provider is to submit the following information on the Form HCFA-701:

1. Patient's Name.—This item indicates the patient's last name, first name, and middle initial as shown on the health insurance Medicare card.

2. Provider Number.—This item indicates the six digit number issued by Medicare to the provider. The number contains two digits, a hyphen, and four digits (e.g., 00-7000).

3. HICN.—This item indicates the numeric plus alpha indicator(s) as shown on the patient's health insurance card, certification award, utilization notice, temporary eligibility notice, or as reported by the SSO.

4. Provider Name.—This item indicates the name of the Medicare billing provider (i.e., the billing provider's facility name that corresponds to the Medicare provider number).

5. Medical Record Number.—This item indicates the patient's medical/clinical record number issued by the billing provider.

6. Onset Date.—This item indicates the onset date of the primary medical diagnosis (DX), if it is a new DX, or the date of the most recent exacerbation of a previous DX. If the exact day is not known, the provider uses "01" for the day (e.g., 120192). This date must match Occurrence Code 11 on the UB-92.

7. SOC (Start of Care) Date.—This item indicates the six digit month, day, and year on which rehabilitation services began at the billing provider (i.e., MMDDYY (061392)). The SOC date is the first Medicare billable visit (normally the date of initial evaluation). This date remains the same on subsequent claims until the patient is discharged or the claim is denied. Services may be suspended and later resumed under the same SOC in accordance with a provider's internal procedures. The SOC date may also reflect a re-initiation after discharge or denial if for an exacerbation. For PT, the SOC date must correspond to Occurrence Code 35 on the UB-92, for OT code 44, for SLP code 45, and for CR code 46.

8. Type.—This item indicates the type of therapy furnished, i.e., PT, OT, SLP, or outpatient hospital, CR, RT, or PS (CORFs may also check SN and/or SW).

9. Primary Diagnosis.—This item indicates the medical DX that has resulted in the therapy disorder and which is most closely related to the current plan of care for therapy. The DX may or may not relate to the patient's most recent hospital stay but must relate to the services furnished by the provider. If the provider treated more than one DX concurrently, the provider enters the DX that represents the most intensive services (over 50 percent of rehabilitation effort for the revenue code billed). The primary DX may change on subsequent forms if the patient develops an acute condition or an exacerbation of a secondary DX requiring intensive services different than established on the initial plan of care. In all such instances, the date treatment started at the billing provider remains the same until the patient is discharged or the claim is denied.

10. Treatment Diagnosis.—This item indicates the DX for which the provider furnished rehabilitative services. For example, while CVA may be the primary medical DX, aphasia might be the SLP treatment DX. If the treatment DX is the same as the medical DX, the provider uses the word "same" in this item.

11. Visits From Start of Care.—This item indicates the cumulative total visits that were completed since the start of service at the billing provider for the diagnosis treated through the last visit on the bill. This total is to correspond to the UB-92, Value Code 50 for PT, 51 for OT, 52 for SLP, or 53 for CR.

12. Current Frequency/Duration.—This item indicates the frequency of treatment the provider expects to furnish per day, week or month. Also, projected is the length of time the services are expected to be furnished per days, weeks, or months (e.g., 3/Wk x 4 Wks).

13. Current Plan Update, Functional Goals.—This item indicates the functional treatment goals for the patient for this billing period. The provider is to state the goals in measurable, objective terms. They are to stress functional short-term goals to reach overall long-term outcomes that the patient is expected to achieve upon discharge (Item 12, HCFA-700). They are to document changes to the initial plan of treatment and effective date(s). Providers must estimate time-frames to reach goals when possible. They are to record procedures or modalities used. If appropriate, they are to describe justification of intensity or any changes to the initial plan in Item 18.

14. Recertification.—This code indicates the six digit month, day, and year, i.e., MMDDYY (061592-071592), that identifies the period covered by the plan of treatment. The "From" date for the initial certification must match the SOC date. The "Through" date can be up to, but never exceed 30 days (60 days for CORFs). The provider is to repeat the "Through" date on a subsequent recertification as the next sequential "From" date. Services delivered on the "Through" date are covered in the next recertification period. On interim CORF claims, "N/A" is used.

> EXAMPLE: Initial certification "From" date 051593
> Initial certification "Through" date 061593
> Recertification "From" date 061593
> Recertification "Through" date 071593

Certification/recertification is required for outpatient PT, OT, and SLP and CORF plans of care. Certification is required for partial hospitalization PS. When certification/recertification is not required, the provider uses "N/A."

There is no requirement that the provider enter the certification on the Forms HCFA-700/701 or handle it in any specific way as long as you can determine, where necessary, that certification/recertification requirements are met.

15. Physician Signature.—If the provider uses the Form HCFA-701 as the physician's recertification, the physician must sign and date the statements. If not, when appropriate, the "On File" box in Item 17 must be checked. Identify the period of recertification in Item 14 on the form. For interim CORF claims and when recertification is not required, the provider must use the "N/A" box.

If the physician established the plan of treatment, the physician must sign both Items 15 and 19. If the plan of treatment is established by a PT, OT, or speech-language pathologist, that therapist or speech-language pathologist must sign the plan (Item 19). A physician who has knowledge of the care signs the certification/recertification.

16. Date.—This item indicates the date the physician signs the certification/recertification in six digits (month, date, and year). The date must be shown even if the provider checks the "On File" box in Item 18.

17. On File.—When the "On File" box is checked, request the certification/recertification in accordance with your internal procedures, that are approved by your Regional Office (RO).

18. Reason(s) for Continuing Treatment This Billing Period.— This item indicates the major reason(s) justifying continued therapy and the need for additional rehabilitation. Safety/medical complications are to be stated when further applicable. In the event of discharge, the provider is to provide the reason.

19. Signature.—The professional who furnishes care or supervises services must enter his/her signature and professional designation.

20. Date.—This item indicates the date of the signature in 6 digits (month, day, and year).

21. Continued or Discontinued.—The provider checks this box to identify whether services are continued, or discontinued (last bill).

22. Functional Level (end of claim period).—This item indicates the functional level(s) and progress made at the end of the billing period. Obtain objective tests and measurements when practical. The providers are to date specific short-term gains when practical (e.g., when the patient is able to consistently perform them in this billing period). Providers are to document pertinent safety problems and/or precautions needed. They are to update the patient's current functional level(s) and progress (or lack of progress with an explanation) achieved as compared to the previous month and/or initial assessment. They are to document assistive devices used. Providers are to submit concise, quality, objective documentation and restrict subjective quantity. They should avoid such terms as "improved strength" or "improved communication." Providers billing 5 or more visits per week should use this space to update progress at 2 weeks and at the end of the claim period.

> NOTE: When relating functional level(s) and progress made, the reviewer considers that a patient might not progress (or progress little) during a part of a claim period and the patient notes will reflect that fact. This should not be interpreted so stringently to result in an impulsive termination of coverage at that point. Medically review the entire period (including the prior month in relation to the full month in question) to determine coverage.

23. Service Dates.—This item indicates the "From and Through" dates which represent the billing period. If the Provider uses the form for certification/recertification, with the exception of CORFs, they are to bill monthly. The "From and Through" dates in field 23 are to match the dates on UB-92. Providers should not use "00" in the date, e.g., 010892 for January 8, 1992.

INSTRUCTIONS FOR COMPLETION OF FORM HCFA-700
(Enter dates as 6 digits month, day, year)

1. **Patient's Name** - Enter the patient's last name, first name and middle initial as shown on the health insurance Medicare card.

2. **Provider Number** - Enter the number issued by Medicare to the billing provider (*i.e., 00-7000*)

3. **HICN** - Enter the patient's health insurance Medicare card, certification award, utilization notice, temporary eligibility notice, or as reported by SSO.

4. **Provider Name** - Enter the name of the Medicare billing provider.

5. **Medical Record No.** - *(optional)* Enter the patient's medical/clinical record number used by the billing provider.

6. **Onset Date** - Enter the date of onset for the patient's primary medical diagnosis, if it is a new diagnosis, or the date of the most recent exacerbation of a previous diagnosis (*i.e., 120191*). The date matches occurrence code 11 on the UB-82.

7. **SOC** *(start of care)* **Date** - Enter the date services began at the billing provider (the date of the first Medicare billable visit which **remains the same on subsequent claims** until discharge or denial corresponds to occurrence code 35 for PT, 44 for OT, 45 for SLP, and 46 for CR on the UB-82).

8. **Type** - Check the type therapy billed i.e., physical therapy (PT), occupational therapy (OT), speech-language pathology (SLP), cardiac rehabilitation (CR), respiratory therapy (RT), psychological services (PS), skilled nursing services (SN), or social services (SW).

9. **Primary Diagnosis** - Enter the pertinent written medical diagnosis resulting in the therapy disorder and relating to 50% or more of effort in the plan of treatment.

10. **Treatment Diagnosis** - Enter the written treatment diagnosis for which services are rendered. For example, for PT the primary medical diagnosis might be Degeneration of Cervical Intervertebral Disc while the PT treatment DX might be Frozen R Shoulder or, for SLP, while CVA might be the primary medical DX, the treatment DX might be Aphasia. If the same as the primary DX enter SAME.

11. **Visits From Start of Care** - Enter the cumulative total visits *(sessions)* completed since services were started at the billing provider for the diagnosis treated, through the last visit on this bill. (*Corresponds to UB-82 value code 50 for PT, 51 for OT, 52 for SLP, or 53 for cardiac rehab on the UB-82*)

12. **Plan of Treatment/Functional Goals** - Enter brief current plan of treatment goals for the patient for this billing period. Enter the major short-term goals to reach overall long-term outcome.

Enter the major plan of treatment to reach stated goals and outcome. Estimate time-frames to reach goals, when possible.

13. **Signature** - Enter the signature (*or name*) and the professional designation of the professional establishing the plan of treatment.

14. **Frequency/Duration** - Enter the current frequency and duration of your treatment, e.g., 3 times per week for 4 weeks is entered 3/Wk x 4Wk.

15. **Physician's Signature** - If the form HCFA-700 is used for certification, the physician enters his/her signature. **If certification is required and the form is not being used for certification, check on ON FILE box in item 18.** If the certification is not required of the type service rendered, check the N/A box.

16. **Date** - Enter the date of the physician's signature only if the form is used for certification.

17. **Certification** - Enter the inclusive dates of the certification, **even if the ON FILE box is checked in item 18.** Check the N/A box if certification is not required.

18. **ON FILE** (Means certification signature and date) - Enter the **typed/printed name of the physician** who certified the plan of treatment that is on file at the billing provider. If certification is not required for the type of service checked in item 8, type/print the name of the physician who referred or ordered the service, **but do not check the ON FILE box.**

19. **Prior Hospitalization** - Enter the inclusive dates of recent hospitalization (*1st to DC day*) **pertinent** to the patient's current plan of treatment. Enter N/A if the hospital stay does not relate to the rehabilitation being rendered.

20. **Initial Assessment** - Enter **only current relevant history** from records or patient interview. Enter the major functional limitations stated, if possible, in objective measurable terms. Include only relevant surgical procedures, prior hospitalization and/or therapy for the same condition. Include only pertinent baseline tests and measurements from which to judge future progress or lack of progress.

21. **Functional Level** (end of billing period) - Enter the pertinent progress made and functional levels obtained at the end of the billing period compared to levels shown on initial assessment. Use objective terminology. Date progress when function can be consistently performed. When only a few visits have been made, enter a note indicating the training/treatment rendered and the patient's response if there is no change in function.

22. **Service Dates** - Enter the from and through dates which represent this billing period (*should be monthly*). Match the From and Through dates in field 22 on the UB-82. DO NOT use 00 in the date. Example: 01 08 91 for January 8, 1991.

DEPARTMENT OF HEALTH AND HUMAN SERVICES
HEALTH CARE FINANCING ADMINISTRATION

FORM APPROVED
OMB NO. 0938-0227

PLAN OF TREATMENT FOR OUTPATIENT REHABILITATION *(COMPLETE FOR INITIAL CLAIMS ONLY)*

1. PATIENT'S LAST NAME	FIRST NAME	M.I.	2. PROVIDER NO.	3. HICN

4. PROVIDER NAME	5. MEDICAL RECORD NO. *(Optional)*	6. ONSET DATE	7. SOC. DATE

8. TYPE: ☐ PT ☐ OT ☐ SLP ☐ CR
☐ RT ☐ PS ☐ SN ☐ SW

9. PRIMARY DIAGNOSIS *(Pertinent Medical D.X.)*	10. TREATMENT DIAGNOSIS	11. VISITS FROM SOC.

12. PLAN OF TREATMENT FUNCTIONAL GOALS

GOALS *(Short Term)*

OUTCOME *(Long Term)*

PLAN

13. SIGNATURE *(professional establishing POC including prof. designation)*

14. FREQ/DURATION *(e.g., 3/Wk x 4 Wk.)*

I CERTIFY THE NEED FOR THESE SERVICES FURNISHED UNDER THIS PLAN OF TREATMENT AND WHILE UNDER MY CARE   ☐ N/A

15. PHYSICIAN SIGNATURE

16. DATE

17. CERTIFICATION
FROM   THROUGH   ☐ N/A

18. ON FILE *(Print/type physician's name)*
☐

20. INITIAL ASSESSMENT *(History, medical complications, level of function at start of care. Reason for referral)*

19. PRIOR HOSPITIALIZATION
FROM   TO   ☐ N/A

21. FUNCTIONAL LEVEL *(End of billing period)*   PROGRESS REPORT   ☐ CONTINUE SERVICES *OR* ☐ DC SERVICES

22. SERVICE DATES
FROM   THROUGH

FORM HCFA-700 (11-91)

*U.S. Government Printing Office: 1993 — 771-86

INSTRUCTIONS FOR COMPLETION OF FORM HCFA-701
(Enter dates as 6 digits month, day, year)

1. **Patient's Name** - Enter the patient's last name, first name and middle initial as shown on the health insurance Medicare card.

2. **Provider Number** - Enter the number issued by Medicare to the billing provider *(i.e., 00-7000)*

3. **HICN** - Enter the patient's health insurance number as shown on the health insurance Medicare card, certification award, utilization notice, temporary eligibility notice, or as reported by SSO.

4. **Provider Name** - Enter the name of the Medicare billing provider.

5. **Medical Record No.** - *(optional)* Enter the patient's medical/clinical record number used by the billing provider. *(This is an item which you may enter for your own records)*

6. **Onset Date** - Enter the date of onset for the patient's primary medical diagnosis, if it is a new diagnosis, or the date of the most recent exacerbation of a previous diagnosis. If the exact date is not known enter 01 for the day *(i.e., 120191)*. The date matches occurrence code 11 on the UB-82.

7. **SOC *(start of care)* Date** - Enter the date services began at the billing provider *(the date of the first Medicare billable visit which **remains the same on subsequent claims** until discharge or denial corresponds to occurrence code 35 for PT, 44 for OT, 45 for SLP, and 46 for CR on the UB-82).*

8. **Type** - Check the type therapy billed i.e., physical therapy (PT), occupational therapy (OT), speech-language pathology (SLP), cardiac rehabilitation (CR), respiratory therapy (RT), psychological services (PS), skilled nursing services (SN), or social services (SW).

9. **Primary Diagnosis** - Enter the pertinent written medical diagnosis resulting in the therapy disorder and relating to 50% or more of effort in the plan of treatment.

10. **Treatment Diagnosis** - Enter the written treatment diagnosis for which services are rendered. For example, for PT the primary medical diagnosis might be Degeneration of Cervical Intervertebral Disc while the PT treatment DX might be Frozen R Shoulder or, for SLP, while CVA might be the primary medical DX, the treatment DX might be Aphasia. If the same as the primary DX enter SAME.

11. **Visits From Start of Care** - Enter the **cumulative total** visits *(sessions)* completed since services were started at the billing provider for the diagnosis treated, through the last visit on this bill. *(Corresponds to UB-82 value code 50 for PT, 51 for OT, 52 for SLP, or 53 for cardiac rehab on the UB-82)*

12. **Current Frequency/Duration** - Enter the urrent frequency and duration on treatment, e.g., 3 times per week for 4 weeks is entered 3/Wk x 4Wk.

13. **Current Plan Update, Functional Goals** – Enter the current plan of treatment goals for the patient for this billing period. *(If the same as shown on the HCFA-700 or previous 701 enter "same").* Enter the short-term goals to reaach overall long-term outcome. Justify intensity if appropriate. Estimate time-frames to meet goals, when possible.

14. **Recertification** - Enter the inclusive dates when recertification is required, **even if the ON FILE box is checked in item 17.** Check the N/A box if recertification is not required for the type of service rendered.

15. **Physician's Signature** - If the form HCFA-701 is used for recertification, the physician enters his/her signature. If recertification is not required for the type of services rendered, check N/A box. **If the form HCFA-701 is not being used for recertification, check the ON FILE box — item 17.**

16. **Date** - Enter the date of the physician's signature only if the form is used for recertification.

17. **ON FILE** (Means certification signature and date) - Enter the **typed/printed name of the physician** who recertified the plan of treatment that is on file at the billing provider. If recertification is not required for the type of services checked in item 8, type/print the name of the physician who referred or ordered the service, **but do not check the ON FILE box.**

18. **Reason(s) For Continuing Treatment This Billing Period** - Enter the **major reason(s)** why the patient needs to continue skilled rehabilitation **for this billing period** *(e.g., briefly state the patient's need for specific functional improvement, skilled training, reduction in complication or improvement in safety and how long you believe this will take, if possible, or state your reasons for recommending discontinuance).* Complete by the rehab specialist prior to physicians' recertification.

19. **Signature** - Enter the signature *(or name)* and the professional designation of the individual justifying or recommending need for care *(or discontinuance)* for this billing period.

20. **Date** - Enter the date of the rehabilitation professional's signature.

21. Check the box if services are continuing or discontinuing at end of this billing period.

22. **Functional Level** *(end of billing period)* - Enter the pertinent progress made through the end of this billing period. Use objective terminology. Compare progress made to that shown on the previous HCFA-701, item 22, or the HCFA-700, items 20 and 21. Date progress when function can be consistently performed or when meaningful functional improvement is made or when significant regression in function occurs. Your intermediary reviews this progress compared to that on the prior HCFA-701 or 700 to determine coverage for this billing period. Send a photocopy of the form covering the previous billing period.

23. **Service Dates** - Enter the from and through dates which represent this billing period *(should be monthly)*. Match the From and Through dates in field 22 on the UB-82. DO NOT use 00 in the date. Example: 01 08 91 for January 8, 1991.

Public reporting burden for this collection of information is estimated to average 15 minutes per response, including time for reviewing instructions, searching existing data sources, gathering and maintaining data needed, and completing and reviewing the collection of information. Send comments regarding this burden estimate or any other aspect of this collection of information, including suggestions for reducing the burden, to HCFA, Office of Financial Management, P.O. Box 26684, Baltimore, MD 21207; and to the Office of Management and Budget, Paperwork Reduction Project (0938-0227), Washington, D.C. 20503.

DEPARTMENT OF HEALTH AND HUMAN SERVICES
HEALTH CARE FINANCING ADMINISTRATION

FORM APPROVED
OMB NO. 0938-0227

UPDATED PLAN OF PROGRESS FOR OUTPATIENT REHABILITATION
(Complete for Interim to Discharge Claims. Photocopy of HCFA-700 or 701 is required)

1. PATIENT'S LAST NAME	FIRST NAME	M.I.	2. PROVIDER NO.	3. HICN

4. PROVIDER NAME	5. MEDICAL RECORD NO. *(Optional)*	6. ONSET DATE	7. SOC. DATE

8. TYPE:
☐ PT ☐ OT ☐ SLP ☐ CR
☐ RT ☐ PS ☐ SN ☐ SW

9. PRIMARY DIAGNOSIS *(Pertinent Medical D.X.)*	10. TREATMENT DIAGNOSIS	11. VISITS FROM SOC.

12. FREQ/DURATION *(e.g., 3/Wk x 4 Wk.)*

13. CURRENT PLAN UPDATE, FUNCTIONAL GOALS *(Specify changes to goals and plan)*

GOALS *(Short Term)*

PLAN

OUTCOME *(Long Term)*

I HAVE REVIEWED THIS PLAN OF TREATMENT AND
RECERTIFY A CONTINUING NEED FOR SERVICES. ☐ N/A ☐ DC

15. PHYSICIAN'S SIGNATURE

16. DATE

14. RECERTIFICATION
FROM   THROUGH   ☐ N/A

17. ON FILE *(Print/type physician's name)*
☐

18. REASON(S) FOR CONTINUING TREATMENT THIS BILLING PERIOD *(Clarify goals and necessity for continued skilled care)*

19. SIGNATURE *(or name of professional, including prof. designation)*

20. DATE

☐ CONTINUE SERVICES *OR* ☐ DC SERVICES

22. FUNCTIONAL LEVEL *(at end of billing period - Relate your documentation to functional outcomes and list problems still present)*

23. SERVICE DATES
FROM   THROUGH

FORM HCFA-701 (11-91)

☆ U.S. GOVERNMENT PRINTING OFFICE: 1993 771-862

PRINTED BY STANDARD REGISTER U.S.A. ZIPSET ®

NovaCare
Helping Make Life a Little Better.

PLAN OF TREATMENT FOR OUTPATIENT REHABILITATION (COMPLETE FOR INITIAL CLAIMS ONLY)

1. PATIENT'S LAST NAME	FIRST NAME / M.I.	2. PROVIDER NO.	3. HICN
Doe	Jane E.	12-3456	123-45-6789A

4. PROVIDER NAME	5. MEDICAL RECORD NO. (Optional)	6. ONSET DATE	7. SOC. DATE
Happy Home Center	123	7/27/97	8/10/97

8. TYPE: ☐ PT ☒ OT ☐ SLP ☐ CR ☐ RT ☐ PS ☐ SN ☐ SW

9. PRIMARY DIAGNOSIS (Pertinent Medical D.X.): s/p acute pneumonia

10. TREATMENT DIAGNOSIS: muscle wkness/disuse atrophy 728.2

11. VISITS FROM SOC.: 22

12. PLAN OF TREATMENT FUNCTIONAL GOALS (to be met within 2 weeks)

GOALS (Short Term)
① Res. will ↑ UE strength to complete UB grooming, bathing and dressing with setup only.
② Res will ↑ postural strength and balance to complete LB bathing and dressing with moderate assistance.

OUTCOME (Long Term)
Res will ↑ strength and balance to complete basic ADLs ① for return to home.
③ Res will ↑ strength to complete bed mobility at ① level for 50% time.
④ Res will ↑ strength/balance and ↓ anxiety to complete functional ADL trnsfrs w/ min ①.

PLAN: ADL retraining, kinetics, functional balance and transfer training, home assessment, environmental modification, pt/family education.

Rehab potential is excellent for stated goals 2° to recent onset, previous history, resident motivation and family support

D/C plan: return to live in senior hi-rise with assistance for home management

13. SIGNATURE (professional establishing POC including prof. designation)

14. FREQ/DURATION (e.g., 3/Wk x 4 Wk.): 5x/wk for 5 weeks

I CERTIFY THE NEED FOR THESE SERVICES FURNISHED UNDER THIS PLAN OF TREATMENT AND WHILE UNDER MY CARE ☐ N/A

17. CERTIFICATION FROM 8/10/97 THROUGH 8/31/97 ☐ N/A

15. PHYSICIAN SIGNATURE | 16. DATE

18. ON FILE (Print/type physician's name): ☐ Dr. Douglas

20. INITIAL ASSESSMENT (History, medical complications, level of function at start of care. Reason for referral.)

19. PRIOR HOSPITALIZATION FROM 7/27/97 TO 8/9/97 ☐ N/A

med hx: s/p acute ① L pneumonia, CAD, DJD, s/p old cataract surgery (10 yrs), mild OBS. DOB: 9/9/19
social hx: prior to onset, resident lived in senior hi-rise apt alone. ① for basic ADLs (sponge bathing) and rec'd assist for shopping, cleaning and meals on wheels; has supportive family. Res leisure interests include bingo and knitting. Res goal thru rehab is to return to previous living status.
UE STATUS: ® hand dominant. PROM/AROM WFL ® UE ⊗ mild arthritic Δ's for end range shoulder flexion + elbow extension. Strength for manual muscle test 3+/5 but sustained strength/endurance severely limited for all sustained activity. GMC = WFL FMC = impaired for ADL fasteners and leisure tasks (ie. knitting)
ADL STATUS: feeding: ① w/ setup grooming: min ① 2° to strength limitations bathing: UB = min ① LB = max ①, ↓'d postural control for forward flexion and ↓'d balance in standing. dressing: UB = min/mod ① LB = max ①. toileting: continent of bowel + bladder mod ① for toilet trnsfrs and dressing but able to ① ly complete personal hygiene. Resident is currently dependent to gather her ADL items 2° to ↓'d mobility associated with overall weakness.
MOBILITY/ POSITIONING: bed: rolling = min ① and use of side rails supine↔sit = mod ① balance: unsupported sit = F+; dyn sit = F- IF; unsupported static standing = poor. Transfers: sit→stand = min ①; stand pivot = mod ② 2° to ↓'d strength and resident's fear/anxiety. OOB in w/c.
cognition: alert, Ox2, demonstrates good attention and follows multistep simple commands, mildly ↓'d memory but fair safety awareness
perception: wears glasses + hearing aid but WFL; body scheme + R/L discrim intact; no gross deficits noted.

21. FUNCTIONAL LEVEL (End of billing period) PROGRESS REPORT ☒ CONTINUE SERVICES OR ☐ DC SERVICES
Excellent progress via skilled OT with notable gains in strength + balance. Res. is less anxious and continues to provide maximum effort towards achievement of goals. Progress per above goals as follows:
① Re: UB ADLs w/ setup. Goal met. Via participation in selective resistive kinetic tasks + ADL retraining, res demonstrates 4/5 strength + can complete tasks with setup only. Res. able to self-pace as needed.
② Re: LB ADLs w/ mod ①. Goal met + upgraded. In addition to ADL retraining, res working via co-treatment w/ PT to ↑ LB strength for dynamic standing balance skills. Postural strength ↑'d from F- → F+ dynamic sitting but continues to impede functional ①. OT currently seeking to introduce adaptive equipment as a compensatory measure 2° to lack of further restoration of function.
③ Re: bed mobility ① IN. Goal met. Res has demon ↑'d UE strength to roll ① ly w/ siderails and can get in/out of bed w/o assistance 100% time.
④ Re: ADL Transfers w/ min ①. Goal met. Via ↑'d strength and activities such as standing table top + anxiety, res. now completing stnd-pivot transfers w/ min ①. Sit→stand ① for moderate height surfaces.

Room #: A1	Patient #: 123	Facility: Happy Home Center	22. SERVICE DATES FROM 8/10/97 THROUGH 8/31/97

FORM HCFA-700 (6-93)

white - original - FACILITY COPY

NovaCare
Helping Make Life a Little Better.

UPDATED PLAN OF PROGRESS FOR OUTPATIENT REHABILITATION
(Complete for Interim to Discharge Claims. Photocopy of HCFA-700 or 701 is required)

1. PATIENT'S LAST NAME	FIRST NAME	M.I.	2. PROVIDER NO.	3. HICN
Doe	Jane		12-3456	123-45-6789 A

4. PROVIDER NAME	5. MEDICAL RECORD NO. *(Optional)*	6. ONSET DATE	7. SOC. DATE
Happy Home Center	123	7/27/97	8/10/97

8. TYPE:	9. PRIMARY DIAGNOSIS *(Pertinent Medical D.X.)*	10. TREATMENT DIAGNOSIS	11. VISITS FROM SOC.
☐ PT ☒ OT ☐ SLP ☐ CR	s/p acute pneumonia)	muscle wkness/ disuse 728.2	31
☐ RT ☐ PS ☐ SN ☐ SW	12. FREQ./DURATION *(e.g., 3/Wk x 4Wk.)* 5x/wk for 2 weeks		

13. CURRENT PLAN UPDATE, FUNCTIONAL GOALS *(Specify changes to goals and plan)*

GOALS (Short Term) (2 wks)

① Resident will ↑ strength/balance to complete UB/LB ADLs ①ly including setup using adaptive equipment as needed.
② Resident will ↑ bal to complete all functional ADL transfers ①ly with adaptive equipment as needed.

OUTCOME (Long Term)

① Resident will ↑ strength + balance to complete basic ADLs ①ly for d/c to home.
② Resident will ↑ activity tolerance to complete simple basic homemaking tasks ①ly using energy conservation strategies

PLAN ADL retraining, kinetics, functional balance + transfer training, home assessment, environmental modification, pt/family education

Rehab potential is excellent for stated goals 2° to recent onset, motivation and family support

D/c plan: return to own apt w/ outside assistance

I HAVE REVIEWED THIS PLAN OF TREATMENT AND RECERTIFY A CONTINUING NEED FOR SERVICES. ☐ N/A ☐ DC	14. RECERTIFICATION FROM 9/1/97 THROUGH 9/30/97 ☐ N/A
15. PHYSICIAN'S SIGNATURE	16. DATE	17. ON FILE *(Print/type physician's name)* ☐ Dr. Douglas

18. REASON(S) FOR CONTINUING TREATMENT THIS BILLING PERIOD *(Clarify goals and necessity for continued skilled care)*

Resident has demonstrated excellent gains in functional ADL performance via skilled OT services thus far. At current state of function, resident would remain unable to return home as ① in ADLs has yet to be achieved. With continued services and appropriate environmental modifications as well as family education, res will return to prior living arrangement.

Current functional levels in summary as follows:

UB ADLs = ① w/ setup Strength 4/5 with continued limitations in endurance.

LB ADLs = minimum assistance. F+ dynamic sitting balance and F-/F dynamic standing balance

bed mobility = ①

Transfers = minimum assistance

toileting = minimum assistance for clothing and transfers

functional mobility = ambulating with wheeled walker and CGA of 1; able to gather self-care items in her room with minimum assistance.

* Family, resident and facility staff have met to discuss d/c plan - resident still plans to go home. Family will provide any and all assistance as needed.

19. SIGNATURE *(or name of professional, including prof. designation)*	20. DATE	21.
	9/1/97	☐ CONTINUE SERVICES OR ☒ DC SERVICES

22. FUNCTIONAL LEVEL *(at end of billing period - Relate your documentation to functional outcomes and list problems still present)*

Resident is d/c'd from skilled OT program 2° to all goals met. Res is being d/c'd to home at this time. Progress per above goals as follows:

① RE: UB/LB ADLs ①ly including setup. **Goal met.** Via resistance training and dynamic balance activities, resident gathers ADL items using wheeled walker. Basket on walker aids in transport of items. Resident using elastic shoelaces, long-handled shoe horn and reacher for ① LB dressing.

② RE: ADL transfers ①. **Goal partially met.** Increased strength noted for ① transfers to bed, lounge chair and toilet (with aid of raised toilet seat). Res continues to require assistance with car and tub transfers - will receive home therapy for further ① in this area.

③ RE: basic homemaking tasks ①. **Goal met.** OTR/L conducted home assessment with resident present. Kitchen area modified for ease and safety of tasks. Res demonstrates ability to perform tasks such as making simple breakfasts and making her bed using strategies such as pacing, sit vs. stand and simplification of task. Family will be supportive in providing assistance for more difficult chores.

At this time, resident has demonstrated sufficient gains in strength, balance and activity tolerance to complete basic ADL tasks ①ly thus meeting OT's primary long term goal. Resident to be d/c'd home as a result of these interventions. D/C OT.

Room #	Patient #	Facility	23. SERVICE DATES
A1	123	Happy Home Center	FROM 9/1/97 THROUGH 9/12/97

FORM HCFA-701 (L-025)

white-original-FACILITY COPY

Effective Documentation for Occupational Therapy

MEDICARE MEDICAL REVIEW PART B
GUIDELINES FOR SPEECH-LANGUAGE PATHOLOGY

A3 3905. MEDICAL REVIEW (MR) OF PART B INTERMEDIARY OUTPATIENT SPEECH-LANGUAGE PATHOLOGY (SLP) BILLS

A. General.—Use the following guidelines for review of SLP services. Base your review of SLP on focused review criteria which you determine to be effective. Implement the HCFA edits only if your data supports their effectiveness in focusing review. These criteria do not apply to SLP services provided under a home health plan of care.

The criteria for MR case selection are based on ICD-9-CM diagnoses, elapsed time from start of care (at the billing provider) and number of visits. (See Exhibit I.)

Do not deny a bill solely on the basis that it exceeds the criteria in the edits.

The edits are only for selecting bills to review or for paying bills without MR if they meet Level I criteria. Do not provide automatic coverage up to these criteria. They neither guarantee minimum nor set maximum coverage limits.

B. Level I Review Process.—SLP edits have been developed for a number of diagnoses which were selected on the basis that, when linked with a recent date of onset, there is a high probability that Medicare patients with these diagnoses will require skilled SLP. The edits do not specify every diagnosis which may require SLP, and therefore, the fact that a given diagnosis does not appear in the edits does not create a presumption that SLP services are not necessary, or are inappropriate. Do not approve or deny claims at Level I for medical necessity. You may pay claims that pass the edits in Exhibit I and any additional edits approved by your RO without being subjected to Level II MR.

For patients receiving SLP services only (V57.3, Speech therapy) during an encounter/visit, the appropriate V code for the service is sequenced first, and, if documented, the diagnosis or problem for which the services are performed is sequenced second. Program your system to read the diagnosis or problem sequenced second to determine if it meets the Level I SLP edits.

> EXAMPLE: SLP services V57.3, for a patient with aphasia 784.3. The V code will be sequenced first, followed by the code for aphasia (V57.3, 784.3). Edit for aphasia not the V code. Use this same procedure for V57.89, other specified rehabilitation procedure, and V57.9, unspecified rehabilitation procedure.

Evaluate bills at Level I based upon each of the following:

1. Facility and Patient Identification.—(Facility name, patient name, provider number, HICN, age.)

2. Diagnosis.—The primary diagnosis for which SLP services were rendered must be listed by ICD-9-CM code first; other Dx(s) applicable to the patient or that influence care must follow.

3. Duration.—The total elapsed time in days that SLP services have been rendered beginning with the date treatment was initiated by the billing provider for the diagnosis being treated (includes the last day in the current billing period).

4. Number of Visits.—The total number of visits completed since SLP services were initiated by the billing provider for the diagnosis being treated. Include the last visit in the billing period in the total visits to date. Do not obtain only the visits for this month's billing period. (Value code 52).

5. Date Treatment Started (Occurrence Code 45).—The date SLP services were initiated by the billing provider for the speech, language and related disorder.

6. Billing Period.—When SLP services began and ended in the billing period (from/through dates).

C. Level II Review Process.—If a bill meets your focused MR criteria, refer it to the Level II MR health professional staff. If possible, have speech-language pathologists review SLP bills.

Once the bill is selected for focused MR, review it in conjunction with medical information submitted by the provider.

1. Payable SLP Services.—Pay SLP services only if they meet applicable Medicare coverage requirements. Each bill for SLP services that is subjected to Level II MR must be supported with adequate medical documentation for you to make a determination. (See 3101.A and 3148.)

2. MR and Documentation.—When a claim is referred to Level II MR, use the following pertinent data elements in addition to those used for Level I review:

   a. Medical History.—Obtain only the medical history which is pertinent to, or influences the SLP treatment rendered, including a brief description of the functional status of the patient prior to the onset of the condition requiring SLP, and any pertinent prior SLP treatment.

   b. Speech, Language and Related Disorder.—The diagnosis or diagnoses established by the speech-language pathologist. Examples are spoken language production disorder (expressive aphasia), dysarthria, and dysphagia.

   c. Date of Onset (Occurrence Code 11).—The date of onset or exacerbation of the speech, language and related disorder diagnosis for which services were rendered by the billing provider.

d. Physician Referral and Date Received by the Billing Provider.

e. Initial Assessment and Date.—The procedure used by the speech-language pathologist to diagnose speech, language, and related disorders, and the date the initial assessment is completed by the billing provider.

f. Plan of Treatment and Date Established.

g. Date of Last Certification.—Obtain the date on which the plan of treatment was last certified by the physician.

h. Progress Notes.—Obtain updated patient status reports concerning the patient's current functional communication abilities/limitation.

3905.1 MEDICAL HISTORY. – If a history of previous SLP treatment is not available, the provider may furnish a general summary regarding the patient's past relevent medical history recorded during the initial assessment with the patient/family (if reliable) or through contact with the referring physician. Information regarding prior treatment for the current condition, progress made, and treatment by the referring physician must be provided when available. The level of function prior to the current exacerbation or onset should be described.

The patient's medical history includes the date of onset and/or exacerbation of the illness or injury. If the patient has had prior therapy for the same condition, use that history in conjunction with the patient's current assessment to establish whether additional treatment is reasonable.

The history of treatments from a previous provider is necessary for patients who have transferred to a new provider for additional treatment. For chronic conditions, the history gives the date of the change or deterioration in the patient's condition and a description of the changes that necessitate skilled care.

3905.2 ASSESSMENT. – Approve the initial assessment when it is reasonable and necessary for the speech-language pathologist to determine if there is an expectation that either restorative services or establishment of a maintenance program will be appropriate for the patient's condition.

Reassessments are covered if the patient exhibits a demonstrable change in motivation, clearing of confusion, or the remission of some other medical condition which previously contraindicated SLP services. Periodic routine reevaluations (e.g., monthly, bimonthly) for a patient undergoing a SLP program are part of the treatment session and are not covered as separate evaluations. An initial assessment or reassessment that is determined reasonable and necessary based on the patient's condition, may be approved even though the expectations are not realized, or when the assessment determines that skilled services are not needed.

The assessment establishes the baseline data necessary for assessing expected rehabilitation potential, setting realistic goals, and measuring communication status at periodic intervals.

The initial assessment must include objective baseline diagnostic testing (standardized or nonstandardized), interpretation of test results, and clinical findings. If baseline testing cannot be accomplished for any reason, note this in the initial assessment or progress notes, along with the reason(s). Include a statement of the patient's expected rehabilitation potential.

3905.3 PLAN OF TREATMENT. – The plan of treatment must contain the following:

- Type and nature of care to be provided;

- Functional goals and estimated rehabilitation potential;

- Treatment objectives;

- Frequency of visits; and

- Estimated duration of treatment.

A. Functional Goals.—Must be written by the speech-language pathologist to reflect the level of communicative independence the patient is expected to achieve outside of the therapeutic environment. The functional goals reflect the final level the patient is expected to achieve, are realistic, and have a positive effect on the quality of the patient's everyday functions.

Assume that certain factors may change or influence the final level of achievement. If this occurs, have the speech-language pathologist document the factors which led to the change of the functional goal. Examples of functional communication goals in achieving optimum communication independence are the ability to:

- Communicate basic physical needs and emotional status;

- Communicate personal self-care needs;

- Engage in social communicative interaction with immediate family or friends; or

- Carry out communicative interactions in the community.

  NOTE: The term "communication" includes speech, language, as well as voice skills.

A functional goal may reflect a small, but meaningful change which enables the patient to function more independently in a reasonable amount of time. For some patients, it may be the ability to give a consistent "yes" and "no" response; for others, it may be the ability to demonstrate a competency in naming objects using auditory/verbal cues. Others may receptively and expressively use a basic spoken vocabulary and/or short phases, and still others may regain conversational language skills.

B. Treatment Objectives.—Specific steps designed to reach a functional goal. When the patient achieves these objectives, the functional goal is met.

C. Frequency of Visits.—An estimate of how often the treatments are to be rendered (e.g., 3x week).

Length of visits are typically 30, 45, or 60 minutes. Sometimes patients are seen for shorter periods several times a day (e.g., three 10 minute sessions, or a total of 30 minutes). Rarely, except during an assessment, are sessions longer than 60 minutes. If so, the provider must justify them, by noting, for example, that the patient is exceptionally alert, the number of appropriate activities needing skilled intervention is greater than average, special staff/family training is required. Post-operative intensive treatment is sometimes required (e.g., tracheoesophageal puncture) or post-onset of disorder (due to intensive family involvement).

D. Estimated Duration of Treatment.—Estimated duration of treatment refers to the total estimated time over which the services are to be rendered, and may be expressed in days, weeks, or months.

3905.4 Progress Reports (Treatment Summary for Billing Period). – Obtain:

- The initial functional communication level of the patient at this provider setting;
- The present functional level of the patient and progress (or lack of progress) specific for this reporting period;
- The patient's expected rehabilitation potential; and
- Changes in the plan of treatment.

Where a valid expectation of improvement existed at the time services were initiated, or thereafter, the services are covered even though the expectation may not be realized. However, in such instances, approve the services up to the time that no further significant practical improvement can be expected. Progress reports must document a continued expectation that the patient's condition will improve significantly in a reasonable and generally predictable period of time.

"Significant," means a generally measurable and substantial increase in the patient's present level of communication, independence, and competence compared to their levels when treatment was initiated. Do not interpret the term "significant" so stringently that you may deny a claim because of a temporary setback in the patient's progress. For example, a patient may experience a new intervening medical complication or a brief period when lack of progress occurs. The medical reviewer may approve the claim if there is still a reasonable expectation that significant improvement in the patient's overall functional ability will occur. However, the speech-language pathologist and/or physician should document such lack of progress and explain the need for continued intervention.

Documentation includes a short narrative progress report and objective information in a clear, concise manner. This provides you with the status on progress in meeting the plan of treatment, along with any changes in the goals or the treatment plan. Request that new plans be forwarded with the original so that you can review the entire plan. However, you must have access to an overall treatment plan with final goals and enough objective information with each claim to determine progress toward meeting the goals.

Consistent reporting is important. For example, if the provider reports that the patient can produce an "m" 25 percent of the time, then reports 40, 60, 90 percent success, you may believe that treatment might be ending. However, if you have the final goal and the objectives, you can see the progress toward that goal and the steps needed to reach it. The speech-language pathologist might state that the final goal is "the ability to converse in a limited environment." One underlying SLP goal might be to "reduce the apraxia sufficiently so the patient can initiate short intelligible phrases with a minimum of errors." Short-term goals may include the patient's ability to initiate easier phonemes before other, more difficult, phonemes. Therefore, the speech-language pathologist has a linguistically and neurologically sound basis for working on one phoneme production before initiating another.

The speech-language pathologist might work on a group of phonemes having a "feature" in common before working on another group. For example, working on all bilabials (since the patient can easily see the movement), might be desirable prior to sounds that are produced more intraorally.

The speech-language pathologist may choose how to demonstrate progress. However, the method chosen, as well as the measures used, generally remain the same for the duration of treatment. The provider must interpret reports of test scores, or comparable measures and their relationship to functional goals in progress notes or reports. Diagnostic testing should be appropriate to the communication disorder.

While a patient is receiving SLP treatment, the speech-language pathologist reassesses the patient's condition and adjusts the treatment. However, if the method used to document progress is changed, the reasons must be documented, including how the new method relates to the previous method. If the speech-language pathologist reports a subtest score for one month, then a score of a different subtest the next month without demonstrating the subtest's interrelationship, you are not able to judge the progress. Return these claims for an explanation/interpretation. Refer to Level III MR if needed.

3905.5 LEVEL OF COMPLEXITY OF TREATMENT. – Base decisions on the level of complexity of the services rendered by the speech-language pathologist, not what the patient is asked to do. For example, the patient may be asked to repeat a word and the speech-language pathologist analyzes the response and gives the patient feedback that the patient uses to modify the response. The speech-language pathologist may ask staff or family to repeat the activity as a reinforcement. It is the speech-language pathologist's analysis that makes the activity skilled.

3905.6 REPORTING ON NEW EPISODE OR CONDITION. – Occasionally, a patient who is receiving, or has previously received SLP services, experiences a secondary or complicating new illness. The provider documents the signficance of any change to the communication capabilities. This may be by pre-and post-episodic objective documentation, through nursing notes or by physician reports. If the patient is receiving treatment, it might have to be lengthened because of his change in condition. If the patient has completed treatment, a significant change in the communication status must be documented to warrant a new treatment plan.

3905.7 QUALIFIED SPEECH-LANGUAGE PATHOLOGIST. – The following information is provided to familiarize you with Medicare requirements for qualifications of speech-language pathologists and specific acronyms commonly used.

- A person who is licensed, if applicable, by the State in which he/she is practicing; and

- Is eligible for a certificate of clinical competence in SLP granted by the American Speech•Language•Hearing Association; or

- Meets the educational requirements for certification, and is in the process of accumulating the supervised experience required for certification.

- Normally indicates certification status by utilizing CCC-SLP or CFY-SLP:

   — CCC-SLP - Certificate of Clinical Competence in SLP; or

   — CFY-SLP - Clinical Fellowship Year in Speech-Language Pathology.

3905.8 SKILLED AND UNSKILLED PROCEDURES. – Certain services are skilled or nonskilled by definition. However, for coverage, the services must be reasonable and necessary based on your medical review of the documentation submitted. The following are examples of specific types of skilled and nonskilled SLP procedures:

A. Skilled Procedures.—

- Diagnostic and assessment services to ascertain the type, causal factor(s) and severity of speech and language disorders. Reassessment is needed if the patient exhibits a change in functional speech or motivation, clearing of confusion, or remission of some other medical condition which previously contraindicated SLP or audiology services.

- Design of a treatment program relevant to the patient's disorder(s). Continued assessment of progress during the implementation of the treatment program, including documentation and professional analysis of the patient's status at regular intervals.

- Establishment of compensatory skills (e.g., air-injection techniques, word finding strategies).

- Establishment of a hierarchy of speech-language tasks and cueing that directs a patient toward communication goals.

- Analysis related to actual progress toward goals.

- Patient and family training to augment restorative treatment or to establish a maintenance program.

B. Unskilled Procedures.—

- Nondiagnostic/nontherapeutic routine, repetitive and reinforced procedures (e.g., the practicing of word drills without skilled feedback).

- Procedures which are repetitive and/or that reinforce previously learned material which the patient or family is instructed to repeat.

- Procedures which may be effectively carried out with the patient by any nonprofessional (e.g., family member, restorative nursing aide) after instruction and training is completed.

- Provision of practice for use of augmentative or alternative assessment communication systems.

    NOTE: It is only after the patient has established a high level of consistency of performance in a task with the speech-language pathologist that unskilled techniques can be implemented.

3905.9 STATEMENTS SUPPORTING AND NOT SUPPORTING COVERAGE. – This is documentation which is objective or subjective and demonstrates whether there is progress toward a stated functional goal.

A. Statements Supporting Coverage.—Typically, these statements have an objective component which is compared to previous reports, and which demonstrate progress toward a stated functional goal.

    EXAMPLES: "Mr. Smith achieved 75 on the Word Subtest on the Johnson Test of Aphasia compared with last month's score of 50 on the same Subtest."

    "Mr. Jones achieved a combined score of 352 on the A, B, C, D, and E subtests this month compared with an overall score of 250 for these same subtests last month."

    "Mrs. Jones achieved the next steps in the treatment plan outlined last month (see attached sheet). If she continues at this rate, she should complete treatment within the next 2 months."

    "Mrs. Jones achieved 75% (7.5 out of 10 or 75 out of 100) on word naming which compares to last month's score of 50% (5.0 out of 10 or 50 out of 100)."

NOTE: Percentages should be based on real number count. Interpretation of scores must be presented in progress notes or summary information. The narrative should also contain reference to objective scoring, comparison of previous scores, or treatment plan with present status compared to previous status. This information may be embedded in narrative or attached, however, the reviewer should have access to this information and stated functional goals.

B. Statements Not Supporting Coverage.—Typically, these statements are subjective, and do not demonstrate progress toward a stated functional goal, or a comparison to previous test scores.

EXAMPLE: "Ms. Jones is very concerned about going home. She has begun smoking again which is causing family as well as physical problems."

"Speech somewhat slurred today."

"Mr. Smith more consistent in responses."

"Mr. Jones has shown significant improvement in his ability to make himself understood."

"Patient is now able to inject air 80% of the time." (No comparison to previous report.)

"Mrs. Smith achieved 75% accuracy on word naming task. (No comparison to previous report)."

"Auditory comprehension improved from moderately impaired to mildly impaired." (By itself, the statement does not offer sufficient objective information.)

C. Resumption of Treatment.—There are conditions and circumstances that justify resuming treatment after it has been delayed. Obtain verification (when needed for coverage decisions). Examples include:

- Patient becomes more alert, attentive, cooperative;

- Patient shows rehabilitation potential;

- Medical complications cleared;

- Environmental change improves motivation or communicative capabilities;

- Progressive nature of disorder warrants further treatment; and

- Drug or other medical treatment is reduced or ended.

3905.10 MR Considerations.—

A. Disorders Typically Not Covered for the Geriatric Patient.

- Stuttering (except neurogenic stuttering caused by brain damage)

  Fluency Disorder

  Cluttering

  Disprosody

  Disfluency;

- Myofunctional Disorders

  Tongue Thrust; and

- Behavioral/Psychological Speech Delay.

B. Maintenance Program.—Approve claims only when the specialized knowledge and judgment of a qualified speech-language pathologist is required to design and establish a maintenance program. By the time the patient's restorative program has been completed, the maintenance program has already been designed, with instructions to patient, supportive personnel, or family. Do not approve a separate charge for establishing the maintenance program immediately after the restorative program has been completed.

Obtain documentation that justifies a provider reestablishing a maintenance program, e.g., loss in previous functional abilities occurs, intervening medical conditions develop, difficulty in communicating with caregivers arises.

The initial assessment should be documented with standardized testing (if possible) to establish base-line data. This is critical if a claim is submitted for care at a future date. Documentation should show that the maintenance program is designed by the speech-language pathologist appropriate to the capacity and tolerance of the patient and the treatment objectives of the physician.

The maintenance program is established when documentation indicates it has been designed for the patient's level of function and instructions to the patient and supportive personnel have been completed for them to safely and effectively carry them out. The documentation must give reasonable assurances that this has occurred. After that point, the services are not reasonable and necessary.

C. Group Treatment.—Generally, group therapy treatment and attendance at social or support groups, such as stroke clubs or lost cord clubs, are not payable. Ensure that the "reasonable and necessary" requirements are met.

D. Total Laryngectomy.—Surgical removal of the larynx. Documentation may involve pre-op/post-op sessions as part of the assessment, to inform the patient, the family, and staff about alternative communication methods, and to provide an immediate means of communication. Documentation includes assessment and any treatment necessary to establish a means of communication using esophageal speech, an artifical larynx (electronic or pneumatic device), a tracheoesophageal puncture prosthesis, and/or other alternate communication methods.

E. Partial Laryngectomy.—Surgical removal of part of the larynx. Documentation includes the voice problems that require assessment and treatment. Documentation may involve pre-op/post-op sessions as part of the assessment, and to inform the patient, the family, and staff about voice problems. Documentation for rehabilitation includes the assessment and type of treatment required for the voice disorders, as well as base-line objective data and progress notes.

F. Total Glossectomy.—Surgical removal of the tongue. Total glossectomy results in articulation problems that require assessment and may require treatment. Documentation may include pre-op/post-op sessions as part of the assessment to inform the patient, the family, and staff about articulation disorders, and to provide an immediate means of communication and/or to establish an effective maintenance program. Documentation includes assessment and type of treatment for the articulation disorders. Documentation for articulation treatment involves instruction of compensatory techniques and alternate communication methods if needed.

G. Partial Glossectomy.—Surgical removal of part of the tongue. Documentation should indicate the articulation problems that require assessment and treatment. Documentation may include pre-op/post-op sessions as part of the assessment to inform the patient, the family, and staff about articulation disorders, and to provide an immediate means of communication following surgery. Documentation includes the assessment and type of treatment for the articulation disorders including base-line objective data and progress notes. Documentation for articulation treatment involves instruction of compensatory techniques and alternate communication methods if needed.

H. Congenital Disorders.—Documentation must always substantiate need, e.g., no previous treatment; the patient's communicative capabilities have recently deteriorated; new, special techniques or instruments have become available; or intervening medical complications have affected SLP communication. Approve claims for maintenance or short-term treatment only if objective documentation supports that need.

I. Alzheimer's Disease (chronic brain syndrome, organic brain syndrome).—Objective documentation must indicate the patient's condition, alertness and mental awareness. Documentation must justify that services are needed to establish a reasonable and necessary maintenance program. Review these claims carefully for medical necessity.

J. Chronic Conditions.—Approve claims for patients with chronic conditions such as MS, ALS, Parkinson's Disease or Myasthenia Gravis if they document a need for reasonable and necessary short-term care or a need to establish a maintenance program. However, clear documentation must be present concerning any prior care or maintenance program designed for the same condition. Approve claims for reasonable and necessary short-term intervention to improve oral and laryngeal strength, speech intelligibility, or vocal intensity, but only when the documentation supports the need to increase function, or to establish a maintenance program.

3905.11 CERTIFICATION AND RECERTIFICATION. − SLP services must be certified and recertified by a physician and furnished while under the care of a physician. They must be furnished under a written plan of treatment established by the physician or a qualified speech-language pathologist providing such services. If the plan is established by a speech-language pathologist, it must be reviewed periodically by the physician. The plan of care must be established (reduced to writing by either professional or the provider when it makes a written record of the oral orders) before treatment is begun. When outpatient SLP services are continued under the same plan of treatment for a period of time, the physician must certify at intervals of at least every 30 days that there is a continuing need for them. Obtain the recertification when reviewing the plan of treatment since the same interval of at least 30 days is required for the review of the plans. Recertification must be signed by the physician who reviewed the plan of treatment. Any changes established by the speech-language pathologist must be in writing and signed by the speech-language pathologist or by the attending physician. The physician may change a plan of treatment established by the speech-language pathologist. The speech-language pathologist may not alter a plan of treatment established by a physician.

3905.12 FOCUSED MR EVALUATION. − The HCFA edits will aid in identifing SLP claims for focused MR. Perform regular evaluations of provider claims which pass or fail the edits. Change your focused review selection based on the results of the evaluation. For example, a provider billing at an aberrantly consistent rate just below the parameters is to be subjected to focused review.

Be on the alert for any of the following trends or characteristics in developing focused MR:

- Edits with high charges per aggregate bill charges;
- Providers billing a higher than average utilization of specific diagnostic codes that fall just below the edit parameters; or
- Specific principal DX codes, such as those with longer visits and duration, those representing the most frequent denials in pre-pay MR, special codes, and/or certain edit groups such as 1, 3, 5 and 8 in one quarter, and others in the next quarter.

3905.13 Speech-Language Pathology Terms.—

Agnosia - Inability to attach meaning to sensory information although the physiologic receptor mechanism is intact.

Agrammatism - Impairment of the ability to produce words in their correct sequence; difficulty with grammar and syntax.

Agraphia - Disorder of writing. It may result from a central nervous system lesion or from lack of muscular coordination.

Anomia - Loss of the ability to identify or to recall and recognize names of persons, places or things.

Aphasia - Communication disorder caused by brain damage and characterized by complete or partial impairment of language comprehension, formulation, and use. It excludes disorders associated with primary sensory deficits, general mental deterioration, or psychiatric disorders. Partial impairment is often referred to as dysphasia.

Aphonia - Loss of voice.

Apraxia - (1) Disruption in the ability to transmit a motor response along a specific modality; involves disruption of voluntary or purposeful programming of muscular movements while involuntary movements remain intact; characterized by difficulty in articulation of speech, formulation of letters in writing, or in movements of gesture and pantomime. (2) In speech, a nonlinguistic sensorimotor disorder of articulation characterized by impaired capacity to program the position of speech musculature and the sequencing of muscle movements (respiratory, laryngeal, and oral) for the volitional production of phonemes.

Dysarthria - Term for a collection of motor speech disorders due to impairment originating in the central or peripheral nervous system. Respiration, articulation, phonation, resonation, and/or prosody may be affected; volitional and automatic actions, such as chewing and swallowing, and movements of the jaw and tongue may also be deviant. It excludes apraxia and functional or central language disorders.

Dysphagia - Difficulty in swallowing. It may include inflammation, compression, paralysis, weakness, or hypertonicity of the esophagus.

Generalization - (1) In conditioning, the eliciting of a conditioned response by stimuli similar to a particular conditioned stimulus. (2) Transfer of learning from one environment to a similar environment; the more similar the environments or situations, the greater transfer takes place.

Hard Glottal Attack - Forceful approximation of the vocal folds during the initiation of phonation.

Intonation - Linguistic system within a language which is concerned with pitch, stress, and juncture of the spoken language; a unit with specific communicative import, such as interrogation, exclamation, and assertion.

Lexicon - Total accumulation of linguistic signs, words or morphemes, or both, in a given language; the list of all the words in a language.

Morphology - Component of grammar concerned with the formation of words, the smallest meaningful unit in a language, as a bridge between phonology and syntax.

Obturator - (l) Any structure which occludes an opening. (2) Prosthetic appliance, similar to a dental plate, that forms an artificial palate to cover a cleft palate, designed so that the musculature of the palate and pharynx are able to contract around it.

Paraphasia - Any error of commission modifying a specific word (sound and morpheme substitution) or of word substitution in the spoken or written production of a speaker or writer.

Perseveration - Tendency to continue an activity, motor or mental, once started, and to be unable to modify or stop even though it is acknowledged to have become inappropriate.

Phoneme - Shortest arbitrary unit of sound in a given language that can be recognized as being distinct from other sounds in the language.

Phonological - Component of grammar determining the meaningful combination of sounds.

Pitch - Acuteness or gravity of a tone, dependent upon the frequency of the vibrations producing it and their intensity and overtone structure. The greater the number of vibrations per unit of time, the higher the pitch and the more acute the tone.

Pragmatics - Functional use of language in context. It includes such factors as intention in communication; sensorimotor actions preceding, accompanying, and following the utterance; knowledge shared in the communicative dyad; and the elements in the environment surrounding the message.

Prosody - (1) Physical attributes of speech that signal linguistic qualities such as stress and intonation. It includes the fundamental frequency intensity of the voice, and the duration of the individual speech sounds. (2) A melody of speech determined primarily by modifications of pitch, quality, strength, and duration; perceived primarily as stress and intonational patterns.

Psychoacoustics - Combined disciplines of psychology and acoustics concerned with the study of man's response to sound.

Semantic - Component of grammar concerned with word meanings and meaningful sentences.

Syntactic - Component of grammar concerned with grammatically well formed structures.

3905.14 ACRONYMS AND ABBREVIATIONS.—

ADL - Activities of Daily Living.

ALPS - Aphasia Language Performance Scales.

ASHA - American-Speech-Language-Hearing Association.

ASL - American Sign Language.

CVC - Consonant-vowel-consonant.

CPS - Cycles per second. Former unit of measurement for the number of successive compressions and rarefactions of a sound wave within one second of time, now replaced with Hertz (Hz).

Dx - Diagnostic therapy.

MLU - Mean Length of Utterance - Average length of oral expressions as measured by a representative sampling of oral language. It is usually obtained by counting the number of morphemes per utterance and dividing by the number of utterances.

VOT - Voice Onset Time - (1) Time between the release of the stop consonant and the beginning of voicing in the vowel. (2) Time required to initiate sound at the vocal folds.

3905.15 SPEECH-LANGUAGE PATHOLOGY TESTS. — These tests include but are not limited to:

A. Widely Used Adult Language Tests.

Ammons Full Range Picture Vocabulary Test
Aphasia Clinical Battery I
Aphasia Language Performance Scales (ALPS)
Appraisal of Language Disturbances (ALD)
Boston Diagnostic Aphasia Examination (BDAE)
Communicative Abilities in Daily Living (CADL)
Examining for Aphasia
Functional Communication Profile
International Test for Aphasia

Language Modalities Test for Aphasia

Language Proficiency Test (LPT)

Minnesota Test for Differential Diagnosis of Aphasia

Porch Index of Communicative Abilities (PICA)

Revised Token Test

Sklar Aphasia Scale

Token Test for Receptive Disturbances in Aphasia

Hodson Phonological Process Analysis

Clinical Evaluation of Language Functions (CELF)

Western Aphasia Battery

B. Widely Used Adult Articulation Tests.

Apraxia Battery for Adults (ABA)

Assessment of Intelligibility of Dysarthric Speech

Compton-Hutton Phonological Assessment

Frenchay Dysarthria Test

The Fisher-Logemann Test of Articulation Competence

Iowa Pressure Articulation Test

Templin Darley Test of Articulation

C. Speech and Language Diagnostic Tests.—An initial assessment (including diagnostic testing, if clinically possible) must be performed prior to the commencement of treatment. If you need assistance in understanding tests used, consult your speech language pathologist consultant or the American Speech•Language•Hearing Association.

3905.16 OUTPATIENT SPEECH-LANGUAGE PATHOLOGY EDITS. – These edits do not represent normative (or average) treatment. Do not deny a bill solely on the basis that it exceeds the edits. The edits are for selecting bills for Level II MR.

A3 3904. MEDICAL REVIEW (MR) OF PART B INTERMEDIARY OPT BILLS

A. General.—These instructions specify the criteria for MR of OPT services. Use the edits listed in Exhibit 1 to assist you in conducting focused review within your budgeted levels. Conduct focused MR using other selection criteria which you determine to be effective. If you choose to use any of the diagnostic edits listed in Exhibit 1, do not change the visits and/or duration parameters without approval from CO. Conform to the MR requirements for all outpatient claims from rehabilitation agencies, SNFs, hospitals, and HHAs that provide OPT in addition to home health services (bill types, hospital-12 and 13, SNF-22 and 23, HHA-34, rehabilitation agency, public health agency or clinic-74 and CORF-75). These criteria do not apply to PT services provided under a home health plan of care.

The criteria for MR case selection are based on ICD-9-CM diagnoses, elapsed time from start of care (at the billing provider) and number of visits. See Exhibit 1. Do not deny a bill solely on the basis that it exceeds the criteria in these edits. The edits are only for assisting you to select bills for focused MR or for paying bills that meet Level I. Also, do not provide automatic coverage up to these criteria. They neither guarantee minimum coverage nor set maximum coverage limits.

B. Use of PT Edits (Exhibit 1) in Level I Review.—PT edits have been developed for a number of diagnoses. The diagnoses were selected on the basis that, when linked with a recent date of onset, there is a high probability that Medicare patients with those diagnoses will require skilled OPT. The edits do not specify every diagnosis which may require PT, and the fact that a given diagnosis does not appear in the edits does not create a presumption that OPT services are not necessary or are inappropriate. Do not approve or deny claims at Level I for reasons of medical necessity. Pay claims that suspend or pass the edits in Exhibit 1 without being subjected to Level II MR. However, refer all claims which meet your focused MR criteria to Level II MR.

For patients receiving other PT services (V57.1) only during an encounter/visit, list the appropriate V code for the service first, and, if documented, the diagnosis or problem for which the services are being performed second. Program your system to read the diagnosis or problem listed second to determine if it meets one of the Level I edits.

> EXAMPLE: Outpatient rehabilitation services, V57.1 (Other PT), for a patient with multiple sclerosis, 340. The V code is listed first, followed by the code for multiple sclerosis (V57.1, 340). Edit for multiple sclerosis not the V code.) Use this same procedure for V57.81 (Orthotic training), V57.89 (Other specified rehabilitation procedure), and V57.9 (Unspecified rehabilitation procedure).

Evaluate bills at Level I based upon each of the following:

- Facility and Patient Identification - (facility name, patient name, provider number, HICN, age).

- Diagnosis - List the primary diagnosis for which OPT services were furnished by ICD-9-CM code first. List other Dx(s) applicable to the patient or that influence care next.

- Duration - The total length of time OPT services have been rendered (in days) from the date treatment was initiated for the diagnosis being treated at the billing provider (including the last day in the current billing period).

- Number of Visits - The total number of patient visits completed since OPT services were initiated for the diagnosis being treated by the billing provider. Enter the total number of visits to date (including the last visit in the billing period) rather than for each separate billing (value code 50).

- Date Treatment Started (Occurrence Code 35) - The date OPT services were initiated by the billing provider for the primary PT Dx being treated.

- Billing Period - When OPT services began and ended in the billing period (from through dates).

C. Level II Review Process.—If a bill is selected for focused MR, refer it to the Level II health professional MR staff. If possible, have physical therapists review OPT bills.

Once the bill is selected for focused MR, review it in conjunction with medical information submitted by the provider. Use this criteria performing MR of OPT claims for the bill types identified in 3904.

1. Payable OPT Services.—Pay for OPT services only if they meet all requirements established by Medicare guidelines and regulations. Ensure that each bill for OPT services that is subjected to Level II or III MR is supported with adequate medical documentation for you to make a determination. The documentation must show that the requirements of 3101.8 and 3148, and in these instructions, are met.

2. MR and Documentation.—When a claim is referred to Level II MR, use the following pertinent data elements in addition to those used for Level I review:

- Medical History - Obtain only the medical history which is pertinent to, or influences the OPT treatment rendered, including a brief description of the functional status of the patient prior to the onset of the condition requiring OPT, and any pertinent prior PT treatment.

- Date of Onset (Occurrence Code 11) - The date of onset of the primary physical therapy diagnosis for which OPT services were being rendered by the billing provider.

- Physician Referral and Date

- PT Initial Evaluation and Date

- Plan of Treatment and Date Established

- Date of Last Certification - Obtain the date on which the plan of treatment was last certified by the physician.

- Progress Notes - Obtain updated patient status reports concerning the patient's current functional abilities/limitations.

Use the above information along with that in subsection B, to assess the appropriateness of the OPT plan of treatment and the patient's progress relative to diagnosis, date of onset, etc. The medical information supporting a bill must be specific. Documentation written in general terms, e.g, "strength appears to have increased" or "can now reach higher overhead" or "medical history-chronic arthritis" is insufficient. To make an informed MR decision request documentation from the provider when incomplete or inadequate documentation is present. The physician's pertinent evaluations, progress notes and opinions about the patient's need for rehabilitation services should also be used (when these are available). Obtain this information from the provider regardless of the document type the provider keeps (i.e., it does not matter whether the baseline evaluation is part of the treatment plan, the progress notes or the medical history, obtain and use this information).

3. Medical History.—If a history of previous OPT treatment is not available, the provider may provide a general summary regarding the patient's past relevent medical history recorded during the initial evaluation with the patient/family (if reliable) or through contact with the referring physician. Information regarding prior history and treatment by the referring physician must be provided when available.

The patient's medical history, as it relates to the OPT, must include the date of onset and/or exacerbation of the illness or injury. If the patient has had prior OPT for the same condition, use that history in conjunction with the patient's current assessment to establish whether additional treatment is reasonable.

The history of treatments from a previous provider is also necessary for patients who have transferred to a new provider for additional treatment. For example, if surgery has been performed, be aware of the type and date of surgery. The date of onset and type of surgical procedure should be specific for diagnoses such as fractured hip. For other diagnoses, such as arthritis, the date of onset may be general and can be established from the date the patient first required medical treatment. For other types of chronic diagnoses, the history must give the date of the change or deterioration in the patient's condition and a description of the changes that necessitate skilled OPT. For example, a patient that had an amputation several years ago might recently have been fitted with a new prosthesis.

4. Evaluation.—A PT initial evaluation, (excluding routine screening) should be approved when it is reasonable and necessary for the therapist to determine if there is an expectation that either restorative or maintenance services will be appropriate for the patient's condition. Approve reevaluations when the patient exhibits a demonstrable change in physical functional ability in order to reestablish appropriate treatment goals, or when required for ongoing assessment of the patient's rehabilitation needs. Initial evaluations or reevaluations that are determined reasonable and necessary based on the patient's condition, may be approved even though the expectations are not realized, or when the evaluation determines that skilled rehabilitation is not needed.

The PT evaluation establishes the baseline data necessary for assessing expected rehabilitation potential, setting realistic goals, and measuring progress. The evaluation of the patient's condition must form the basis for the physical therapy treatment goals.

The evaluation must (when possible) include objective tests and measurements which normally will include functional, strength, and range of motion (ROM) assessments. However, for patients with certain neurological conditions (such as upper motor neuron conditions) assessment of strength may not be valid. Where the above tests are not applicable, the physical therapist should document the patient's functional loss and the need for skilled OPT intervention resulting from conditions such as:

- Self-Care Dependence - The individual is dependent upon skilled assistance or supervision from another person in self-care activities. These activities include, but are not limited to, signficant functional loss or loss of previous functional gains in the ability to:

    — Drink;

    — Feed;

    — Dress; or

    — Maintain personal hygiene.

Additionally, this could include care of braces or other adaptive devices.

- Mobility Dependence - The individual is dependent upon another person for skilled OPT assistance or supervision in such areas as transfer, gait training, stair climbing, and wheelchair maneuvering activities due to, but not limited to:

    — Decreased strength;

    — Marked muscle spasticity;

    — Moderate to severe pain;

— Contractures;

— Incoordination;

— Perceptual motor loss;

— Orthotic need; or

— Need for ambulatory or mobility device.

This could involve patients with or without impairment of the lower leg who are partially independent with wheelchair and/or who have significant architectural or environmental barriers.

- Safety Dependence/Secondary Complications - A safety problem exists when a patient without skilled assistance cannot handle him/herself in a manner that is physically safe. This may extend to the performance of activities of daily living or to acquired secondary complications which could potentially intensify medical sequelae such as fracture nonunion, or decubiti. Some examples of safety dependence may be demonstrated by high probability of falling, swallowing difficulties, severe pain, loss of skin sensation, progressive joint contracture, and infection requiring skilled PT intervention to protect the patient from further complication.

Each patient's condition calls for assessments which are unique to specific impairments. For example, documentation in the treatment of open wounds or ulcerations require other objective and subjective documentation, such as size and depth of the wound, amount and frequency of drainage, signs of granulation, or evidence of infection, etc.

If the goal for any patient is to increase functional abilities, range of motion, or strength, the initial evaluation must measure (if possible) the patient's starting functional abilities, range of motion and strength. If the assessment indicates that joint range of motion or strength is normal, there should be evidence of this assessment in the initial evaluation or progress notes, e.g., "within normal limits." If objective documentation cannot be accomplished for any reason, this should be noted in the inital evaluation or progress notes along with the reason(s).

5. Plan of Treatment.—The PT plan of treatment must include specific functional goals and a reasonable estimate of when they will be reached (e.g., 6 weeks). It is not adequate to estimate "1 to 2 months on an ongoing basis." The plan of treatment must include specific modalities/procedures, frequency, and duration of treatment. Changes in the plan of treatment should be submitted with the progress notes.

The plan of treatment must contain the following information concerning the OPT treatment:

- Type of Modalities/Procedures - Should describe he specific nature of the therapy to be provided. Some examples of PT modalities/procedures are deep heat (e.g., diathermy, ultrasound), superficial heat (e.g., hot packs, whirlpool), and therapeutic exercises and gait training.

- Frequency of Visits - An estimate of the frequency of treatment to be rendered (e.g., 3x week).

- Estimated Duration - Identifies the length of time over which the services are to be rendered and may be expressed in days, weeks, or months.

- Diagnoses - Should include the OPT diagnosis if different from the medical diagnosis. For example, the medical diagnosis might be "rheumatoid arthritis." However, the shoulder might be the only area being treated, so the PT diagnosis might be "adhesive capsulitis." In order to establish the OPT diagnosis, diagnostic tests must be used whenever possible.

- Functional Goals - Should reflect the physical therapist's and/or physician's description of what the patient is expected to achieve as a result of therapy.

- Rehabilitation Potential - The therapist's and/or physician's expectation concerning the patient's ability to meet the goals at initiation of treatment.

6. Progress Reports (Status Summary(s) Related to the Billing Period). —The physical therapist must provide treatment information regarding the current status of the patient during the course of the billing period. The PT progress notes and any needed reevaluation(s) must update the baseline information provided at the initial evaluation. If there is a change in the plan of treatment, it must be documented in accordance with 3148.3. Additionally, when a patient is continued from one billing period to another, the progress report(s) must reflect comparison between the patient's current functional status and that obtained during the previous billing and/or at the initial evaluation.

Where a valid expectation of improvement exists at the time OPT services are initiated, or thereafter, reasonable and necessary services would be covered even though the expectation may not be realized. However, in such instances, the OPT services are covered only up to the point in time that no further significant functional improvement can be reasonably expected. Progress reports or status summaries by the physician and/or physical therapist must document a continued expectation that the patient's condition will continue to improve significantly in a reasonable and generally predictable period of time. "Significant," in this context, means a generally measurable and substantial increase in the patient's present level of physical functional abilities compared to their level at the time treatment was initiated.

Do not interpret the term "significant" so stringently that you deny a claim simply because of a temporary setback in the patient's progress. For example, a patient may experience a new intervening medical complication or a brief period when lack of progress occurs. The medical reviewer should approve the claim if the services are considered reasonable and necessary and if there is still a reasonable expectation that significant improvement in the patient's overall safety or functional ability will occur. However, the physical therapist and/or physician should document such lack of progress and briefly explain the need for continued skilled PT intervention.

MR of rehabilitation claims must be conducted with an understanding that skilled intervention may be needed, and improvement in a patient's condition may occur, even where a patient's full or partial recovery is not possible. For example, a terminally ill patient may begin to exhibit self care, mobility and/or safety dependence requiring PT services. The fact that full or partial recovery is not possible or rehabilitation potential is not present, must not affect MR coverage decisions. The deciding factor is always based on whether the services are considered reasonable, effective, treatment for the patient's condition and they require the skills of a physical therapist, or whether they can be safely and effectively carried out by nonskilled personnel, without physical therapy supervision. The reasons for physical therapy intervention must be clear to you, as well as their goals, prior to a coverage determination. These claims often require review at Level III.

It is essential that the physical therapist document the updated status in a clear, concise, and objective manner. Objective tests and measurements are stressed when these are practical. The physical therapist selects the appropriate method to demonstrate current patient status. However, the method chosen, as well as the measures used, should be consistent during the treatment duration. If the method used to demonstrate progress is changed or comparable measures are used; the reasons for the change should be documented, including how the new method relates to the old. You must have an overview of the purpose of treatment goals in order to compare the patient's current functional status to that in previous reporting periods.

While objective documentation often necessitates range of motion, strength, and other objective measurements; documentation of the patient's current functional status compared to previous reporting period(s) is of paramount importance. The deficits in functional ability should be clear.

Physical therapists must document functional improvements (or lack thereof) as a result of their treatments. Documentation of functional progress must be stated whenever possible in objective, measurable terms. The following illustrates these principles:

- Pain - Documentation describing the presence or absence of pain and its effect on the patient's functional abilities must be considered in MR decisions. A description of its intensity, type, changing pattern, and location at specific joint ranges of motion will materially aid correct MR decisions. Documentation should describe the limitations placed upon the patient's self care, mobility and/or safety, as well as the subjective progress made in the reduction of pain through treatment.

Transcutaneous electrical nerve stimulation (TENS) uses surface electrodes and electrical current to interrupt pain pathways and sensation of pain through peripheral nerves. Generally, it is covered on a trial basis for up to 1 month. Any trial period extending beyond 1 month must be documented as to reason and medical necessity. Approve such claims only when the documentation supports the need to assess the patient's suitability for continued treatment with TENS. When it is determined that TENS should be continued as therapy and the patient has been trained to use the stimulator, it is expected that the stimulator will be employed by the patient at home. Payment may be made under the prosthetic devices benefit for the TENS stimulator. Payment may not be approved for continued OPT treatments with TENS. (See Coverage Issues Manual 35-46 and 65-8.)

- Therapeutic Exercise - The objective documentation should support the skilled nature of the exercise program, and/or the need for design and establishment of a maintenance exercise program. The goals should be to increase functional abilities in self care, mobility or patient safety. Documentation should indicate the goals and type of exercise provided and the major muscle groups treated.

Approve claims when the therapeutic exercise, because of documented medical complications, the condition of the patient, or complexity of the exercise employed, must be rendered by, or under, the supervision of a physical therapist. For example, while passive and active assistive exercise may often be performed safely and effectively by non-skilled personnel, the presence of fracture nonunion, severe joint pain, or other medical or safety complications may warrant skilled PT intervention to render the service and/or to establish a safe maintenance program. In these cases, the complications and the skilled services they require, must be documented by physician orders and/or physical therapy notes. To make correct MR decisions, the patient's losses and/or dependencies in self care, mobility and safety must also be documented. The possibility of adverse effects from the improper performance of an otherwise unskilled service does not make it a skilled service unless there is documentation to support why skilled PT is needed for the patient's medical condition and/or safety.

Approve establishment and design of a maintenance exercise program to fit the patient's level of ADL, function, and any instructions supportive personnel and/or family members need to safely and effectively carry out the program. Reevaluation may be approved when reasonable and necessary to readjust the maintenance program to meet the changing needs of the patient. There must be adequate justification for readjusting a maintenance program, e.g., loss of previous functional gain.

- Cardiac Rehabilitation Exercise - PT is not covered when furnished in connection with cardiac rehabilitation exercise program services unless there also is a diagnosed noncardiac condition requiring it, e.g., where a patient who is recuperating from an acute phase of heart disease may have had a stroke which requires PT. (See Coverage Issues Manual 35-25.) While the cardiac rehabilitation exercise program may be considered by some a form of PT, it is a specialized program conducted and/or supervised by specially trained personnel whose services are formed under the direct supervision of a physician. Restrictions on PT coverage do not affect rules regarding coverage or noncoverage of such services when furnished in a hospital inpatient or outpatient setting.

- Gait Training - The documentation must support the need for skilled gait training to restore functional abilities (or to design and establish a safe maintenance program) which can reasonably be expected to improve the patient's ability to walk or walk more safely. Documentation should clarify the patient's gait deviation, current functional abilities and limitations, and/or safety dependence during gait. Documentation should identify the gait problem being treated, e.g., to correct a balance/incoordination and safety problem or a specific gait deviation, such as a Trendelenberg gait. The type of gait deviation requiring skilled intervention, the functional limitations in mobility, the patient's understanding or lack of understanding of the gait training, and the amount of assistance needed during training is needed to make correct review decisions. The documentation must differentiate skilled gait training rendered from assistive walking, when the patient is walking repetitiously and merely improving distance or endurance (assistive or nonassistive).

- Transfer Training - The documentation should describe the patient's functional limitations in transfer ability that warrant skilled PT intervention. Documentation should include the special transfer training needed and rendered, and any training needed by supportive personnel and/or family members to safely and effectively carry it out. Approve transfer training when the documentation supports a skilled need for evaluation, design and effective monitoring and instruction of the special transfer technique for safety and completion of the task.

Documentation that supports only repetitious carrying out of the transfer method, once established, and monitored for safety and completion of the task is noncovered care.

- Electrical Nerve Stimulation - Approve reasonable and necessary electrical stimulation to delay or prevent disuse atrophy, but only where the documentation indicates that the nerve supply (including brain, spinal cord and peripheral nerves) to the muscle is intact, and other nonneurological reasons for disuse are causing atrophy. (See Coverage Issues Manual 35-77.)

Electrotherapy for the treatment of facial nerve paralysis, e.g., Bell's palsy is not a covered service. (See Coverage Issues Manual 35-72.)

Approve functional electrical stimulation (FES) used to test the suitability for improving the patient's functional ability, e.g., stimulating the dorsiflexors of the ankle to reduce toe drag during the swing-through phase of gait. Documentation must indicate the patient's functional limitation.

- Biofeedback Therapy - Approve claims when the documentation indicates that biofeedback therapy is reasonable and necessary for the patient for muscle reeducation of specific muscle groups or for treating pathological muscle abnormalities of spasticity, incapacitating muscle spasm, or weakness.

Deny claims where the documentation supports treatment for ordinary muscle tension states or for psychosomatic conditions. (See Coverage Issues Manual 35-27.)

- Fabrication of Temporary Prostheses, Braces, and Splints - Approve reasonable and necessary fabrication of temporary prostheses, braces and splints, and any reasonable and necessary skilled training needed in their safe and effective use. The documentation must indicate the need for the device and training.

D. Certification and Recertification.—To meet Medicare guidelines, PT services must be certified and recertified by a physician. They must be furnished while the patient is under the care of a physician. The OPT services may be furnished under a written plan of treatment established by the physician or a qualified physical therapist providing them; however, if the plan is established by a physical therapist, it must be reviewed periodically by the physician.

The plan of care must be established (reduced to writing by either professional or the provider when it makes a written record of the oral orders) before treatment is begun. When OPT services are continued under the same plan of treatment for a period of time, the physician must certify at least every 30 days that there is a continuing need for them. Obtain the recertification at the time the plan of treatment is reviewed since the same 30 day interval is required for the plan's review. Any changes to the treatment plan established by a physical therapist must be in writing and signed by the physical therapist or by the attending physician. Recertifications must be signed by the physician who reviewed the plan of treatment. The physician may change a plan of treatment established by the physical therapist, but the physical therapist may not alter a plan of treatment established by a physician.

E. Physical Therapy Forms.—Documentation may be submitted on a specific form or copies of the provider's record. Require a specific form if you find it more efficient than using provider records; however, it must capture the MR information required by these instructions. If you choose to require one, show the OMB clearance number. The information must be complete. If it is not, request the missing information and return the bill for the additional information. The information you require to review the bill is that required by a physical therapist to properly treat a patient.

F. Evaluation of PT Edits.—Perform regular evaluations of provider utilization of PT services if you are using the HCFA edits to assist you in identifying PT claims for focused MR. Change your focused review claims selection based on the results of the evaluation. For example, a provider billing at an aberrantly consistent rate just below the edit parameters or providers billing aberrantly high utilization for specific diagnostic codes may be subject to focused review.

VIRGINIA COMMONWEALTH UNIVERSITY
Medical College of Virginia Hospitals
Richmond, Virginia 23298
REHABILITATION INTERDISCIPLINARY EVALUATION

DATE:_____   TIME:_____

OCCUPATIONAL THERAPY EVALUATION

DATE OF REFERRAL:_____
OCCUPATIONAL HISTORY EVALUATION:
FAMILY CONSTELLATION: Patient lives: [ ] alone [ ] with someone
[ ] Someone is home during day to assist patient   [ ] Someone is home evenings and nights to assist patient
[ ] Patient provides primary care for another person   Comments:_____
_____

HOME ACCESSIBILITY: Dwelling:[ ] house [ ]apartment   [ ] trailer   [ ] other:_____
Levels [ ] one   [ ] two   [ ] other:_____
Entrance: # of steps: Front:___   Back:___   Side:____   Handrails: Front: +/-   Back: +/-   Side: +/-
Interior Steps: + / - Number of steps:_____   Handrails: +/-
Utilities: [ ] electricity   [ ] plumbing   [ ] telephone:_____
Available DME:_____
_____

Other comments regarding accessibility:_____
_____

PRE-HOSPITALIZATION LIFE SKILL RESPONSIBILITIES:
(KEY: (-) = none (+) = partial (++) = full (n/a) = not applicable)

Meal Planning:	_____	Driving:	_____	Cleaning:	_____
Yardwork:	_____	Care of Others:	_____	Shopping:	_____
Money Management:	_____	Clothing Care:	_____	Household Maintenance:	_____
Pet Care:	_____	Other/ Comments:			

_____

WORK HISTORY:_____
_____

PATIENT'S ROUTINES/HABITS PRIOR TO ADMISSION:_____
_____

PATIENT'S INTERESTS/ VALUES:_____

PATIENT/FAMILY GOALS FOR REHABILITATION:
1._____
2._____
3._____

ACTIVITIES OF DAILY LIVING EVALUATION
(Key: FIM/FAM SCALE)
7 Complete Independence (timely and safely)   6 Modified Independence (extra time and/or device needed)   5 Supervision (cueing)
4 Minimal Assist (performs 75% or more of task)   3 Moderate Assist (performs 50-74% of task)
2 Maximal Assist (performs 25-49% of task)   1 Dependent (performs less than 25% of task)

FEEDING AND EATING:	Level	Comments:	DRESSING/ UNDRESSING:	Level	Comments:
Prepares all items on tray			t-shirt/ pull-over shirt		
Chews/swallows safely			shirt/blouse		
Eats prescribed diet			bra		
Appropriately uses utensils			underwear		
Brings food to mouth with precision			pants		
Drinks from cup or glass skillfully			socks/ shoes		
Eats/drinks neatly			fasteners		
Uses proper safety judgment			splints/slings		
Uses acceptable dining pragmatics					

DATE:_____ TIME:_____

OCCUPATIONAL THERAPY EVALUATION (continued)

GROOMING:

			BATHING:		
washes face/hands			washes upper extremities		
performs oral care			washes L.E.'s/ back		
combs/styles hair			washes hair		
shaves face			dries hair		
applies makeup			transfers to/from tub		
applies deodorant					

TOILETING ACTIVITIES:

			VOCATIONAL ACTIVITIES:		
performs toilet hygiene			recognizes area of skill/ interest		
adjusts clothing			makes vocational contact		
transfers to/from toilet					

FUNCTIONAL COMMUNICATION:

			HOME MANAGEMENT:		
writes name			performs clothing care		
writes shopping list			performs household cleaning		
manages telephone			plans meal		
uses phone book			prepares/ cleans up after meal		
turns pages/opens mail			performs survival cooking		
uses call bell/radio & tv control			demonstrates home safety		
does simple math			provides care for another		
performs money management			driving		

VISUAL-PERCEPTUAL-MOTOR SCREENING: [] not indicated [] screening complete; findings below:_____

_____
_____
_____

FUNCTIONAL COGNITIVE SCREENING: [] not indicated [] screening complete; findings below:_____

_____
_____
_____

ASSESSMENT OF PERFORMANCE IN ADL' S AND POTENTIAL FOR IMPROVEMENT:_____

_____
_____
_____
_____
_____

LONG TERM GOALS:
1) Patient will perform self care at _____ level of function.
2) Patient will perform advanced living skills at _____ level of function.
3) Patient /family will complete training/education/ preparations for discharge from hospital.
SHORT TERM GOALS:

_____
_____
_____
_____

TREATMENT PLAN: Projected frequency of treatment:_____
[ ] Individual Treatment   [ ] Dressing Program   [ ] Cognitive Group   [ ] Reality Orientation Group   [ ] Feeding Program
[ ] Interdisciplinary Group   [ ] Social Skills Group   [ ] Cooking Group   [ ] Craft Group   [ ] Breakfast Group
[ ] Grocery Shopping Grp   [ ] Patient/Family Education   [ ] Other:_____

         Occupational Therapist:_____

         Others Contributing to Evaluation:_____

DATE:_____ TIME:_____

VISUAL-PERCEPTUAL-MOTOR EVALUATION

EVALUATIONS ADMINISTERED:
[ ] SANTA CLARA PERCEPTUAL MOTOR EVALUATION FOR ADULTS

[ ] LOWENSTEIN OCCUPATIONAL THERAPY COGNITIVE ASSESSMENT

[ ] CLINICAL VISION ASSESSMENT

[ ] VISUAL SCREENING

[ ] FUNCTIONAL TASK ANALYSIS

[ ] BEHAVIORAL HEMI-INATTENTION TEST

[ ] OTHER:_____

VISUAL FUNCTION:
[ ] WEARS GLASSES   [ ] HAS GLASSES AT HOSPITAL

TYPE OF GLASSES:_____

PATIENT'S REPORT OF VISUAL FUNCTION/ VISUAL CHANGES:_____

_____

CLINICAL OBSERVATIONS OF VISUAL FUNCTION:_____

_____

VISUAL ACUITY: [] WNL [] IMPAIRED:_____

_____

PERIPHERAL VISION: [] WNL [] IMPAIRED:_____

_____

OCULOMOTOR FUNCTION: [] WNL [] IMPAIRED:_____

_____

OTHER COMMENTS:_____

_____

_____

(continued on next page)

DATE:_____ TIME:_____

VISUAL-PERCEPTUAL-MOTOR EVALUATION (continued)

VISUAL-PERCEPTUAL-MOTOR FUNCTION:

PRAXIS/MOTOR PLANNING: [] WNL [] IMPAIRED:_____

CONSTRUCTIONAL PRAXIS: [] WNL [] IMPAIRED:_____
_____

BODY SCHEME: [] WNL [] IMPAIRED:_____

DEPTH PERCEPTION: [] WNL [] IMPAIRED:_____

FORM PERCEPTION: [] WNL [] IMPAIRED:_____

SIZE DISCRIMINATION: [] WNL [] IMPAIRED:_____

FIGURE-GROUND PERCEPTION: [] WNL [] IMPAIRED:_____

RIGHT/LEFT DISCRIMINATION: [] WNL [] IMPAIRED:_____

FORM CONSTANCY: [] WNL [] IMPAIRED:_____

PART/WHOLE INTEGRATION: [] WNL []IMPAIRED:_____
POSITION-IN-SPACE: [] WNL [] IMPAIRED:_____

SPATIAL RELATIONS: [] WNL [] IMPAIRED:_____

SPATIAL AWARENESS [] WNL [] IMPAIRED: _____
OTHER/COMMENTS:_____
_____

ASSESSMENT OF VISUAL-PERCEPTUAL-FUNCTION AND PROGNOSIS:_____
_____
_____
_____

RECOMMENDATIONS:_____
_____
_____

OCCUPATIONAL THERAPIST_____

OTHERS CONTRIBUTING TO EVALUATION:_____ ___

	VIRGINIA COMMONWEALTH UNIVERSITY
	Medical College of Virginia Hospitals
	Richmond, Virginia 23298
	REHABILITATION INTERDISCIPLINARY EVALUATION

DATE:_____   TIME:_____

PHYSICAL THERAPY/OCCUPATIONAL THERAPY
SENSORI-MOTOR EVALUATION

	INITIALS
MENTAL STATUS DURING EVALUATION:	

	INITIALS
TONE/REFLEXES:	
HEAD/NECK:	
UPPER LIMBS:	
LOWER LIMBS:	

	INITIALS
PAIN:	

	INITIALS
ORTHOPEDIC DEVICES/ PRECAUTIONS	
SKIN INTEGRITY/CONDITION	
[ ]W/C CUSHION ISSUED:	

		INITIALS
RESPIRATORY/PULMONARY FUNCTION:		
RESPIRATION RATE AT REST:		
SUPPLEMENTAL 02	[ ] NO [ ] YES	
WHEN:		
COMPLAINTS OF SOB:	[ ] NO [ ] YES	
EXERTIONAL DYSPNEA:	[ ] NO [ ] YES	
FUNCTIONAL/PRODUCTIVE COUGH:	[ ] NO [ ] YES	
OTHER:		
RESPIRATORY PRECAUTIONS:		

	INITIALS:
CARDIOVASCULAR FUNCTION:	
RESTING HEART RATE:	
RESTING BP:	
RESPONSE TO EXERCISE:	
CARDIAC PRECAUTIONS:	

(continued on next page)

DATE:_____   TIME:_____

PHYSICAL THERAPY/OCCUPATIONAL THERAPY SENSORI-MOTOR EVALUATION (continued)

Physical Therapy measurements in shaded areas
Occupational Therapy measurements in unshaded areas.

UPPER EXTREMITY RANGE OF MOTION :

(NRML ROM)	LEFT UE		RIGHT UE		COMMENTS:
	A	P	A	P	
SHOULDER FLEXION (0-180)					
SHOULDER ABDUCTION (0-180)					
SHOULDER EXT. ROTATION (0-90)					
SHOULDER INT. ROTATION (0-70)					
ELBOW FLEX/EXTENSION (0-160)					
PRONATION (0-90)					
SUPINATION (0-90)					
WRIST EXTENSION (0-70)					
WRIST FLEXION (0-80)					
THUMB					
FINGERS					

LOWER EXTREMITY RANGE OF MOTION:

(NRML ROM)	LEFT LE		RIGHT LE		COMMENTS:
	A	P	A	P	
HIP EXTENSION (0-30)					
HIP FLEXION (1-150)					
HIP ABDUCTION (0-40)					
HIP ADDUCTION (0-35)					
HIP EXT. ROTATION (0-45)					
HIP INT. ROTATION (0-45)					
KNEE EXT/FLEX (0-135)					
SLR					
ANKLE DORSIFLEX (SOLEUS) - KNEE FLEXED					
ANKLE DORSIFLEX - KNEE EXTENDED					
ANKLE PLANTARFLEX (0-50)					

COMMENTS: _____

_____

_____

(continued on next page)

DATE:_____   TIME:_____

PHYSICAL THERAPY/OCCUPATIONAL THERAPY SENSORI-MOTOR EVALUATION (continued)

Physical Therapy measurements in shaded area
Occupational Therapy measurements in unshaded area

UPPER EXTREMITY MUSCLE STRENGTH :

KEY: 5   Normal   4   Good   3   Fair
        2   Poor   1   Trace   0   Zero

	LEFT UE	RIGHT UE	COMMENTS:
SHOULDER FLEXION			
SHOULDER ABDUCTION			
SHOULDER EXT ROTATION			
SHOULDER INT ROTATION			
ELBOW FLEXION			
ELBOW EXTENSION			
SUPINATION			
PRONATION			
WRIST FLEXION			
WRIST EXTENSION			

HAND AND FINGER FUNCTION:

	LEFT UE	RIGHT UE	COMMENTS:
DOMINANCE			
GRIP			
PINCH			

LOWER EXTREMITY MUSCLE STRENGTH:

KEY: 5   Normal   4   Good   3   Fair
        2   Poor   1   Trace   0   Zero

	LEFT LE	RIGHT LE	COMMENTS:
HIP FLEXION			
HIP EXTENSION			
HIP ABDUCTION			
HIP EXT. ROTATION			
HIP INT. ROTATION			
KNEE FLEXION			
KNEE EXTENSION			
ANKLE DORSIFLEXION			
ANKLE PLANTARFLEXION			

(continued on next page)

DATE:_____ TIME:_____

PHYSICAL THERAPY/OCCUPATIONAL THERAPY SENSORI-MOTOR EVALUATION (continued)

QUALITY OF U.E. MOVEMENT:(synergy patterns, ataxia, dysmetria, tremor, rigidity. etc)

_____

_____

_____

_____ INITIALS:

QUALITY OF L.E. MOVEMENT:(synergy patterns, ataxia, dysmetria, tremor, rigidity. etc)

_____

_____

_____

_____ INITIALS:

SENSATION:

KEY:
WNL = NORMAL   IMP = IMPAIRED   ABS = ABSENT   UNK = UNABLE TO TEST   N/T = NOT TESTED

	SHARP/DULL	LIGHT TOUCH	TEMP	PROPRIO-CEPTION	STEREO-GNOSIS	COMMENTS:
RT UE						
LT UE						
RIGHT HAND						
LEFT HAND						
TRUNK						INITIALS:
RT LE						
LT LE						
RT FOOT						
LT FOOT						INITIALS:

COMMENT:_____INITIALS:_____

PHYSICAL THERAPIST_____

OCCUPATIONAL THERAPIST:_____

OTHERS CONTRIBUTING TO EVALUATION:_____

<table>
<tr><td colspan="2"></td><td>Medical College of Virginia Hospitals
VIRGINIA COMMONWEALTH UNIVERSITY
Richmond, Virginia 23298
Rehabilitation Occupational Therapy
REEVALUATION NOTE</td></tr>
</table>

PATIENT INFORMATION STAMP (Stamp patient plate-front and back   Page 1 of 3 pages

DATE	TIME	NOTES
		Rehabilitation Occupational Therapy Reevaluation Note:
		S:
		O: Pt. was seen this week for reevaluation/treatment including:

Date							
Consult/Screen							
Eval/Re-evaluation							
Treatment							
Group Treatment							
Splints/Aids							
Missed Treatment							

☐ Reevaluation completed

   Please see for long and short term goals.

☐ O.T./P.T. have conferred on proper w/chair and cushion for this patient,
   and these items have been loaned to the patient:

☐ Skin Integrity Issues Noted   ☐ yes   ☐ No

Referral Date: Reeval Dates:

Diagnosis: Physician:

Relevant Medical History:

Noted Precautions:

		Medical College of Virginia Hospitals
		VIRGINIA COMMONWEALTH UNIVERSITY
		Richmond, Virginia 23298
		Rehabilitation Occupational Therapy
		REEVALUATION NOTE

PATIENT INFORMATION STAMP (Stamp patient plate-front and back

DATE	TIME	NOTES		
		ACTIVITIES OF DAILY LIVING: FIMs	Comments:	
		Feeding		
		Dressing/Undressing		
		Grooming		
		Bathing		
		Toileting		
		Functional Communication		
		Functional Mobility		
		Home Management		
		Vocational Activities		
		SENSORY MOTOR SKILLS :		
		LUE		RUE
			Upper Extremity Range of Motion	
			Upper Extremity Strength	
			Grip/Pinch	
			Coordination	
			Sensation	
		Comments of Upper Extremity Function:		
		VISUAL/PERCEPTUAL :	[] WNL, testing not indicated	
			[] Impaired, same as on previous admission	
			[] testing indicated, scheduled and results to follow	
		COGNITION:	[] WNL, testing not indicated	
			[] Impaired, same as on previous admission	
			[] testing indicated, scheduled and results to follow	

| | | Medical College of Virginia Hospitals
VIRGINIA COMMONWEALTH UNIVERSITY
Richmond, Virginia 23298
Rehabilitation Occupational Therapy
REEVALUATION NOTE |

PATIENT INFORMATION STAMP (Stamp patient plate-front and back

DATE	TIME	NOTES
		A: GENERAL IMPRESSIONS AND RECOMMENDATIONS:
		LONG TERM GOALS:
		Patient will perform activities of daily living to a level of:
		Patient will perform work skills to a level of:
		Patient and/or family will complete preparations to permit discharge from hospital
		setting.
		SHORT TERM GOALS:
		P:PLAN: Patient will be seen times daily to accomplish goals.

_____   _____

DATE   **OCCUPATIONAL THERAPIST**

<table>
<tr><td colspan="2"></td><td>Medical College of Virginia Hospitals
VIRGINIA COMMONWEALTH UNIVERSITY
Richmond, Virginia 23298
Rehabilitation Occupational Therapy
PATIENT PROGRESS NOTE</td></tr>
</table>

| PATIENT INFORMATION STAMP (Stamp patient plate-front and back | | Page ___ of ___ pages |

DATE	TIME	NOTES

		Medical College of Virginia Hospitals
		VIRGINIA COMMONWEALTH UNIVERSITY
		Richmond, Virginia 23298
		Rehabilitation Occupational Therapy
		PATIENT PROGRESS NOTE

PATIENT INFORMATION STAMP (Stamp patient plate-front and back   Page 1 of 2 pages

DATE	TIME	NOTES							
		Rehabilitation Occupational Therapy Progress Note:							
	S:								
	O:	Pt. was seen this week for treatment including:							
		Date							
		Consult/Screen							
		Eval/Re-evaluation							
		Treatment							
		Group Treatment							
		Splints/Aids							
		Missed Treatment							

Goal is:

Met	Not Met	Progress toward last week's goals:	Con't.	D/Ced	Modfd
		Summary of Functional Status:			

		Medical College of Virginia Hospitals
		VIRGINIA COMMONWEALTH UNIVERSITY
		Richmond, Virginia 23298
		Rehabilitation Occupational Therapy
		PATIENT PROGRESS NOTE

PATIENT INFORMATION STAMP (Stamp patient plate-front and back   Page 2 of 2 pages

DATE	TIME	*Rehabilitation Occupational Therapy Progress Note Continued:*
		Summary of Discharge Planning Issues:
	A:	Assessment and Recommendations:
	P:	Plan is to follow patient times daily to address the following STGs.:

Rehabilitation Occupational Therapy Progress Note Continued on the next page(s): +/–

DATE:_____ TIME: _____

OCCUPATIONAL THERAPY DISCHARGE SUMMARY

DATE OF ADMISSION TO MCVH/RRC: _____

DATE OF DISCHARGE FROM MCVH/RRC: _____

SUMMARY OF REHABILITATION COURSE: _____

_____

_____

_____

ACTIVITIES OF DAILY LIVING:

KEY:
7 = Complete Independence (timely and safely)   6 = Mod. Independence (extra time and /or device needed)   5 = Supervision (cueing)
4 = Minimal Assist (completes 75% of task)   3 = Moderate Assist (completes 50-74% of task)
2 = Maximal Assist (completes 25-49& of task)   1 = Dependent (completes less than 25% of task)

PERFORMANCE AREA	INITIAL	D/C	COMMENTS
Feeding			
Grooming			
UE Dressing			
LE Dressing			
Bathing			
Toileting			
Tub Transfers			
Toilet Transfers			

SUMMARY OF CURRENT FUNCTIONAL STATUS: _____

_____

_____

_____

AREAS OF CONTINUED IMPAIRMENT:

KEY: CHECK MARK INDICATES CURRENT AREA OF IMPAIRMENT

[_] Basic Self Care _____

[_] Instrumental ADL's _____

[_] Functional Mobility _____

[_] Functional Communication _____

[_] Visual-Perceptual-Motor Function _____

[_] Functional Cognition _____

CURRENT SAFETY ISSUES/ PRECAUTIONS:

KEY: CHECK MARK INDICATES CURRENT AREA OF SAFETY CONCERN

[_] Fall risk _____

[_] Supervision needed _____

[_] Dietary precautions _____

[_] Operation of motor vehicle _____

[_] Other _____

Comments: _____

_____

_____

(continued on next page)

DATE:_____ TIME: _____

OCCUPATIONAL THERAPY DISCHARGE SUMMARY(continued)

DISCHARGE PREPARATION:

IF RESPONSE IS "NO", EXPLANATION IS OFFERED IN SPACES PROVIDED

Caregiver training was provided for therapeutic leave: [ ] YES [ ] NO_____

Caregiver training was provided for discharge: [ ] YES [ ] NO _____

Caregiver/ patient training provided in the following areas: [ ] ADL's [ ] Transfers [ ] Safety issues
[ ] other: _____

Therapeutic leave was granted: [ ] YES [ ] NO _____

Home evaluation was conducted: [ ] YES [ ] NO _____

DME evaluation was conducted & equipment prescribed: [ ] YES [ ] NO _____

DME prescribed was procured/ will be procured by family: [ ] YES [ ] NO _____

Home program was designed and provided: [ ] YES [ ] NO _____
Discharge information form was completed: [ ] YES [ ] NO _____

LONG TERM GOAL ACHIEVEMENT:

1. Patient will perform self care at the _____ level of function.   Achieved   Not Achieved
2. Patient will perform advanced living skills at the _____ level of function.   Achieved   Not Achieved
3. Patient/family will complete training/education/ preparation for discharge from hospital. Achieved   Not Achieved
Comments: _____

_____

ASSESSMENT:_____

_____

PLAN: Discharge patient to day rehab/ outpatient OT/ home health / other:_____

FOLLOW-UP RECOMMENDATIONS: _____

_____

Occupational Therapist:_____
Phone Number: _____

THE INSTITUTE OF LIVING
Hartford Hospital's Mental Health Network

Department of Rehabilitation Services
OCCUPATIONAL THERAPY
INITIAL GERIATRIC EVALUATION SUMMARY

1. ASSESSMENT TOOL:

☐ Interview   ☐ Allen Cognitive Level   ☐ Family/Caregiver Interview

☐ Chart Review   ☐ Functional Task

2. ALLEN COGNITIVE LEVEL

☐ ACL 3 Attention focused on repetitive motor actions, not goal directed, unaware of end product.

☐ ACL 4 Needs assistance with tasks requiring new learning. Unable to self-correct errors.

☐ ACL 5 Uses trial and error problem-solving. Needs assistance with planning. Unable to anticipate potential problems

☐ ACL 6 Able to pre-plan, initiate and sustain tasks.

3. PERFORMANCE CONTEXTS

a) Pre-hospitalization environment_____

b) Recent Loss_____

c) Physical Limitations_____

d) Recent Changes In Routine_____

e) Other_____

4. PERFORMANCE COMPONENTS/COGNITIVE SKILLS

MODERATE ASSIST: Not goal directed, errors are not recognized
MINIMAL ASSIST: Errors are recognized, but not independently corrected
STANDBY ASSIST: Uses trial and error problem solving
INDEPENDENT: Pre-plan, initiate and sustain tasks

PERFORMANCE AREA	MODERATE ASSIST	MINIMAL ASSIST	STANDBY ASSIST	INDEPENDENT	UNABLE TO ASSESS
Safety Procedures					
Leisure Performance					
Attention Span					
Problem Solving					
Self-Concept					
Interpersonal Skills					
Coping Skills					
Time Management					
Self Control					

5. Strengths: _____
_____
_____

6. Leisure Interests:

Past: _____
_____

Present: _____
_____

7. Comments: _____
_____
_____

TREATMENT RECOMMENDATIONS	MODALITY/GROUP
☐ Monitor and assess cognitive level	
☐ Develop and maintain involvement in physical activity	
☐ Facilitate and develop socialization/interpersonal skills	
☐ Provide success oriented activities to enhance self concept	
☐ Develop and reinforce the pursuit of leisure interests and skills	
☐ Develop and utilize appropriate coping skills	
☐ Encourage increased activity level and/or arousal	
☐ Provide an outlet for appropriate expression of feelings	
☐ Provide feedback to encourage self control	
☐ Recommend Physical Therapy consultation	
☐ Recommend Life Skills evaluation	
☐ Other	

SEE MTP FOR GOALS AND INTERVENTIONS

☐ Treatment Plan Discussed With Patient

Patient education to include:

☐ coping skills   ☐ safety procedures

☐ time management   ☐ interpersonal skills

☐ other:_____   ☐ other:_____

_____   _____
Occupational Therapist Signature   Date

THE INSTITUTE OF LIVING
Hartford Hospital's Mental Health Network

Department of Rehabilitation Services
OCCUPATIONAL THERAPY
ADULT EVALUATION SUMMARY

1. ASSESSMENT TOOL:

☐ Interview   ☐ Allen Cognitive Level   ☐ Other _____
☐ Chart Review   ☐ Functional Task

2. ALLEN COGNITIVE LEVEL

☐ ACL 3 - Attention focused on repetitive motor actions, not goal directed, unaware of end product.

☐ ACL 4 - Needs assistance with tasks requiring new learning. Unable to self-correct errors.

☐ ACL 5 - Uses trial and error problem-solving. Needs assistance with planning. Unable to anticipate potential problems.

☐ ACL 6 - Able to pre-plan, initiate and sustain tasks.

3. PERFORMANCE CONTEXTS:

Living Situation _____

Vocational Status _____

Social Supports _____

Physical Limitations _____

Other _____

4. PERFORMANCE COMPONENTS/COGNITIVE SKILLS

MODERATE ASSIST: Not goal directed, errors are not recognized
MINIMAL ASSIST: Errors are recognized, but not independently corrected
STANDBY ASSIST: Uses trial and error problem solving
INDEPENDENT: Pre-plan, initiate and sustain tasks

PERFORMANCE AREA	MODERATE ASSIST	MINIMAL ASSIST	STANDBY ASSIST	INDEPENDENT	UNABLE TO ASSESS
Safety Procedures					
Leisure Performance					
Attention Span					
Problem Solving					
Self-Concept					
Interpersonal Skills					
Coping Skills					
Time Management					
Self Control					

H DEPT JOBS ADLTEVAL.doc (5) 11-96

5. STRENGTHS _____

_____

_____

6. LEISURE INTERESTS: _____

_____

_____

7. COMMENTS _____

_____

_____

TREATMENT RECOMMENDATIONS   **MODALITY/GROUP**

☐ Encourage increased activity level or arousal _____

☐ Improve concentration and attention _____

☐ Provide feedback to encourage development of self control _____

☐ Monitor and assess cognitive function _____

☐ Evaluate/enhance ability to perform valued life roles. _____

☐ Enhance, maintain and develop interpersonal/communication skills. _____

☐ Increase awareness of assertive behavior and assertiveness skills. _____

☐ Enhance and develop stress management skills. _____

☐ Recommend further assessment _____

☐ Other _____

Occupational Therapy Treatment Recommendations discussed with patient ☐ yes ☐ no

SEE MTP FOR GOALS AND INTERVENTIONS

PATIENT EDUCATION TO INCLUDE:

☐ coping skills _____   ☐ safety procedures_____
☐ time management_____   ☐ interpersonal skills_____
☐ other: _____   ☐ other: _____

_____   _____
Occupational Therapist Signature   Date

HH DEPT JOBS ADLTEVAL.doc side 2 (5) 11-96

The Institute of Living
Hartford Hospital's Mental Health Network

DEPARTMENT OF REHABILITATION SERVICES
OCCUPATIONAL THERAPY PROGRESS NOTE

_____WEEKLY _____BI-WEEKLY _____ MONTHLY

MODERATE ASSIST: Constant cognitive assistance such as intermittant 1:1 demonstrations or physical or verbal cuing are needed to sustain and complete simple, repetitive tasks safely.

MINIMAL ASSIST: Periodic cognitive assistance is needed to correct repeated mistakes, check for safety compliance, or solve problems presented by unexpected hazards.

STANDBY ASSIST: Supervision by one person is needed to perform new procedure adapted by practioner for safe and effective performance. Does not use safety precautions and demonstrates errors in performance.

INDEPENDENT: No assistance is needed.

PERFORMANCE AREA	MODERATE ASSIST	MINIMAL ASSIST	STANDBY ASSIST	INDEPENDENT	NOT OBSERVED
SAFETY PROCEDURES					
LEISURE PERFORMANCE					
ATTENTION SPAN					
INITIATION OF ACTIVITY					
MEMORY					
SEQUENCING					
PROBLEM SOLVING					
INTERPERSONAL SKILLS					
COPING SKILLS					
TIME MANAGEMENT					
SELF CONTROL					

EVALUATION OF PROGRESS IN MEETING TREATMENT GOALS:

1. MTP PROBLEM #_____
   - ☐ ACHIEVED SHORT TERM GOAL (S)
   - ☐ PARTIALLY ACHIEVED SHORT TERM GOAL(S)
   - ☐ REFUSED TO WORK ON SHORT TERM GOAL(S)
   - ☐ DID NOT ACHIEVE SHORT TERM GOAL(S)
   - ☐ NEW SHORT TERM GOAL DEVELOPED (MTP UPDATED)

2. MTP PROBLEM #_____
   - ☐ ACHIEVED SHORT TERM GOAL(S)
   - ☐ PARTIALLY ACHIEVED SHORT TERM GOAL(S)
   - ☐ REFUSED TO WORK ON SHORT TERM GOAL(S)
   - ☐ DID NOT ACHIEVE SHORT TERM GOAL(S)
   - ☐ NEW SHORT TERM GOAL DEVELOPED (MTP UPDATED)

EDUCATION: THE PATIENT WAS INSTRUCTED IN:
- ☐ COMMUNITY RESOURCE_____
- ☐ NEW ACTIVITY/SKILL_____
- ☐ OTHER_____

- ☐ COGNITIVE STRATEGY_____
- ☐ COPING STRATEGY_____
- ☐ SAFETY TECHNIQUES_____
- ☐ OTHER_____

COMMENTS
_____
_____
_____
_____
_____
_____

SEE INDIVIDUAL GROUP ATTENDANCE SHEET FOR GROUPS ATTENDED

_____
OCCUPATIONAL THERAPIST SIGNATURE

DATE

HH FORMS **573149**.doc 2-97

The Institute of Living
Hartford Hospital's Mental Health Network

DEPARTMENT OF REHABILITATION SERVICES
OCCUPATIONAL THERAPY PROGRESS NOTE

_____WEEKLY _____BI-WEEKLY _____ MONTHLY

MODERATE ASSIST: Constant cognitive assistance such as intermittant 1:1 demonstrations or physical or verbal cuing are needed to sustain and complete simple, repetitive tasks safely.

MINIMAL ASSIST: Periodic cognitive assistance is needed to correct repeated mistakes, check for safety compliance, or solve problems presented by unexpected hazards.

STANDBY ASSIST: Supervision by one person is needed to perform new procedure adapted by practioner for safe and effective performance. Does not use safety precautions and demonstrates errors in performance.

INDEPENDENT: No assistance is needed.

PERFORMANCE AREA	MODERATE ASSIST	MINIMAL ASSIST	STANDBY ASSIST	INDEPENDENT	NOT OBSERVED
SAFETY PROCEDURES					
LEISURE PERFORMANCE					
ATTENTION SPAN					
INITIATION OF ACTIVITY					
MEMORY					
SEQUENCING					
PROBLEM SOLVING					
INTERPERSONAL SKILLS					
COPING SKILLS					
TIME MANAGEMENT					
SELF CONTROL					

EVALUATION OF PROGRESS IN MEETING TREATMENT GOALS:

1. MTP PROBLEM #_____
- ☐ ACHIEVED SHORT TERM GOAL (S)
- ☐ PARTIALLY ACHIEVED SHORT TERM GOAL(S)
- ☐ REFUSED TO WORK ON SHORT TERM GOAL(S)
- ☐ DID NOT ACHIEVE SHORT TERM GOAL(S)
- ☐ NEW SHORT TERM GOAL DEVELOPED (MTP UPDATED)

2. MTP PROBLEM #_____
- ☐ ACHIEVED SHORT TERM GOAL(S)
- ☐ PARTIALLY ACHIEVED SHORT TERM GOAL(S)
- ☐ REFUSED TO WORK ON SHORT TERM GOAL(S)
- ☐ DID NOT ACHIEVE SHORT TERM GOAL(S)
- ☐ NEW SHORT TERM GOAL DEVELOPED (MTP UPDATED)

EDUCATION: THE PATIENT WAS INSTRUCTED IN:
- ☐ COMMUNITY RESOURCE_____
- ☐ NEW ACTIVITY/SKILL_____
- ☐ OTHER_____

- ☐ COGNITIVE STRATEGY_____
- ☐ COPING STRATEGY_____
- ☐ SAFETY TECHNIQUES_____
- ☐ OTHER_____

COMMENTS
_____
_____
_____
_____
_____
_____

SEE INDIVIDUAL GROUP ATTENDANCE SHEET FOR GROUPS ATTENDED

_____

OCCUPATIONAL THERAPIST SIGNATURE   *DATE*

HH FORMS **573149**.doc 2-97

Uniform Terminology for Occupational Therapy— Third Edition

This is an official document of The American Occupational Therapy Association. This document is intended to provide a generic outline of the domain of concern of occupational therapy and is designed to create common terminology for the profession and to capture the essence of occupational therapy succinctly for others.

It is recognized that the phenomena that constitute the profession's domain of concern can be categorized, and labeled, in a number of different ways. This document is not meant to limit those in the field, formulating theories or frames of reference, who may wish to combine or refine particular constructs. It is also not meant to limit those who would like to conceptualize the profession's domain of concern in a different manner.

Introduction

The first edition of Uniform Terminology was approved and published in 1979 (AOTA, 1979). In 1989, *Uniform Terminology for Occupational Therapy—Second Edition* (AOTA, 1989) was approved and published. The second document presented an organized structure for understanding the areas of practice for the profession of occupational therapy. The document outlined two domains. **Performance areas** (activities of daily living [ADL], work and productive activities, and play or leisure) include activities that the occupational therapy practitioner emphasizes when determining functional abilities (*occupational therapy practitioner* refers to both registered occupational therapists and certified occupational therapy assistants). **Performance components** (sensorimotor, cognitive, psychosocial, and psychological aspects) are the elements of performance that occupational therapists assess and, when needed, in which they intervene for improved performance.

This third edition has been further expanded to reflect current practice and to incorporate contextual aspects of performance. **Performance areas**, **performance components**, and **performance contexts** are the parameters of occupational therapy's domain of concern. *Performance areas* are broad categories of human activity that are typically part of daily life. They are activities of daily living, work and productive activities, and play or leisure activities. *Performance components* are fundamental human abilities that—to varying degrees and in differing combinations—are required for successful engagement in performance areas. These components are sensorimotor, cognitive, psychosocial, and psychological. *Performance contexts* are situations or factors that influence an individual's engagement in desired and/or required performance areas. Performance contexts consist of *temporal* aspects (chronological age, developmental age, place in the life cycle, and health status) and *environmental* aspects (physical, social, and cultural considerations). There is an interactive relationship among performance areas, performance components, and performance contexts. Function in performance areas is the ultimate concern of occupational therapy, with performance components considered as they relate to participation in performance areas. Performance areas and performance components are always viewed within performance contexts. Performance contexts are taken into consideration when determining function and dysfunction relative to performance areas and performance components, and in planning intervention. For example, the occupational therapist does not evaluate strength (a performance component) in isolation. Strength is considered as it affects necessary or desired tasks (performance areas). If the individual is interested in homemaking, the occupational therapy practitioner would consider the interaction of strength with homemaking tasks. Strengthening could be addressed through kitchen activities, such as cooking and putting groceries away. In some cases, the practitioner would employ an adaptive approach and recommend that the family switch from heavy stoneware to lighter-weight dishes, or use lighter-weight pots on the stove to enable the individual to make dinner safely without becoming fatigued or compromising safety.

Occupational therapy assessment involves examining performance areas, performance components, and performance contexts. Intervention may be directed toward elements of performance areas (e.g., dressing, vocational exploration), performance components (e.g., endurance, problem solving), or the environmental aspects of performance contexts. In the latter case, the physical and/or social environment may be altered or augmented to improve and/or maintain function. After identifying the performance areas the individual wishes or needs to address, the occupational therapist assesses the features of the environments in which the tasks will be performed. If an individual's job requires cooking in a restaurant as opposed to leisure cooking at home, the occupational therapy practitioner faces several challenges to enable the individual's success in different environments. Therefore, the third critical aspect of performance is the performance context, the features of the environment that affect the person's ability to engage in functional activities.

This document categorizes specific activities in each of the performance areas (ADL, work and productive activities, play or leisure). This categorization is based on what is considered "typical," and is not meant to imply that a particular individual characterizes personal activities in the same manner as someone else. Occupational therapy practitioners embrace individual differences, and so would document the unique pattern of the individual being served, rather than forcing the "typical" pattern on him or her and family. For example, because of experience or culture, a particular individual might think of home management as an ADL task rather than "work and productive activities" (current listing). Socialization might be considered part of a play or leisure activity instead of its current listing as part of "activities of daily living," because of life experience or cultural heritage.

Examples of Use in Practice

Uniform Terminology—Third Edition defines occupational therapy's domain of concern, which includes performance areas, performance components, and performance contexts. While this document may be used by occupational therapy practitioners in a number of different areas (e.g., practice, documentation, charge systems, education, program development, marketing, research, disability classifications, and regulations), it focuses on the use of uniform terminology in practice. This document is not intended to define specific occupational therapy programs or specific occupational therapy interventions. Examples of how performance areas, performance components, and performance contexts translate into practice are provided below.

• An individual who is injured on the job may have the potential to return to work and productive activities, which is a performance area. In order to achieve the outcome of returning to work and productive activities, the individual may need to address specific performance components, such as strength, endurance, soft tissue integrity, time management, and the physical features of performance contexts, like structures and objects in his or her environment. The occupational therapy practitioner, in collaboration with the individual and other members of the vocational team, uses planned interventions to achieve the desired outcome. These interventions may include activities such as an exercise program, body mechanics instruction, and job site modifications, all of which may be provided in a work-hardening program.

• An elderly individual recovering from a cerebrovascular accident may wish to live in a community setting, which combines the performance areas of ADL with work and productive activities. In order to achieve the outcome of community living, the individual may need to address specific performance components, such as muscle tone, gross motor coordination, postural control, and self-management. It is also necessary to consider the sociocultural and physical features of performance contexts, such as support available from other persons, and adaptations of structures and objects within the environment. The occupational therapy practitioner, in cooperation with the team, utilizes planned interventions to achieve the desired outcome. Interventions may include neuromuscular facilitation, practice of object manipulation, and instruction in the use of adaptive equipment and home safety equipment. The practitioner and individual also pursue the selection and training of a personal assistant to ensure the completion of ADL tasks. These interventions may be provided in a comprehensive inpatient rehabilitation unit.

• A child with learning disabilities is required to perform educational activities within a public school setting. Engaging in educational activities is considered the performance area of work and productive activities for this child. To achieve the educational outcome of efficient and effective completion of written classroom work, the child may need to address specific performance components. These include sensory processing, perceptual skills, postural control, motor skills, and the physical features of performance contexts, such as objects (e.g., desk, chair) in the environment. In cooperation with the team, occupational therapy interventions may include activities like adapting the student's seating in the classroom to improve postural control and stability, and practicing motor control and coordination. This program could be developed by an occupational therapist and supported by school district personnel.

• The parents of an infant with cerebral palsy may ask to facilitate the child's involvement in the performance areas of activities of daily living and play. Subsequent to assessment, the therapist identifies specific performance components, such as sensory awareness and neuromuscular control. The practitioner also addresses the physical and cultural features of performance contexts. In collaboration with the parents, occupational therapy interventions may include activities such as seating and positioning for play, neuromuscular facilitation techniques to enable eating, facilitating parent skills in caring for and playing with their infant, and modifying the play space for accessibility. These interventions may be provided in a home-based occupational therapy program.

• An adult with schizophrenia may need and want to live independently in the community, which represents the performance areas of activities of daily living, work and productive activities, and leisure activities. The specific performance categories may be medication routine, functional mobility, home management, vocational exploration, play or leisure performance, and social interaction. In order to achieve the outcome of living independently, the individual may need to address specific performance components, such as topographical orientation; memory; categorization; problem solving; interests; social conduct; time management; and sociocultural features of performance contexts, such as social factors (e.g., influence of family and friends) and roles. The occupational therapy practitioner, in cooperation with the team, utilizes planned interventions to achieve the desired outcome. Interventions may include activities such as training in the use of public transportation, instruction in budgeting skills, selection and participation in social activities, instruction in social conduct, and participation in community reintegration activities. These interventions may be provided in a community-based mental health program.

• An individual with a history of substance abuse may need to reestablish family roles and responsibilities, which represent the performance areas of activities of daily living, work and productive activities, and leisure activities. In order to achieve the outcome of family participation, the individual may need to address the performance components of roles; values; social conduct; selfexpression; coping skills; self-control; and the sociocultural features of performance contexts, such as custom, behavior, rules, and rituals. The occupational therapy practitioner, in cooperation with the team, utilizes planned interventions to achieve the desired outcomes. Interventions may include roles and values exercises, instruction in stress management techniques, identification of family roles and activities, and support to develop family leisure routines. These interventions may be provided in an inpatient acute care unit.

Person–Activity–Environment Fit

Person–activity–environment fit refers to the match among the skills and abilities of the individual; the demands of the activity; and the characteristics of the physical, social, and cultural environments. It is the interaction among the performance areas, performance components, and performance contexts that is important and determines the success of the performance. When occupational therapy practitioners provide services, they attend to all of these aspects of performance and the interaction among them. They also attend to each individual's unique personal history. The personal history includes one's skills and abilities (performance components), the past performance of specific life tasks (performance areas), and experience within particular environments (performance contexts). In addition to personal history, anticipated life tasks and role demands influence performance.

When considering the person–activity–environment fit, variables such as novelty, importance, motivation, activity tolerance, and quality are salient. Situations range from those that are completely familiar to those that are novel and have never been experienced. Both the novelty and familiarity within a situation contribute to the overall task performance. In each situation, there is an optimal level of novelty that engages the individual sufficiently and provides enough information to perform the task. When too little novelty is present, the individual may miss cues and opportunities to perform. When too much novelty is present, the individual may become confused and distracted, inhibiting effective task performance.

Humans determine that some stimuli and situations are more meaningful than others. Individuals perform tasks they deem important. It is critical to identify what the individual wants or needs to do when planning interventions.

The level of motivation an individual demonstrates to perform a particular task is determined by both internal and external factors. An individual's biobehavioral state (e.g., amount of rest, arousal, tension) contributes to the potential to be responsive. The features of the social and physical environments (e.g., persons in the room, noise level) provide information that is either adequate or inadequate to produce a motivated state.

Activity tolerance is the individual's ability to sustain a purposeful activity over time. Individuals must not only select, initiate, and terminate activities, but they must also attend to a task for the needed length of time to complete the task and accomplish their goals.

The quality of performance is measured by standards generated by both the individual and others in the social and cultural environments in which the performance occurs. Quality is a continuum of expectations set within particular activities and contexts (see Figure 1).

Figure 1

UNIFORM TERMINOLOGY FOR OCCUPATIONAL THERAPY
THIRD EDITION OUTLINE

I. Performance Areas	II. Performance Components	III. Performance Contexts
A. Activities of Daily Living 　1. Grooming 　2. Oral Hygiene 　3. Bathing/Showering 　4. Toilet Hygiene 　5. Personal Device Care 　6. Dressing 　7. Feeding and Eating 　8. Medication Routine 　9. Health Maintenance 　10. Socialization 　11. Functional Communication 　12. Functional Mobility 　13. Community Mobility 　14. Emergency Response 　15. Sexual Expression B. Work and Productive Activities 　1. Home Management 　　a. Clothing Care 　　b. Cleaning 　　c. Meal Preparation/Cleanup 　　d. Shopping 　　e. Money Management 　　f. Household Maintenance 　　g. Safety Procedures 　2. Care of Others 　3. Educational Activities 　4. Vocational Activities 　　a. Vocational Exploration 　　b. Job Acquisition 　　c. Work or Job Performance 　　d. Retirement Planning 　　e. Volunteer Participation C. Play or Leisure Activities 　1. Play/Leisure Exploration 　2. Play/Leisure Performance	A. Sensorimotor Component 　1. Sensory 　　a. Sensory Awareness 　　b. Sensory Processing 　　　(1) Tactile 　　　(2) Proprioceptive 　　　(3) Vestibular 　　　(4) Visual 　　　(5) Auditory 　　　(6) Gustatory 　　　(7) Olfactory 　　c. Perceptual Processing 　　　(1) Stereognosis 　　　(2) Kinesthesia 　　　(3) Pain Response 　　　(4) Body Scheme 　　　(5) Right-Left Discrimination 　　　(6) Form Constancy 　　　(7) Position in Space 　　　(8) Visual-Closure 　　　(9) Figure Ground 　　　(10) Depth Perception 　　　(11) Spatial Relations 　　　(12) Topographical Orientation 　2. Neuromusculoskeletal 　　a. Reflex 　　b. Range of Motion 　　c. Muscle Tone 　　d. Strength 　　e. Endurance 　　f. Postural Control 　　g. Postural Alignment 　　h. Soft Tissue Integrity 　3. Motor 　　a. Gross Coordination 　　b. Crossing the Midline 　　c. Laterality 　　d. Bilateral Integration 　　e. Motor Control 　　f. Praxis 　　g. Fine Coordination/Dexterity 　　h. Visual-Motor Integration 　　i. Oral-Motor Control B. Cognitive Integration and Cognitive Components 　1. Level of Arousal 　2. Orientation 　3. Recognition 　4. Attention Span 　5. Initiation of Activity 　6. Termination of Activity 　7. Memory 　8. Sequencing 　9. Categorization 　10. Concept Formation 　11. Spatial Operations 　12. Problem Solving 13. Learning 　14. Generalization C. Psychosocial Skills and Psychological Components 　1. Psychological 　　a. Values 　　b. Interests 　　c. Self-Concept 　2. Social 　　a. Role Performance 　　b. Social Conduct 　　c. Interpersonal Skills 　　d. Self-Expression 　3. Self-Management 　　a. Coping Skills 　　b. Time Management 　　c. Self-Control	A. Temporal Aspects 　1. Chronological 　2. Developmental 　3. Life Cycle 　4. Disability Status B. Environmental Aspects 　1. Physical 　2. Social 　3. Cultural

Uniform Terminology for Occupational Therapy—Third Edition

Occupational therapy is the use of purposeful activity or interventions to promote health and achieve functional outcomes. *Achieving functional outcomes* means to develop, improve, or restore the highest possible level of independence of any individual who is limited by a physical injury or illness, a dysfunctional condition, a cognitive impairment, a psychosocial dysfunction, a mental illness, a developmental or learning disability, or an adverse environmental condition. *Assessment* means the use of skilled observation or evaluation by the administration and interpretation of standardized or nonstandardized tests and measurements to identify areas for occupational therapy services.

Occupational therapy services include, but are not limited to

> 1. the assessment, treatment, and education of or consultation with the individual, family, or other persons; or
>
> 2. interventions directed toward developing, improving, or restoring daily living skills, work readiness or work performance, play skills or leisure capacities, or enhancing educational performance skills;
>
> 3. providing for the development, improvement, or restoration of sensorimotor, oral-motor, perceptual or neuromuscular functioning; or emotional, motivational, cognitive, or psychosocial components of performance.

These services may require assessment of the need for and use of interventions such as the design, development, adaptation, application, or training in the use of assistive technology devices; the design, fabrication, or application of rehabilitative technology such as selected orthotic devices; training in the use of assistive technology, orthotic or prosthetic devices; the application of physical agent modalities as an adjunct to or in preparation for purposeful activity; the use of ergonomic principles; the adaptation of environments and processes to enhance functional performance; or the promotion of health and wellness (AOTA, 1993, p. 1117).

I. Performance Areas

Throughout this document, activities have been described as if individuals performed the tasks themselves. Occupational therapy also recognizes that individuals arrange for tasks to be done through others. The profession views independence as the ability to self-determine activity performance, regardless of who actually performs the activity.

> A. *Activities of Daily Living*—Self-maintenance tasks.
>   1. *Grooming*—Obtaining and using supplies; removing body hair (use of razors, tweezers, lotions, etc.); applying and removing cosmetics; washing, drying, combing, styling, and brushing hair; caring for nails (hands and feet), caring for skin, ears, and eyes; and applying deodorant.

2. *Oral Hygiene*—Obtaining and using supplies; cleaning mouth; brushing and flossing teeth; or removing, cleaning, and reinserting dental orthotics and prosthetics.

3. *Bathing/Showering*—Obtaining and using supplies; soaping, rinsing, and drying body parts; maintaining bathing position; and transferring to and from bathing positions.

4. *Toilet Hygiene*—Obtaining and using supplies; clothing management; maintaining toileting position; transferring to and from toileting position; cleaning body; and caring for menstrual and continence needs (including catheters, colostomies, and suppository management).

5. *Personal Device Care*—Cleaning and maintaining personal care items, such as hearing aids, contact lenses, glasses, orthotics, prosthetics, adaptive equipment, and contraceptive and sexual devices.

6. *Dressing*—Selecting clothing and accessories appropriate to time of day, weather, and occasion; obtaining clothing from storage area; dressing and undressing in a sequential fashion; fastening and adjusting clothing and shoes; and applying and removing personal devices, prostheses, or orthoses.

7. *Feeding and Eating*—Setting up food; selecting and using appropriate utensils and tableware; bringing food or drink to mouth; cleaning face, hands, and clothing; sucking, masticating, coughing, and swallowing; and management of alternative methods of nourishment.

8. *Medication Routine*—Obtaining medication, opening and closing containers, following prescribed schedules, taking correct quantities, reporting problems and adverse effects, and administering correct quantities by using prescribed methods.

9. *Health Maintenance*—Developing and maintaining routines for illness prevention and wellness promotion, such as physical fitness, nutrition, and decreasing health risk behaviors.

10. *Socialization*—Accessing opportunities and interacting with other people in appropriate contextual and cultural ways to meet emotional and physical needs.

11. *Functional Communication*—Using equipment or systems to send and receive information, such as writing equipment, telephones, typewriters, computers, communication boards, call lights, emergency systems, Braille writers, telecommunication devices for the deaf, and augmentative communication systems.

12. *Functional Mobility*—Moving from one position or place to another, such as in-bed mobility, wheelchair mobility, transfers (wheelchair, bed, car, tub, toilet, tub/shower, chair, floor). Performing functional ambulation and transporting objects.

13. *Community Mobility*—Moving self in the community and using public or private transportation, such as driving, or accessing buses, taxi cabs, or other public transportation systems.

14. *Emergency Response*—Recognizing sudden, unexpected hazardous situations, and initiating action to reduce the threat to health and safety.

15. *Sexual Expression*—Engaging in desired sexual and intimate activities.

B. *Work and Productive Activities*—Purposeful activities for self-development, social contribution, and livelihood.

1. *Home Management*—Obtaining and maintaining personal and household possessions and environment.
    a. *Clothing Care*—Obtaining and using supplies; sorting, laundering (hand, machine, and dry clean); folding; ironing; storing; and mending.
    b. *Cleaning*—Obtaining and using supplies; picking up; putting away; vacuuming; sweeping and mopping floors; dusting; polishing; scrubbing; washing windows; cleaning mirrors; making beds; and removing trash and recyclables.
    c. *Meal Preparation and Cleanup*—Planning nutritious meals; preparing and serving food; opening and closing containers, cabinets and drawers; using kitchen utensils and appliances; cleaning up and storing food safely.
    d. *Shopping*—Preparing shopping lists (grocery and other); selecting and purchasing items; selecting method of payment; and completing money transactions.
    e. *Money Management*—Budgeting, paying bills, and using bank systems.
    f. *Household Maintenance*—Maintaining home, yard, garden, appliances, vehicles, and household items.
    g. *Safety Procedures*—Knowing and performing preventive and emergency procedures to maintain a safe environment and to prevent injuries.

2. *Care of Others*—Providing for children, spouse, parents, pets, or others, such as giving physical care, nurturing, communicating, and using age-appropriate activities.

3. *Educational Activities*—Participating in a learning environment through school, community, or work-sponsored activities, such as ex-

ploring educational interests, attending to instruction, managing assignments, and contributing to group experiences.

4. *Vocational Activities*—Participating in work-related activities.
    a. *Vocational Exploration*—Determining aptitudes; developing interests and skills, and selecting appropriate vocational pursuits.
    b. *Job Acquisition*—Identifying and selecting work opportunities, and completing application and interview processes.
    c. *Work or Job Performance*—Performing job tasks in a timely and effective manner; incorporating necessary work behaviors.
    d. *Retirement Planning*—Determining aptitudes; developing interests and skills; and selecting appropriate avocational pursuits.
    e. *Volunteer Participation*—Performing unpaid activities for the benefit of selected individuals, groups, or causes.

C. *Play or Leisure Activities*—Intrinsically motivating activities for amusement, relaxation, spontaneous enjoyment, or self-expression.

1. *Play or Leisure Exploration*—Identifying interests, skills, opportunities, and appropriate play or leisure activities.

2. *Play or Leisure Performance*—Planning and participating in play or leisure activities. Maintaining a balance of play or leisure activities with work and productive activities, and activities of daily living. Obtaining, utilizing, and maintaining equipment and supplies.

II. Performance Components

A. *Sensorimotor Component*—The ability to receive input, process information, and produce output.

1. *Sensory*
    a. *Sensory Awareness*—Receiving and differentiating sensory stimuli.
    b. *Sensory Processing*—Interpreting sensory stimuli:
        (1) *Tactile*—Interpreting light touch, pressure, temperature, pain, and vibration through skin contact/receptors.
        (2) *Proprioceptive*—Interpreting stimuli originating in muscles, joints, and other internal tissues that give information about the position of one body part in relation to another.
        (3) *Vestibular*—Interpreting stimuli from the inner ear receptors regarding head position and movement.
        (4) *Visual*—Interpreting stimuli through the eyes, including peripheral vision and acuity, and awareness of color and pattern.
        (5) *Auditory*—Interpreting and localizing sounds, and discriminating background sounds.
        (6) *Gustatory*—Interpreting tastes.
        (7) *Olfactory*—Interpreting odors.

c. *Perceptual Processing*—Organizing sensory input into meaningful patterns.

    (1) *Stereognosis*—Identifying objects through proprioception, cognition, and the sense of touch.

    (2) *Kinesthesia*—Identifying the excursion and direction of joint movement.

    (3) *Pain Response*—Interpreting noxious stimuli.

    (4) *Body Scheme*—Acquiring an internal awareness of the body and the relationship of body parts to each other.

    (5) *Right–Left Discrimination*—Differentiating one side from the other

    (6) *Form Constancy*—Recognizing forms and objects as the same in various environments, positions, and sizes.

    (7) *Position in Space*—Determining the spatial relationship of figures and objects to self or other forms and objects.

    (8) *Visual-Closure*—Identifying forms or objects from incomplete presentations.

    (9) *Figure Ground*—Differentiating between foreground and background forms and objects.

    (10) *Depth Perception*—Determining the relative distance between objects, figures, or landmarks and the observer, and changes in planes of surfaces.

    (11) *Spatial Relations*—Determining the position of objects relative to each other.

    (12) *Topographical Orientation*—Determining the location of objects and settings and the route to the location.

2. *Neuromusculoskeletal*

    a. *Reflex*—Eliciting an involuntary muscle response by sensory input.

    b. *Range of Motion*—Moving body parts through an arc.

    c. *Muscle Tone*—Demonstrating a degree of tension or resistance in a muscle at rest and in response to stretch.

    d. *Strength*—Demonstrating a degree of muscle power when movement is resisted, as with objects or gravity.

    e. *Endurance*—Sustaining cardiac, pulmonary, and musculoskeletal exertion over time.

    f. *Postural Control*—Using righting and equilibrium adjustments to maintain balance during functional movements.

    g. *Postural Alignment*—Maintaining biomechanical integrity among body parts.

    h. *Soft Tissue Integrity*—Maintaining anatomical and physiological condition of interstitial tissue and skin.

3. *Motor*

    a. *Gross Coordination*—Using large muscle groups for controlled, goal-directed movements.

    b. *Crossing the Midline*—Moving limbs and eyes across the midsagittal plane of the body.

c. *Laterality*—Using a preferred unilateral body part for activities requiring a high level of skill.

d. *Bilateral Integration*—Coordinating both body sides during activity.

e. *Motor Control*—Using the body in functional and versatile movement patterns.

f. *Praxis*—Conceiving and planning a new motor act in response to an environmental demand.

g. *Fine Coordination/Dexterity*—Using small muscle groups for controlled movements, particularly in object manipulation.

h. *Visual-Motor Integration*—Coordinating the interaction of information from the eyes with body movement during activity.

i. *Oral-Motor Control*—Coordinating oropharyngeal musculature for controlled movements.

B. *Cognitive Integration and Cognitive Components*—The ability to use higher brain functions.

1. *Level of Arousal*—Demonstrating alertness and responsiveness to environmental stimuli.

2. *Orientation*—Identifying person, place, time, and situation.

3. *Recognition*—Identifying familiar faces, objects, and other previously presented materials.

4. *Attention Span*—Focusing on a task over time.

5. *Initiation of Activity*—Starting a physical or mental activity.

6. *Termination of Activity*—Stopping an activity at an appropriate time.

7. *Memory*—Recalling information after brief or long periods of time.

8. *Sequencing*—Placing information, concepts, and actions in order.

9. *Categorization*—Identifying similarities of and differences among pieces of environmental information)

10. *Concept Formation*—Organizing a variety of information to form thoughts and ideas.

11. *Spatial Operations*—Mentally manipulating the position of objects in various relationships.

12. *Problem Solving*—Recognizing a problem, defining a problem, identifying alternative plans, selecting a plan, organizing steps in a plan, implementing a plan, and evaluating the outcome.

13. *Learning*—Acquiring new concepts and behaviors.

14. *Generalization*—Applying previously learned concepts and behaviors to a variety of new situations.

C. *Psychosocial Skills and Psychological Components*—The ability to interact in society and to process emotions.

1. *Psychological*
   a. *Values*—Identifying ideas or beliefs that are important to self and others.
   b. *Interests*—Identifying mental or physical activities that create pleasure and maintain attention.
   c. *Self-Concept*—Developing the value of the physical, emotional, and sexual self.

2. *Social*
   a. *Role Performance*—Identifying, maintaining, and balancing functions one assumes oracquires in society (e.g., worker, student, parent, friend, religious participant).
   b. *Social Conduct*—Interacting by using manners, personal space, eye contact, gestures, active listening, and self-expression appropriate to one's environment.
   c. *Interpersonal Skills*—Using verbal and nonverbal communication to interact in a variety of settings.
   d. *Self-Expression*—Using a variety of styles and skills to express thoughts, feelings, and needs.

3. *Self-Management*
   a. *Coping Skills*—Identifying and managing stress and related factors.
   b. *Time Management*—Planning and participating in a balance of self-care, work, leisure, and rest activities to promote satisfaction and health.
   c. *Self-Control*—Modifying one's own behavior in response to environmental needs, demands, constraints, personal aspirations, and feedback from others.

III. Performance Contexts

Assessment of function in performance areas is greatly influenced by the contexts in which the individual must perform. Occupational therapy practitioners consider performance contexts when determining feasibility and appropriateness of interventions. Occupational therapy practitioners may choose interventions based on an understanding of contexts, or may choose interventions directly aimed at altering the contexts to improve performance.

A. *Temporal Aspects*
   1. *Chronological*—Individual's age.

2. *Developmental*—Stage or phase of maturation.

3. *Lifecycle*—Place in important life phases, such as career cycle, parenting cycle, or educational process.

4. *Disability status*—Place in continuum of disability, such as acuteness of injury, chronicity of disability, or terminal nature of illness.

B. *Environment*

1. *Physical*—Nonhuman aspects of contexts. Includes the accessibility to and performance within environments having natural terrain, plants, animals, buildings, furniture, objects, tools, or devices.

2. *Social*—Availability and expectations of significant individuals, such as spouse, friends, and caregivers. Also includes larger social groups which are influential in establishing norms, role expectations, and social routines.

3. *Cultural*—Customs, beliefs, activity patterns, behavior standards, and expectations accepted by the society of which the individual is a member. Includes political aspects, such as laws that affect access to resources and affirm personal rights. Also includes opportunities for education, employment, and economic support.

References

American Occupational Therapy Association. (1979). *Occupational therapy product output reporting system and uniform terminology for reporting occupational therapy services.* Bethesda, MD: Author.

American Occupational Therapy Association. (1989). Uniform terminology for occupational therapy—Second edition. *American Journal of Occupational Therapy, 43,* 808–815.

American Occupational Therapy Association. (1993). Association policies—Definition of occupational therapy practice for state regulation (Policy 5.3.1). *American Journal of Occupational Therapy, 47,* 1117–1121.

Prepared by

The Terminology Task Force
Winifred Dunn, PhD, OTR, FAOTA
Chairperson; Mary Foto, OTR, FAOTA
Jim Hinojosa, PhD, OTR, FAOTA
Barbara Schell, PhD, OTR/L, FAOTA
Linda Kohlman Thomson, MOT, OTR, FAOTA
Sarah D. Hertfelder, MEd, MOT, OTR/L, Staff Liaison

for
Commission on Practice
Jim Hinojosa, PhD, OTR, FAOTA, Chairperson

Adopted by the Representative Assembly July 1994

This document replaces the following documents, all of which were rescinded by the 1994 Representative Assembly: *Occupational Therapy Product Output Reporting System* (1979), *Uniform Terminology for Reporting Occupational Therapy Services—First Edition* (1979), "Uniform Occupational Therapy Evaluation Checklist" (1981, *American Journal of Occupational Therapy, 35,* 817–818), and "Uniform Terminology for Occupational Therapy—Second Edition" (1989, *American Journal of Occupational Therapy, 43,* 808–815).

Uniform Terminology —Third Edition: Application to Practice

Introduction

This document was developed to help occupational therapists apply *Uniform Terminology—Third Edition* to practice. The original grid format (Dunn, 1988) enabled occupational therapy practitioners to systematically identify deficit and strength areas of an individual and to select appropriate activities to address these areas in occupational therapy intervention (Dunn & McGourty, 1990). For the third edition, the profession is highlighting *contexts* as another critical aspect of performance. A second grid provides therapy practitioners with a mechanism to consider the contextual features of performance in activities of daily living (ADL), work and productive activity, and play or leisure. *Performance Areas* and *Performance Components* (see Figure A)focus on the individual. These features are imbedded in the *Performance Contexts* (see Figure B).

On the original grid (Dunn, 1988), the horizontal axis contains the Performance Areas of Activities of Daily Living, Work and Productive Activities, and Play or Leisure Activities (see Figure A). These Performance Areas are the functional outcomes that occupational therapy addresses. The vertical axis contains the Performance Components, including Sensorimotor components, Cognitive Components, and Psychosocial Components. The Performance Components are the skills and abilities that an individual uses to engage in the Performance Areas. During an occupational therapy assessment, the occupational therapy practitioner determines an individual's abilities and limitations in the Performance Components and how they affect the individual's functional outcomes in the Performance Areas.

The first application document (Dunn & McGourty, 1989) described how to use the original *Uniform Terminology* grid with a variety of individuals. It is quite useful to introduce these concepts. However, the third edition of *Uniform Terminology* contains some changes in the Performance Areas and Performance Components lists. Be sure to check for the terminology currently approved in the third edition before applying this information in current practice environments.

With the addition of Performance Contexts into *Uniform Terminology*, occupational therapy practitioners must consider how to interface what the individual wants to do (i.e., performance area) with the contextual features that may support or block performance. Figure B illustrates the interaction of Performance Areas and Performance Contexts as a model for therapists' planning.

The grid in Figure B can be used to analyze the contexts of performance for a particular individual. For example, when working with a toddler with a developmental disability who needs to learn to eat, the occupational therapy practitioner would consider all the Performance Contexts features as they might affect this toddler's ability to master eating. Unlike the grid in Figure A, in which the occupational therapy practitioner selects both Performance Areas (i.e., what the individual wants or needs to do) and the Performance Component (i.e., a person's strengths and needs), in this grid (Figure B) the occupational therapy practitioner only selects the Performance Area. After the Performance Area is identified through collaboration with the individual and significant others, the occupational therapy practitioner considers *all* Performance Contexts features as they might affect performance of the selected task.

Intervention Planning

Intervention planning occurs both within the general domain of concern of occupational therapy (i.e., uniform terminology) and by considering the profession's theoretical frames of reference that offer insights about how to approach the problem. In Figure A, the occupational therapy practitioner considers the Performance Areas that are of interest to the individual and the individual's strengths and concerns within the Performance Components. The intervention strategies would emerge from the cells on the grid that are placed at the intersection of the Performance Areas and the targeted Performance Components (strength and/or concern). For example, if a child needed to improve sensory processing and fine coordination for oral hygiene and grooming, an occupational therapy practitioner might select a sensory integrative frame of reference to create intervention strategies, such as adding textures to handles and teaching the child sand and bean digging games. Dunn and McGourty (1989) discuss this in more detail.

When using Figure B, the occupational therapy practitioner considers the Performance Contexts features in relation to the desired Performance Area. The occupational therapy practitioner would analyze the individual's temporal, physical, social, and cultural contexts to determine the relevance of particular interventions. For example, if the child mentioned above was a member of a family in which having messy hands from sand play was unacceptable, the occupational therapy practitioner would consider alternate strategies that are more compatible with their life-style. For example, perhaps the family would be more interested in developing puppet play. This would still provide the child with opportunities to experience the textures of various puppets and the hand movements required to manipulate the puppets in play context, without adding the messiness of sand. When occupational therapy practitioners consider contexts, interventions become more relevant and applicable to individual's lives.

Case Example 1

Sophie is a 75-year-old woman who was widowed 3 years ago, is recovering from a cerebrovascular accident (CVA), and has been transferred from an acute care unit to an inpatient medical rehabilitation unit. Prior to her admission, she was living

Figure A–Uniform Terminology Grid
(Performance Areas and Performance Components)

PERFORMANCE AREAS

PERFORMANCE COMPONENTS

A. Sensorimotor Component

	Activities of Daily Living	Grooming	Oral Hygiene	Bathing/Showering	Toilet Hygiene	Personal Device Care	Dressing	Feeding and Eating	Medication Routine	Health Maintenance	Socialization	Functional Communication	Functional Mobility	Community Mobility	Emergency Response	Sexual Expression	Work and Productive Activities	Home Management	Care of Others	Educational Activities	Vocational Activities	Play or Leisure Activities	Play/Leisure Exploration	Play/Leisure Performance
Sensory																								
Sensory Awareness																								
Sensory Processing																								
(1) Tactile																								
(2) Proprioceptive																								
(3) Vestibular																								
(4) Visual																								
(5) Auditory																								
(6) Gustatory																								
(7) Olfactory																								
Perceptual Processing																								
(1) Stereognosis																								
(2) Kinesthesia																								
(3) Pain Response																								
(4) Body Scheme																								
(5) Right-Left Discrimination																								
(6) Form Constancy																								
(7) Position in Space																								
(8) Visual-Closure																								
(9) Figure Ground																								
(10) Depth Perception																								
(11) Spatial Relations																								
(12) Topographical Orientation																								
Neuromusculoskeletal																								
Reflex																								
Range of Motion																								
Muscle Tone																								
Strength																								
Endurance																								
Postural Control																								
Postural Alignment																								
Soft Tissue Integrity																								
Motor																								
Gross Coordination																								
Crossing the Midline																								
Laterality																								
Bilateral Integration																								
Motor Control																								
Praxis																								
Fine Coordination/Dexterity																								
Visual-Motor Integration																								
Oral-Motor Control																								

Figure A–Uniform Terminology Grid Continued
(Performance Areas and Performance Components)

PERFORMANCE AREAS

PERFORMANCE COMPONENTS

B. Cognitive Integration and Cognitive Components

	Activities of Daily Living	Grooming	Oral Hygiene	Bathing/Showering	Toilet Hygiene	Personal Device Care	Dressing	Feeding and Eating	Medication Routine	Health Maintenance	Socialization	Functional Communication	Functional Mobility	Community Mobility	Emergency Response	Sexual Expression	Work and Productive Activities	Home Management	Care of Others	Educational Activities	Vocational Activities	Play or Leisure Activities	Play/Leisure Exploration	Play/Leisure Performance
1. Level of Arousal																								
2. Orientation																								
3. Recognition																								
4. Attention Span																								
5. Initiation of Activity																								
6. Termination of Activity																								
7. Memory																								
8. Sequencing																								
9. Categorization																								
10. Concept Formation																								
11. Spatial Operations																								
12. Problem Solving																								
13. Learning																								
14. Generalization																								

C. Psychosocial Skills and Psychological Components

1. Psychological
   a. Values
   b. Interests
   c. Self-Concept
2. Social
   a. Role Performance
   b. Social Conduct
   c. Interpersonal Skills
   d. Self-Expression
3. Self-Management
   a. Coping Skills
   b. Time Management
   c. Self-Control

in a small house in an isolated location and has no family living nearby. She was driving independently and frequently ran errands for her friends. She is adamant in her goal to return to her home after discharge. All of her friends are quite elderly and are not able to provide many resources for support.

Sophie and the team collaborated to identify her goals. Sophie decided that she wanted to be able to meet her daily needs with little or no assistance. Almost all of the Performance Areas are critical in order to achieve the outcome of community living in her own home. Being able to cook all of her meals, bathe independently, and have alternative transportation available is necessary. Because of their significant impact on the patient's function in the Performance Areas, some of the Performance Components that may need to be addressed are figure ground, muscle tone, postural control, fine coordination, memory, and self management.

In the selection of occupational therapy interventions, it is critical to analyze the elements of Performance Contexts for the individual. The physical and social elements of her home environment do not support returning home without modifications to her home and additional social supports being established. Railings must be added to the front steps, and provision of and instruction in the use of a tub seat and instruction in the use of specialized transportation may need to occur. If this same individual had been living in an apartment in a retirement community prior to her CVA, the contexts of performance would support a return home with fewer environmental modifications being needed. Being independent in cooking might not be necessary due to meals being provided, and the bathroom might already be accessible and safe. If the individual had friends and family available, the social support network might already be established to assist with shopping and transportation needs. The occupational therapy interventions would be different due to the contexts in which the individual will be performing. Interventions must be selected with the impact of the Performance Contexts as an essential element.

Case Example 2

Malcolm is a 9-year-old boy who has a learning disability that causes him to have a variety of problems in the school. His teachers complain that he is difficult to manage in the classroom. Some of the Performance Components that may need to be addressed are his self-control, such as interrupting, difficulty sitting during instruction, and difficulty with peer relations. Other children avoid him on the playground, because he does not follow rules, does not play fair, and tends to anger quickly when confronted. The Performance Component impairment with concept formation is reflected in his sloppy and disorganized classroom assignments.

The critical elements of the Performance Contexts are the temporal aspect of age appropriateness of his behavior and the social environmental aspect of his immature socialization. The significant cultural and temporal aspects of his family are that they place a high premium on athletic prowess.

Figure B–Uniform Terminology Grid
(Performance Areas and Performance Contexts)

PERFORMANCE AREAS

Performance Areas (column headers): Activities of Daily Living, Grooming, Oral Hygiene, Bathing/Showering, Toilet Hygiene, Personal Device Care, Dressing, Feeding and Eating, Medication Routine, Health Maintenance, Socialization, Functional Communication, Functional Mobility, Community Mobility, Emergency Response, Sexual Expression, Work and Productive Activities, Home Management, Care of Others, Educational Activities, Vocational Activities, Play or Leisure Activities, Play/Leisure Exploration, Play/Leisure Performance

PERFORMANCE CONTEXTS

A. Temporal Aspects

Chronological
Developmental
Life Cycle
Disability Status

B. Environment

Physical
Social
Cultural

The occupational therapy practitioner intervenes in several ways to address his behavior in the school environment. The occupational therapy practitioner focuses on structuring the classroom environment and facilitating consistent behavioral expectations for Malcolm by educational personnel. She also consults with the teachers to develop ways to structure activities that will support his ability to relate to other children in a positive way.

In contrast, another child with similar learning disabilities, but who is 12 years old and in the 7th grade might have different concerns. Elements of the Performance Contexts are the temporal aspect of the age appropriateness of his behavior and the social environmental context of school where bullying behavior is unacceptable and in which completing assignments is expected. In addressing the cultural Performance Contexts, the occupational therapy practitioner recognizes from meeting with parents that they have only average expectations for academic performance but value athletic accomplishments.

Since teachers at his school consider completion of home assignments to be part of average performance, the occupational therapy practitioner works with the child and parents on time management and reinforcement strategies to meet this expectation. After consultation with the coach, she works with the father to create activities to improve his athletic abilities. When occupational therapy practitioners consider family values as part of the contexts of performance, different intervention priorities may emerge.

Prepared by

The Terminology Task Force
Winifred Dunn, PhD, OTR, FAOTA, Chairperson
Mary Foto, OTR, FAOTA
Jim Hinojosa, PhD, OTR, FAOTA
Barbara A. Boyt Schell, PhD, OTR/L, FAOTA
Linda Kohlman Thomson, MOT, OTR, OT (C), FAOTA
Sarah D. Hertfelder, MEd, MOT, OTR/L, Staff Liaison
for
The Commission on Practice
Jim Hinojosa, PhD, OTR, FAOTA, Chairperson

This document replaces the 1989 document *Application of Uniform Terminology to Practice* that accompanied the *Uniform Terminology for Occupational Therapy—Second Edition* (*American Journal of Occupational Therapy, 43,* 808–815).

Index

underlying factors, 77–78, 81
Functional history, clinical reasoning, 55
Functional maintenance program, 104–105
Functional mobility, 379
Functional outcome, 120–121
Functional outcome statement, documentation
  review, 154

G

Gait training, 345
Goal, 3. See also Specific type
  training, 2
Grant program, payment, 6
Grief process, clinical reasoning, 55
Grooming, 377

H

Hardware, 212–214
  CD drives, 214
  interface, 213–214
  memory, 212
  modems, 213
  processor, 212
  scanners, 213
  sound cards, 214
  storage, 212, 213
HCFA Common Procedure Coding System (HCPCS),
    19, 20
  Level I HCPCS, 20
  Level II HCPCS, 20
  Level III HCPCS, 20
Health care delivery system, future directions, 117–119
Health Care Financing Administration, 7
Health information privacy, 233–235, 249–250
  Medicare, 234–235
  state laws, 234
Health Insurance Portability and Accountability Act,
    227, 232
Health maintenance, 378
Healthcare Informatics Standards Board, 209
Home exercise program. See Functional maintenance
    program
Home health
  discharge notes, 94

documentation, 92–93
  duplication of services, 97
  guidelines, 94–97
  maintenance, 95–96
  record contents, 94
  red flag areas, 95–97
  target audience, 100–101
initial evaluation, 94
Medicare, 7–8
payment, 92–93
  assumptions for reimbursement, 113
progress notes, 94, 100–113
  assumptions for reimbursement, 113
  avoiding double-level status reporting, 103–104
  case example, 111, 112
  coordination with other disciplines, 111
  details supporting medical necessity, 105
  direct intervention, 110
  evaluations, 110
  explaining slow progress or lack of progress, 109
  focus on function, 102–105
  focus on meaningful activities, 102
  focus on safety, 108
  functional maintenance program, 104–105
  identify meaningful activities, 102
  instruction, 110–111
  long-term goals, 102–103
  prior level of function, 102
  progress focus, 106–108
  relating performance component deficits to
      functional outcomes, 103
  relating performance component goals to
      functional outcomes, 103
  reports organized by performance areas, 103
  short-term goals, 102–103
  stating expectations for progress, 108
  summarizing skilled services delivered, 109–111
  underlying factors, 105–106
safety, 108
Home management, 379
Home program. See Functional maintenance program
Hospice, Medicare, 8
Hospital rates, workers' compensation, 16
Household maintenance, 379

I

J

L

M

Q

R

S

NOV